Ageless MirrorAthlete™

Ageless MirrorAthlete™

Overweight and Unfit No More

Marc T. Woodard, MBA, BS, Exercise Science
Fitness and Healthy Lifestyle Consultant

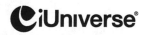

AGELESS MIRRORATHLETE™
OVERWEIGHT AND UNFIT NO MORE

iUniverse books may be ordered through booksellers or by contacting:

iUniverse
1663 Liberty Drive
Bloomington, IN 47403
www.iuniverse.com
1-800-Authors (1-800-288-4677)

ISBN: 978-1-5320-5371-9 (sc)
ISBN: 978-1-5320-5372-6 (hc)
ISBN: 978-1-5320-5373-3 (e)

Library of Congress Control Number: 2018907889

Print information available on the last page.

iUniverse rev. date: 01/18/2019

Contents

Preface

Years ago, at the age of forty-three, physical adversity struck.

At that time, I dusted off a unique, fit, healthy lifestyle manuscript I'd planned to publish one day. I always knew the principled information could provide anyone the knowledge needed to achieve any fitness goal or heal what ailed him or her naturally—and that included myself. This would be especially true when the mind, body, and spirit were broken and in need of mending.

The principled, fit, healthy lifestyle philosophy MirrorAthlete is founded on is uniquely presented in a way that's academically and intuitively relatable and applicable for anyone—young and old. And it will positively motivate any person to become more progressively active and to improve health, fitness levels, and well-being, regardless of the current lifestyle, mobility, and medical condition or environment in which he or she lives.

The plethora of citations, client consultation, personal experience, and other examples within the book provide relatable building blocks that can show anyone how to plan and develop a customized fitness-and-healthy-habits program to remain *forever ageless* and to sustain those results safely and naturally for a lifetime.

If weight loss, strength, cardio-muscular endurance, flexibility, mobility, healthy longevity, wellness, increased energy, or competitive sport or athletic and physical performance enhancement is your number one goal, then MirrorAthlete has the information you need and want now. The consumer truths are presented and revealed in a relatable way you've never seen before.

Rest assured that all aspects of safe diet and weight loss, antiaging, physical enhancement and consumer safety awareness, and more are covered in full detail. You'll learn all this without spending hundreds of dollars on related products and services that don't work and can't be sustained. Plus, you'll understand why they make you sick.

The MirrorAthlete Principled Fitness and Healthy Lifestyle Philosophy first evolved long ago from a love of sport and traditional family and social events with recreational activities experienced during childhood.

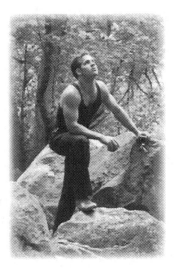

As a young adult, I was ultimately led by those early activities and passions to an undergraduate degree in exercise science from Portland State University (PSU) in Oregon (attained in 1988).

I coined this principled, fit, healthy lifestyle philosophy MirrorAthlete Science. The context of the book is based in science and connected with a fit, healthy lifestyle ideology formed through personal and consulting knowledge, education, and experience. The philosophy enables each person to determine what he or she needs to achieve well-being and live life to the fullest.

The ideology then evolved through academics, client consults, and training experiences into a philosophy on how anyone can live a healthier and happier lifestyle. The *Ageless MirrorAthlete* philosophy is built on eighteen fit, healthy lifestyle principles worth their weight in gold. Soon you'll understand why the marketplace hopes that you never get your hands on this powerful information.

One principle is covered at a time and listed under each chapter title. The information within each chapter is related to the principle and presented in a very unique and personal way that you'll identify with. Each chapter also provides relevant tools that will increase your fitness levels, improve your mobility and health, and give you the quality of life you need and deserve now!

The making of MirrorAthlete

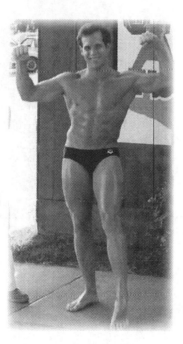

Prior to and after graduating college, I served in the active duty US Air Force from 1982 to 1985 as an administrative specialist and trained to compete in bodybuilding at Castle Air Force Base, California, representing the 93 AMS (Avionics Maintenance Squadron). This is where I met my future wife Beth.

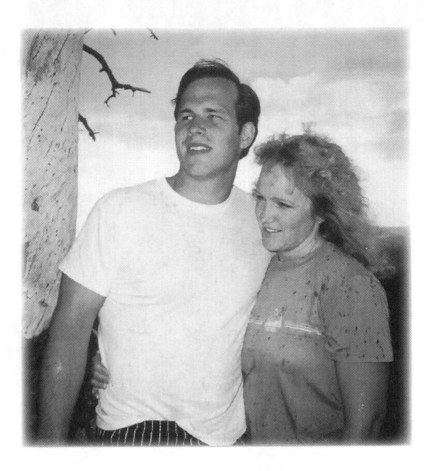

Thereafter, I served within the Air National Guard at Portland International Airport, Oregon, as an NCOIC (noncommissioned officer in charge). I also worked as a civilian employee at the base fitness center from 1986 to 1988. From this point forward, I served in the Air Force Reserves (AFRES) at the same base as a MWR (Morale, Welfare and Recreation) specialist and a civilian recreation director from 1989 to 1991.

Both my wife, Elizabeth, and I secured employment at PIAP (Portland International Airport), Oregon, Air National Guard and Reserve base. At separate times, we each served as MWR fitness center manager and recreation director.

Elizabeth remained a recreation director for some time, while I pursued a change in military career to seek other professional interests and opportunities.

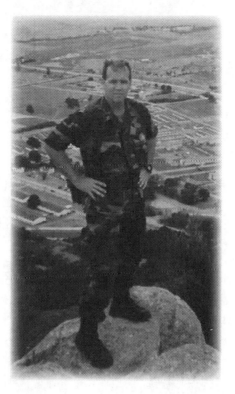

As such, I earned an army commission through the OMA (Oregon Military Academy) at Western University in Monmouth, Oregon, while serving in the Army National Guard. I graduated with the OMA class 36 in July 1993. Then I was commissioned a second lieutenant in the United States Army. Shortly thereafter, I entered into the Medical Services Corp (MSC).

I also wrote and developed fitness-health-and-nutrition course materials and applied exercise science as a fitness consultant and instructor for the Air Force Reserve Command Morale, Welfare and Recreation (AFRC MWR) HQ's Warner Robins Air Force Base in Georgia from 1989 to 1996.

Outside of those things, I owned and operated a fitness-consulting-and-supplement business named Dynamic Dimensions (1987 to 1996). Yep, I had a lot going on. I'm one of those types that burned the candle at both ends.

My wife and I also served as subject matter experts for MWR's fitness-health-and-nutrition book, which we cowrote. I used it as a guide to develop an instructor's curriculum, with course materials for circulation within the military reserve and guard branches. Thereafter, I was contracted by the air force reserve headquarters in Macon, Georgia, to instruct fitness certification courses annually that contained exercise science, fitness, health, and nutrition information.

After instructing the successful completion of the four-day fitness-and-nutrition-course seminars, I'd provide a certification of fitness course completion after student airmen had passed written and practical exams.

As a subject matter expert in exercise science, also known as exercise physiology, I coauthored *Working on Wellness, Fitness and Nutrition, Keys to Good Health*. The book was published, and around 190,000 copies were circulated to all air force reservists, as well as to other military branches of service, during the midnineties. My wife and I received full subject-matter-expert recognition and credit for the publication.

I also used the instructor curriculum course information as a guideline for years during one-on-one client consults in private sessions. I used it mostly to profile and assess client fitness levels and develop custom fitness and healthy habits programs.

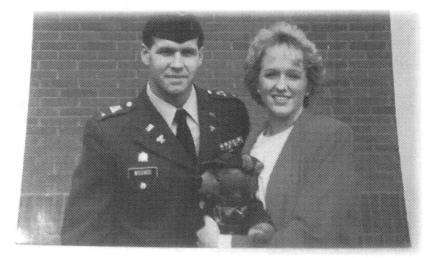

After being commissioned second lieutenant, I served as an Army National Guard treatment platoon leader for the 141st Support Battalion, C-Med Company, Portland, Oregon. Then later I served as a materials health officer (S-4, staff officer, logistician of medical supplies), STARC (state area command), detachment 8, Sacramento, California. I retired with just over twenty years of combined active air force and then nonactive air guard reserve and army guard military service.

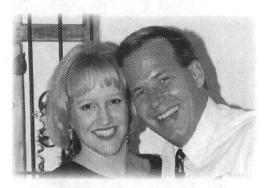

Within these years, I recall a major milestone in 1999 that led to the creation of MirrorAthlete. While on a seven-day Mexican Riviera cruise, I wrote the first manuscript draft, which identified and defined the construct of a principled, fit, healthy lifestyle philosophy based in exercise science.

However, I put the idea of completing and publishing the book on hold to complete a master's in business administration (MBA) from 2000 to 2002, while employed with a large high-tech corporation. Simultaneously, Elizabeth completed her master's in education (MEd) and graduated within the same timeline. She currently works for a large nonprofit corporation that provides services for seniors.

To complete this book project was anything but easy. It literally took nearly two decades to write and get published. Once you understand my full backstory and physical adversity challenge, you'll quickly realize why it took so long and how these hard-earned truths motivated me to complete the book. Without the passage of time and unique lifestyle experiences and education, this book would probably read like any other fitness or health book found on a bookshelf. I assure you this is not the case.

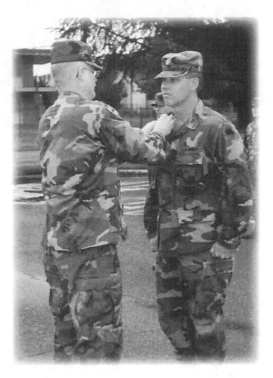

After retiring 03E (captain with prior enlisted time) from the US Army National guard in 2003 and retiring from corporate employment in 2007, I began giving back to community. First, I provided free fitness, nutrition, and health information, which I published online at www.mirrorathlete.com. This is where I really learned how to write. But there's always room for improvement. Forever editing was a huge time sink for me, and editing was a skill set I needed to get better at if I was ever going to get a book published.

I was really good at technical writing but not so good at storytelling, let alone writing a book of this caliber. I began trying to write a factual, fit, healthy narrative manuscript in 2007 from the 1999 outline. By 2013, I submitted it to a publishing company. It was returned with 540 change requests. I damn near stopped writing. Talk about a blow to the ego. I'm glad I didn't give up.

Four years later, I completed the change requests and wrote the book I never thought possible.

In between this time, I also won elected office as a City Councilor in Tigard, OR and began serving the first four-year term in January

2011. I won a second term for another four years, which began January 2014 and ended 31 December 2018.

I set two very important goals for our city—city recreation (2012) and economic development (2013). Both goals won unanimous support from city leaders as priorities. Before these goals were set, those programs and services were nonexistent. Soon you'll understand how environment, city recreation, and economic development are connected in healthy city design and development. And why these things matter if you hope to achieve your fitness goals. You'll also see how these things, when combined, help people live healthier, happier, and more productive lifestyles while bringing community together.

It is within public service that I championed, challenged, and influenced the development of a healthy, walkable city vision. I established goals, priorities, policies, and community engagement. And I brought to the forefront the importance of investing in and planning for more exercise activities, supporting recreational community facilities, and developing more parks and city trail ways throughout neighborhoods.

Recreation facilities located in communities can offer a variety of childhood and adult indoor and outdoor fitness activities that motivate people to move more. These relatively inexpensive and innovative, fit and healthy civic projects support ideals that fight childhood and adult obesity—both of which greatly plague the health of the financially disparaged population living in all communities.

US Surgeon General Dr. Vivek Murthy stated during the annual 2015 National Recreation and Parks Association (NRPA) conference, "We live in a time where health disparity continues to grow." The theme was that city recreation should be of highest priority, alongside policing services, as both save lives in various ways and must be resourced to the fullest extent possible during the city budget process. He stated in various ways and flat-out said, "City recreation saves lives."

How does a healthy city environment apply to fitness and healthy habit and lifestyle programming? If the place you live is stressful or has bad air and/or water quality—or if it provides few safe public use recreation facilities and fitness activities or makes you or your children feel ill for whatever reason—it will be harder to achieve fitness, health, and well-being goals.

This book's focus is not on healthy city development. However, I've sprinkled in just enough on the topic so the reader can appreciate and relate to what a healthy city environment should look and feel like, especially if the reader is considering a move.

Each customized fitness and healthy habits program example shows anyone how to create and apply a personalized fit healthy lifestyle within any environment. *Seeing is also believing.* Your fitness levels will increase as you work toward your fitness goals; you'll physically see and feel the change. These results are measureable and sustainable long term when provided truthful information.

These chapters also have the potential to change young lives dramatically. For example, if this principled philosophy in its basic form was educationally valued and applied in all K–12 schools, its truths would be immediately relatable and applicable for future generations to follow. This, in turn, would spare the nation from a childhood obesity problem and related disease that's sure to become epidemic if something doesn't change.

By the end of the book, you will have applied at least one major lifestyle change if not more. This I guarantee. You'll never look at the old you in the mirror the same way again after absorbing the knowledge shared in this book.

At the end of each chapter, I provide my "Personal Fitness Challenge" adversity story related to each chapter's context. These lessons learned can be applied to any physical adversity or fitness challenge you may face anytime within your lifetime.

My physical adversity challenge began once I was diagnosed with AVN (avascular necrosis) of both hips. If you don't know what that is, you'll know very soon.

Acknowledgments

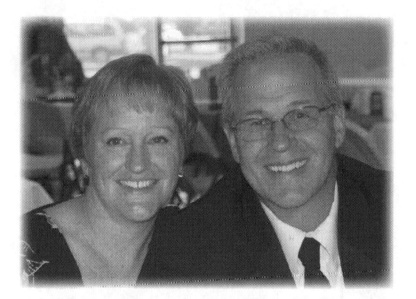

To my wife, Elizabeth Gunn-Woodard, love of my life, friend, life partner, and toughest critic. I'm very appreciative of her support in finishing this book, which would not have been possible without it. Thank you for everything you did to help ease the burden—including all those great meals you made to ensure I didn't starve to death while spending thousands of hours tucked away in creative writer's mode. And thank you especially for sharing your insight and ideals for the book, which added invaluable perspective and insight.

I'd also like to extend a big thanks to a good friend of mine for all the art found throughout the book and of course to his wife, Carol, in support of the long hours he dedicated to making the book extra special.

Within each chapter, I know you'll enjoy the humor of the cartoons and caricatures that are so artfully created by cartoonist John Fiedler. If you'd like to see other creative works by John or send inquiries, he can be found and contacted through Olefuzzcartoons.com.

Introduction

Nothing in life is guaranteed, especially being blessed with good health and mobility. Regardless, feeling well and living life to the fullest is possible no matter what the image in the mirror and mind's eye shows and tells you.

Finding your MirrorAthlete active lifestyle potential and sustaining it naturally is the antiaging and longevity truth the marketplace hopes you never figure out. And soon you'll know why.

When you hold the marketplace consumer truths and difficult-to-find fitness and healthy habit information in your hand, you can achieve any wellness, physical-performance, or healthy-lifestyle-and-longevity goal you set.

Many have asked me during client consults, Why do diets and fitness programs work for some but not others? Truth be told, there's a lot of half-truths and flat-out lies sold to the consumer.

Also, we're all at different stages of life. This includes our age, fitness level, health condition, mobility and productivity capacity, environmental situation, and so on. Each of these factors puts stress on us in various ways and can lead to any number of illnesses or diseases.

No man-made diet, fitness, well-being, antiaging, or longevity gimmick, product, or program will work—or work the same way—for every individual. And in some cases, these products or programs won't work at all for any individual. Most are not sustainable, and they almost always increase health risk eventually.

The fact of the matter is we're all physically, mentally, and spiritually wired differently and experiencing stress at various levels daily. Therefore, we each require unique lifestyle changes relative to our individual fitness and health goals that will help us to feel well and live life to the fullest.

The contents of this book are a gold mine of powerful consumer truths, with powerful stories and useful examples that'll motivate anyone to believe that *overweight and unfit no more* is actually an achievable goal that can be sustained for life. Once these hard-to-find natural science and consumer truths are defined, you will be able to relate to and apply them, and you will be able to unlock your full fit healthy lifestyle potential.

During client consults, I learned many had lost hope that fitness goals and good health could be achieved naturally and sustained over the long term. This is a mind-set. I know I can convince you the opposite is true through truthful marketplace information, client consult examples, and exercise science insight.

Through personal experience, I know it is possible to bounce back from physical adversity to achieve what at first feels or appears to be impossible. This is especially the case after a traumatic injury, illness, or disease.

Read the MirrorAthlete descriptor below. I'm sure you'll understand, in concept, how this principled philosophy evolved first as an ideology based on how unique each one of us is. And as a unique individual, you'll also see what healthy lifestyle choices you must make to improve an unhealthy situation and get fitter!

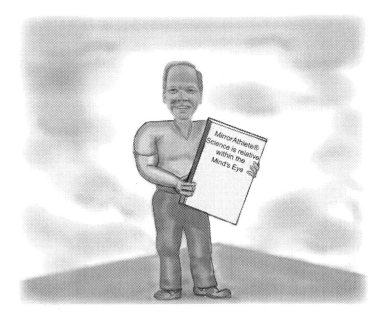

For instance, how do you see yourself in your reflective mind's eye standing in front of the mirror? What do you see? When I look into the mirror, even though I'm slightly overweight for my age and my hair is now white, I still see myself as an athlete and work out daily to sustain the best fitness and health condition possible. I am a "MirrorAthlete." And you can be too. No matter how old I get, I will always be motivated to sustain my mirror athlete image in the best way possible *for me*. I'll teach you how to apply the same principles to sustain a similar mind-set and make the healthy lifestyle changes you need and want now.

I'm not looking for physical or performance perfection; that's an impossible goal, especially as we age. And remember that we're living in bodies that are each genetically wired differently than any other. Although age is only a number, it is important to remain mindful that changing metabolisms mean fifty- or sixty-year-old bodies require different maintenance agreements than do twenty- or thirty-year-old bodies.

Like you, I want to stay well and look good and be competitive, with the physical capacity to participate in as many social and recreational events and activities as possible and live life to the fullest—no matter my age. *Age is only a number.*

But to experience the best physical and well-being state per decade requires an educated and motivated mind-set to sustain the course. If you are missing a passion to actively participate in some form of exercise activity, it will be more challenging to conjure the willpower to change bad habits and behavior, but not impossible!

No worries. This is a major reason I wrote *Ageless MirrorAthlete*™ I'm here to help you find the willpower, motivation, and passion you need to heal what ails you, became more mobile, lose excess body fat, and have more energy—so you'll feel better and live up to your full potential.

What exactly is a "mirror athlete"? It is a person who sees his or her mirror reflection and, within the mind's eye, recognizes and applies the fitness and healthy lifestyle truths in a way that sustains the best fitness levels and health condition possible while aging gracefully.

No matter how you appear in the mirror, if you're happy, healthy, and experience well-being daily, you are living a fit, healthy lifestyle. At some point, I stress to fellow mirror athletes—give back to others by sharing this knowledge. In doing so, you help others live to their full potential in a total state of well-being.

Indulge in learning the fitness, health, and antiaging truths—the best-kept industry secrets. They have changed my life and will change yours forever!

Be patient as you read through the chapters. There is a lot of information. As you work through each one, write notes and highlight what's relative to your situation. Then plan, develop, and apply a relevant fitness and healthy habit and lifestyle change program that'll motivate you to stay the course.

Also, don't be shy about sharing this information with your primary care physician. MirrorAthlete, Inc., recommends cross-sharing of information as a principled healthy lifestyle practice to ensure safe participation in any exercise activity, balanced nutrition, or healthy habit lifestyle change program.

Personal Fitness Challenge: "Believe"

I know many of you have tried to lose that stubborn belly fat and have attempted every diet and exercise gimmick under the sun to improve appearance or simply to feel better and become more fit. Some of you have even quit trying to find a program that will work. I'm here asking you to believe in something I know will change your life by getting you fit and healthy once and for all.

If you apply even a tenth of the knowledge I'm sharing, you'll feel and see results immediately. This will be especially true if you've been suffering from sedentary habits, depression, anxiety, phantom pain, obesity, illness, injury, or disease.

At some point in our lives, each one of us looks into the mirror and thinks, *I'm too old, too fat, too broken to continue on. What's the use?* Instead of seeing yourself this way why not start thinking about new beginnings and possibilities? After all, you now have the tools in hand to make positive lifestyle changes that will stick once and for all.

At one point in my life, I looked into the mirror and saw something I believed too broken to repair. If it wasn't for the combined information you now have in your fitness and healthy lifestyle change arsenal, I'm not so sure I could have bounced back from the physical adversity challenges that plagued me for a long period of time.

From 2004 to 2007, I went through service-connected hip surgeries while suffering with previous back injuries over a period of thirty years.

Within this four-year period, I also put on thirty pounds and was at a low point in my life, battling the stress of mobility challenges, financial burdens, complex body pain, anxiety and depression, and mind-numbing pills.

I was facing the prospect of lifelong mobility issues and unrelenting body pain. At first, I surrendered to the new circumstances. Then I eventually rejected the notion of long-term immobility and disability.

This was my reality and a tough pill to swallow at first, but I was determined to get back what I had lost. An internal drive beckoned me to develop a program—a self-healing process—based on my unique fitness programming knowledge. I immediately recalled that, to begin healing, I first needed to apply the science to stop the weight gain.

To be honest, losing that thirty pounds was no easy accomplishment. After all, I was operating in a broken body that required years of physical rehabilitation and recovery after surgeries. Even after a four-year period of recovery, I wasn't mobility whole and still needed to continue managing pain daily and attend physical therapy in order to exercise on my own and on a limited basis.

With all the education, life experiences, client consults, and fitness programming skill sets I had in my toolbox, you'd think I would have been better prepared for physical adversity. Well, I have to tell you, nothing prepares anyone to self-manage depression, anxiety, chronic pain, and immobility for a long period of time.

The educational institution in which I earned my exercise science degree focused mostly on improving fitness levels, athletic motor skills, biomechanics, kinesiology, sports and fitness performance, and so on— for those without physical injury and pain and mobility challenges. However, through time, I learned that *pain management is* also *a mind-set on how to tolerate a certain amount of it if you want to heal sooner than later.*

Without pain management knowledge and a mind-set of tolerance, it's awfully hard to bounce back from sedentary habits, serious disease or injury, surgery, or physical recovery of a long duration.

Sedentary habits do form rapidly. Thus, to expedite recovery, you don't want to procrastinate on physical therapy and other exercise activity if at all possible. This is exactly what I did. I procrastinated. But eventually, I learned from my mistakes. Hopefully, after reading my physical adversity challenge story (continued at the end of each chapter), you won't make the same ones I did.

Ultimately, it was my fitness programming experience as a military fitness trainer that provided the skill sets I needed to develop a modified exercise program to lose weight and become more mobile and alleviate pain. Ultimately, these recalled experiences provided the knowledge and motivational drivers I needed to heal and move on with life.

I recalled customizing fitness programs while serving in the air force guard back in 1988. This is where I really learned how to define, relate, and apply programming for any physical activity and to improve mobility, fitness levels, and unique healing programs that complemented physical therapy with a treating physician.

A base commander requested I customize fitness programs for fighter pilots and navigators who had lost their flying status due to injury. He also wanted to reduce neck and back stress injuries as a result of g-forces experienced during jet fighter maneuvers by applying my customized fitness programs.

Other squadron commanders then began to request other fitness programs related to occupation to minimize injuries in the workplace. So I developed all types of customized fitness programs in support of military occupations during the late eighties and midnineties. I also learned a great deal about injury prevention, pain tolerance, health risk, diet, weight loss, and well-being during one-on-one consultations.

As you now know, I was seriously injured at one point in my life while in the army. What you don't know is the injury was caused by an insidious bone disease known as AVN (avascular necrosis). The disease weakened my right hip, causing it to collapse during advanced army officer training school. I also suffer with AVN of the left hip, saved by a bone graft, and a previous broken back with degenerative spine disease.

I could personally relate to past military personnel who'd overcome much more serious illness, disease, and injury than I had. Many of them pulled through by applying programs I custom built and managed for them at the time.

I reasoned that, by the same logic, this programming process should work on me, right?

However, as painfully learned, it's much easier to relate and apply principled fitness programs on others than on self.

It's really a matter of *believing* there is a truthful programming process that can heal what ails you. You simply need to be provided the right information that's relatable and applicable for the situation. Then find the willpower and motivation to apply it.

But first you must believe the impossible is possible—especially now that you have all the truthful fitness and healthy lifestyle programming information at the tip of your fingers in a digestible format, provided to you by someone who spent decades accumulating and applying it. Apply it immediately and see positive change now.

You'll not go it alone. I'm here to teach, advise, instruct, and guide you in finding and achieving your MirrorAthlete image. Then you'll experience life to the fullest, regardless of your current fitness or health condition or physical adversity challenge.

Chapter 1

Relatable Knowledge Produces Superior Fitness Results

Optimize fitness results by defining and relating to applied fitness practices.

—MirrorAthlete Principled Fitness and
Healthy Lifestyle Philosophy

Right out the gate, I'm going to show you how to think like a fitness and healthy lifestyle coach and consumer safety advocate. But in order to get you there, it is necessary to start with some basic well-being and fitness terminology to help connect the dots. Then we'll address the number one fitness goal for many Americans—weight loss.

By the end of this book, you'll know the truths, half-truths, and flat-out lies when it comes to consumer weight-loss and health and fitness products. You'll also have the skill sets to customize a fitness program and leverage healthy habit change relevant and applicable to your daily needs and wants.

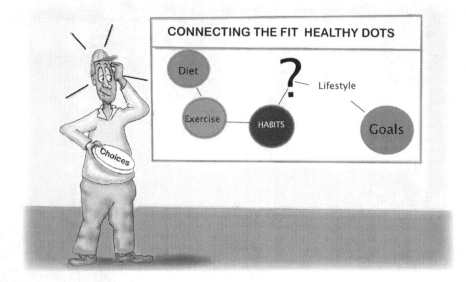

Why are healthy habit checks and balances important to include within a fitness program?

When healthy habits are valued, then one is better able to cope with stress and maintain a positive state of being (in other words, happy, energized, active, in a good mood, and so on). Sustaining fit healthy habits and behaviors is good for your holistic health (mind, body, and spirit). When your holistic health (or, as I often refer to it, encompassing being) is maintained, then the state of well-being is sustained (Georgetown University n.d.).

There is no singular consensus around a definition for *well-being*. However, the Centers for Disease Control and Prevention says, "In simple terms, 'well-being can be described as judging life positively and feeling good.'" Various public health disciplines research and examine many components of well-being—among them physical, economic, social, emotional, and psychological aspects; activity level; workplace and life satisfaction; participation in engaging activities; and many more (CDC 2016).

Feeling well and positive about life may require losing a little weight, especially if the "extra" weight makes you feel bad or overly conscientious about yourself. This makes sense, right? If you're overweight and uncomfortable, how well do you feel or how positively do you see yourself? All too often when overweight problems occur, people go on fad diets to lose weight quickly.

I personally don't refer to a weight-loss program as going on a diet. Going on a diet is not an exciting prospect for most of us because it is perceived as a sacrifice—doing without foods we love to eat. And as you'll soon learn, you don't have to give up the foods you love.

The word *diet*, for me, has a horrible connotation; I see it closely associated with marketplace gimmicks that have repeatedly failed too many clients in their weight-loss efforts.

To think, *I need to go on a weight-loss diet*, does not make one feel warm and fuzzy about changing eating habits. And it certainly doesn't fulfill a sense of well-being—especially since food is a big part of our social and cultural experience.

I do use the term *diet* throughout this book in a nutritional sense. Understand that I use the term to mean learning how to balance healthy food groups or macronutrients and calories and understanding how this balance is important to healthy body weight, good fitness levels and mood, and overall well-being.

Please do keep in mind, and don't forget, you're not on a diet. You're simply learning how to make better food choices and changing a few unhealthy habits.

The format in which you'll learn how to create a customized fitness and healthy habits program is based on MirrorAthlete science.

The fitness and healthy lifestyle principles for each chapter are defined, relatable, and applied in unique ways that progressively take the reader deeper into the mind-set of how fitness and healthy lifestyle consultants engage and program their clients. Then connect the marketplace products and services dots that help achieve a desired result.

As a lifelong fitness consultant and wellness expert, I understand many believe a nonflexible diet and grueling exercise regimen is required to achieve the weight-loss goal. The reality of this belief is that *it's not true*.

Weight-loss failures often occur because consumers don't understand or make a connection between what the organic brain and body need and achieving the goal. Once these connections are made, there's no limit to the fit, healthy results possible without using unsafe man-made products.

The following client examples illustrate how fitness trainers apply their programming skill sets to clients. As you progress through each chapter, you'll learn more advanced fitness programming skill sets that can be applied to yourself.

To begin, the two examples below simply referred to as "Client A" and "Client B" are short summary case studies from client archives. Throughout the learning process, remain mindful that there are no two fitness consultants or trainers who operate under the same principled, fit healthy lifestyle philosophy umbrella. What you are beginning to absorb is a unique training and programming skill set not typically taught in colleges or applied in most gyms or fitness centers or one-on-one client sessions.

The basic principles and programming foundations found throughout the book are important concepts to master. Understanding them will help you begin the process of absorbing the advanced materials covered throughout the book.

I provide two basic client consult summary note examples taken during sessions to get you into the fitness programming mind-set. After this, you'll be able to absorb the more inclusive and advanced materials to follow like a sponge absorbs water.

I use to tell my students "make like a sponge." It worked for them. This mind-set can work for you.

Client A (forty-eight-year-old female)

Fitness goal: Client A wants weight loss and expectation of having the body and energy level of a thirty-year-old.

General notes: During the consult it was determined that more than half of Client A's food consumption appeared to come from processed foods. I didn't note any severe obsessive eating disorders. Instead, it appeared she more or less consumed too many processed foods of low-nutrient quality. What sold her on eating certain diet foods was the "lower calorie per serving" statements on food boxes.

This led her to believe she'd have a significant weight loss in a short period of time if she only consumed these premade meals. These foods were not low-calorie foods; they just had fewer calories than some competing brands. When I asked what type of exercise she participated in daily, she stated she did twenty minutes on an aerobics cycle five days per week. She did not want to lift weights for fear of developing muscular bulk and adding to her body weight.

She also stated an interest in liposuction to remove body fat in her belly and thighs. I provided no recommendations in this area other than mentioning that I believed she could do this naturally once she knew how. However, if she was determined to get the surgery, she should understand the health risks. A doctor could describe those risks.

Exercise modification recommendation: Increase aerobic workout time to thirty minutes on the bike and "add" thirty minutes walking, three to five days per week (chapter 18, "Customized Fitness Programming").

Food habits or behavioral change recommendations: Consume no processed foods, only whole foods for a four- to six-week period. Eat three balanced meals a day. Attempt to stay within 1,500 to 1,800 calories per day (chapter 5, "Caloric Exchange: A Balancing Act"). Consume fruit and vegetable snacks. Drink no less than three liters of water per day.

Applied results: Eight-pound loss within a four-week window.

Follow-up: Client A is no longer interested in liposuction. She intends to stay on this fitness plan until she loses twenty-five pounds and will then follow up to reassess her fitness goals and modify the fitness program.

Is fitness programming really this easy? To be honest, no it's not. And results vary significantly for each individual using similar programs. But what you'll take away from more detailed client examples is an ability to create a program that's uniquely designed to work for you.

Client B (twenty-eight-year-old male)

Fitness goal: Client B is interested in losing belly fat and maintaining his muscle bulk and strength.

General notes: He wants to lose twelve pounds. During the consult, it was revealed that aerobic exercise was not his thing. His daily calorie intake included three to five beers. I can't say his food choices were great. He did agree to focus on two habit changes that would help reduce body fat.

Exercise modification recommendation: Include four to five days per week any aerobic exercise of choice for no less than twenty to thirty minutes between strength-training activities.

Food habits or behavioral change recommendations: Recommend he watch sports over the weekend at home, not in his buddy's man cave—which will help limit beer consumption. He also agreed to choose two days a week to consume no more than two to three beers before 8:00 p.m. I explained that a continuous drinking habit is not good for anyone—especially later in the evening after the metabolism slows down. The ideal is that he'd limit beer and drink more water throughout the day.

Applied results: Client B lost ten pounds in four to five weeks.

Sometimes it's just better to allow clients to choose a degree of habit and fitness effort modification, instead of programming ridged conformity. Once clients begin to see positive results, eventually they learn to strike a balance of healthier habit change (chapter 12, "Many Habits Were Formed Day One").

Follow-up: He is happy to sustain his current fitness program. I did note he appeared more toned with increased muscle definition after applying most of the habit change recommendations.

He has stuck to the aerobics program, even though it wasn't his thing. And he views more sporting events at home and is eating less junk foods. He has not done as well with the beer habit. He cut in half his overall carbohydrate intake and drinks fewer beers throughout the week.

He requested no further client follow-up.

***

Typical fitness trainer services often include one-on-one exercise training orientation, fitness assessments, basic exercise programs, discussions on how to improve fitness levels, and review of medical history. Then the client is provided a basic fitness form designed to track results.

During consultation, I often provided awareness to marketplace product deceptions relevant to a fitness goal. Why is this important? Certain products and services can sabotage your results. If you become ill or develop disease using something unnatural and bad for you, what good is it if it destroys your health, state of wellness, or well-being? And what do those terms actually mean?

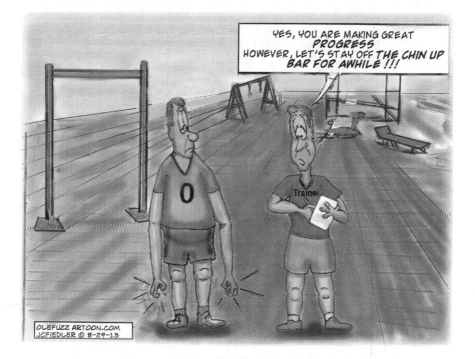

Good health can be defined by the quality of life lived free from illness, injury, or pain or by the quality of wellness. The state of wellness or the state of well-being is dependent upon healthy habits that include balanced nutrition, exercise, adequate rest, good relationships, and activity that also defines quality of lifestyle. Health is also described as an active lifestyle that supports the physical, mental, and spiritual needs of the holistic or encompassing being (Center for Reintegration, n.d.).

Now, let's get down to the nuts and bolts of defining fitness and commonly used assessment terminology and how this understanding will help get the fitness and wellness results you need and want now.

Fitness is defined by many as being the proper shape and size or measured by some medical standard—in other words, height-weight or the body mass index (BMI) Table as seen in chapter 5.

The American College of Sports Medicine measures five components of physical fitness that lead to good health. These fitness measurements are used by fitness trainers to assess fitness levels, overall health, and program exercise activity to achieve specific fitness results. These assessments measure body fat composition, cardiorespiratory fitness, flexibility, muscular strength, and muscular endurance (Percia, Davis, and Dwyer 2012).

The five fitness assessment components below are defined and will help you understand the fitness level relationships related to personal goals.

Throughout the book, I provide the tools you need to assess your current fitness level and set new baselines. Similar to working with a client, I show you how to monitor and improve your fitness levels. Once you learn these things, you're well on your way to achieving positive fitness results without paying for the services.

Body fat is determined by calculating the fat and fat-free "lean" tissue (muscle, bone, organs, and fluids) percentages. The combined lean body and fat weight equal total body weight. Through assessment analysis, it is possible to determine an approximate percentage of body fat with a specialized body fat caliper, impedance, or hydrostatic equipment.

There are various ways fitness trainers assess body fat for clients. The most popular and cost-effective way is to measure body fat using a skin fold caliper or taping the circumference of various sites on the body to approximate a percentage of body fat weight. Measuring and limiting unhealthy body fat is important to understand because of the connection to obesity, illness, and disease.

A fitness trainer will also use a treadmill, stairs, or cycling protocols to test and measure *cardio or aerobic endurance* capacity and prescribe an aerobic exercise program that's relevant to the fitness goal.

It is low-impact aerobic exercise activity that can melt away fat, and as you increase exercise intensity up to a certain point, the fat-burning engine can operate at 100 percent capacity. Advanced aerobics knowledge includes how to use THR (target heart rate) efficiently to burn more body fat naturally (chapter 18, "Customized Fitness Programming"). Soon you'll understand how powerful this fat-burning knowledge is and how intuitively easy it is to apply.

Flexibility testing measures the degree to which (or range of motion) a joint can articulate or move. Flexibility is a measurement that determines the range of motion (ROM) needed to perform activities of daily living (ADL).

In other words, to live an independent lifestyle is highly dependent on ROM and mobility to perform ADLs. Certified fitness trainers and physical therapy professionals typically use a sit-and-reach box or protractor that measures range of various joint articulation or segments of body movement—for example, back, hips, shoulders, neck, wrists, fingers, and so on. Without good flexibility, limited range of motion can make daily tasks and walking more difficult, painful, and challenging.

Muscular strength and endurance can be tested on muscle groups using the one-rep max (1RM) rule and other fitness protocols.

Muscular strength, or force, measurement assesses maximum weight lifted one time (known as the one-rep max, or 1RM), whereas muscular endurance measures a number of repetition(s) completed at an exercise station. Muscular endurance can also be measured during competitive events or completion of personal tasks, such as getting daily work done.

Muscular endurance, unlike muscular strength, is assessed by using timed protocol tests, where the subject typically performs push-ups, bench presses, leg squats at a set weight, or sit-ups doing as many repetitions as possible within a one-minute period. Results are compared against a like average of similar demographics performing the same task.

A lack of good muscular endurance makes it difficult for the body, especially as we age, to maintain healthy weight and perform endurance activities for long periods of time. Muscular endurance is the ability of muscle to perform an activity task that's long in endurance. Examples include walking, jogging, running, yard work, rowing, biking, dancing, household, chores, and so on.

Muscular strength is necessary to get out of a chair, pick up a box, or move an object, and so on. Without good strength, though, muscular-skeletal health is more likely to be compromised during the aging process. Sustaining ROM and good mobility becomes more essential as we age. Through low-stress daily exercise activity, quality well-being experiences are more likely to continue.

There are literally hundreds of ways you could approach *nutrition and fitness tactics and strategies* to sustain decent fitness levels even as they decline.

This knowledge is especially important for our elderly—illustrated by this population. A huge need exists to assist this demographic with relevant fitness information that would keep them mobile and healthy as long as possible. Census Bureau 2010 figures show forty million people age sixty-five and over living in the United States (Internicola 2013). These numbers are not decreasing.

It is also true that health literacy within our children's schools and consumer marketplace need much improvement. "Health literacy is defined as the degree to which individuals have the capacity to obtain, process, and understand basic health information needed to make appropriate health decisions and services needed to prevent or treat illness" (HRSA 2015).

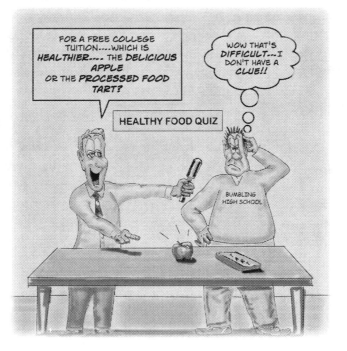

The necessity of health literacy, in my mind, relates directly to what I coined "ill-health prevention education." It's basically health prevention and health literacy education, which is desperately needed if we hope to get a handle on childhood obesity and associated illness and disease.

Today's generation, more than any before, needs to know how poor consumer choices, bad habits, and bad behavior impact health, lifestyle, and well-being. It's what we don't know about our bodies and environment that has an immediate impact on quality of life.

If our children don't learn to value healthy lifestyle choices early on, it's likely they won't value these things as adults. When K–12 schools, city leaders, and marketplaces don't prioritize or see the value of health literacy and the connection between health and recreational activity investments in communities, it does not bode well for the health of future generations. Nor does it bode well for the health and productivity of a nation.

Personal Fitness Challenge: "Embrace Pain"

Within a four-year period, I became overweight after disease and injury held me hostage with limited mobility. The BMI standard (chapter 5, table 5.4) showed I was at 30 percent body fat and in a state of obesity. This is a body fat percentage I never thought I'd personally reach, but it happened. Then I had to find a way to reduce that number. Otherwise, further injury and disease would eventually ravage my mind, body, and spirit.

For most obese or overweight individuals, the techniques found within this book will safely and painlessly allow them to lose one to two pounds a week naturally. This is provided the physical disability, injury, illness, or disease isn't serious enough to completely prevent exercise activity.

I highly recommend, when beginning an exercise program, to make a plan to increase aerobics activity. Plan to lose no more than one to two pounds a week if grossly obese or sedentary for a long period of time. Also seek approval from a medical doctor to participate in low-impact aerobics. It is through my experience that I have learned that losing weight more quickly than this is neither a sustainable nor healthy habit for most (chapter 13, "Leverage Healthy Habit Change").

The techniques offered within this book certainly won't limit you from losing more weight. That decision is entirely up to you. However, keep in mind, there's a right way to lose weight safely, just like there's a right way to build muscle or increase aerobic endurance and so on.

If you're in a disabled mobility state like I was for a long period of time, it may take twenty-four months or more to lose thirty pounds. But if you're overweight and take the time to lose the extra weight naturally, it most likely will be a result you can sustain long-term.

During rehabilitation after surgeries, the weight gain also contributed to disabling chronic back and hip pain, which "I knew" could only be alleviated through increased physical activity.

It seems counterintuitive to increase physical activity when in pain, but doing so is essential to speed up the healing process, which includes weight loss.

What I learned during this particular adversity challenge is that the mind must be prepared to embrace some pain to get well.

And without focus on a rehabilitative plan to move forward, the willingness to accept a certain level of discomfort to heal sooner rather than later declines. Embracing the pain becomes more difficult the longer you wait.

A well-defined fitness plan and program can positively increase mobility while reducing pain and healing sooner rather than later.

This is especially true when applied relative to any physical adversity situation.

Chapter 2

Selfish Interests Impact the Health of Our Kids

Ill-health prevention through health literacy education can save a nation in pain.

—MirrorAthlete Principled Fitness and
Healthy Lifestyle Philosophy

I've learned after years of client consults and working within the fitness industry that the marketplace as a whole is rife with selfish interests. Many private and public goods and services are promotionally hyped, formulated, and promoted in ways that often don't meet consumer expectations and negatively impact health, habits, and behavior starting at a young age.

I know for some it's hard to believe it's possible to achieve a fitness or well-being goal without specialized foods, supplements, enhancement drugs, and intense exercise activity. But it is possible, and you'll learn how.

Through years of experience and education I've learned that many natural, fit healthy truths are hidden within academia's science and cultures, where people live long healthy lives without illness and disease (chapter 17, "Longevity Secrets Divulged"). In many ways, I've realized, the marketplace and, yes, our government hope these well-kept secrets remain secrets. Soon you'll understand why our marketplace operates the way it does.

I've seen charlatans in the fitness industry prey upon those who are desperate to overhaul their bodies, fix what ails them, and even reverse the aging process. Then, once a client is addicted to an unhealthy fad, product, or service—and gets sick—it's not their problem. They already have your money. How sick is that!?

To be honest, not everyone in the marketplace has deceitful intentions. What I'm saying is you will find in the marketplace some less-than-honest folks who care nothing about you or your children's health and well-being. Although they appear to care, their actions speak louder than their words.

This is not such a crazy concept, is it? By understanding human behavior and connecting the consumer and marketplace dots, you decide if there's an ounce of truth and a case to be made here. If there is an ounce of selfish interest, you must call it what it is—"selfish interest truth."

If communities are serious about reversing childhood obesity and related disease, at a minimum, why aren't the basic fit, healthy lifestyle truths taught in our K–12 schools? And why is there no national fitness policy effort to include such coursework into school curriculums? The short answer, it's really about the interests of our government, the marketplace, and what community leaders value and prioritize. And these things are driven by personal agendas and interests, which include job security, profit, power, and control.

It's no secret habits and behaviors are mostly formed during childhood. And if children are to value fit, healthy habits and apply them as adults, early education during the developmental years, in my opinion, is key. This would be the best time for children to learn, value, and apply healthy lifestyle choices throughout their formative years.

Unfortunately, I don't believe the marketplace or our government wants the next generation to become educated consumers and voters. Instead, they need a majority to drink the marketplace Kool-Aid to sustain the current economic supply and demand model, the current socio-politico-economic engine (more easily chalked up as Western culture).

As a fitness consultant, I sprinkle little bits of Western culture into the context of discussions. That way, my clients understand how their healthy lifestyle goals can be sabotaged, without their knowledge, by others' interests. It is this insight that helped my clients make healthier lifestyle choices for themselves. And when they shared what they'd learned, their family and friends benefited.

The marketplace doesn't want consumers to be educated on the differences between pseudoscientific and preventative medicine, for example, diet and fitness fads that don't work long term versus daily exercise activity and healthy eating habits that will work. Nor does it want consumers who are knowledgeable about risky antiaging hormone therapy and supplements commonly used to increase functions like sexual stamina or strength and muscular endurance. The same applies to unproven products that offer pain relief—pain that could otherwise be alleviated by living a healthier lifestyle without increasing health risk.

The reality is what consumers don't know is causing harm to their health, productivity, and ability to live life to the fullest.

Through healthy living education, our children would also understand that, "in the scientific community anti-aging research refers exclusively to slowing, preventing, or reversing the aging process ... In the medical and reputable business community, anti-aging medicine means the early detection, prevention, and treatment of age-related diseases" (Reason 2013). It can become very difficult for consumers to understand and dissect the antiaging message truth and health risks versus the benefits associated with voodoo science sold in the marketplace.

"The American Academy of Anti-Aging Medicine (A4M) [is] an organization created in 1992 to advance technologies that prevent and treat age-related disease as well as support research on extending life. Anti-aging medicine is not recognized as a specialty by the American Board of Medical Specialties. Doctors who practice antiaging medicine use a range of treatments and therapies, including bioidentical hormones and supplements that continue to be the subject of debate in the medical community" (Rhone 2012). Although antiaging prevention has come a long way in support of increased lifespan, living past ninety in good health is still reserved for a few.

I believe sedentary habits, obesity, and related disease could mostly be reversed if our government, community leaders, educational institutions, and parents prioritized and valued ill-health prevention and healthy lifestyle literacy education for our children. Inclusion of this knowledge would improve fitness levels, health, and well-being for life.

But a national fitness policy to fund such a program would be a tough pill to swallow for politicians, government officials, and organized teacher unions; within these organizations, our children's health interests don't align with theirs. Therefore, it is not likely the Department of Education will be lobbied by politicians, school boards, and union executives to put our children's interest first.

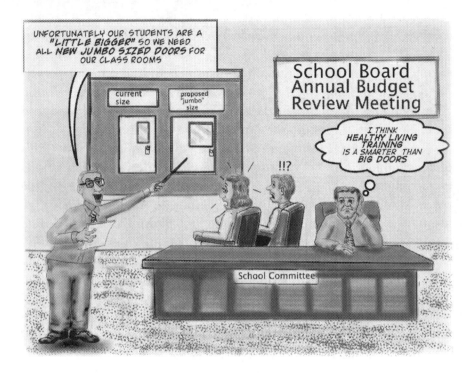

When children are deprived of these educational experiences, their mental, physical, and spiritual growth is not fully developed or realized. Hence, the encompassing being is partially developed. And what they have not experienced—that missing wisdom—can't be passed on to the next generation. Therefore, that generation conforms to Western culture's unhealthy habits and behaviors, which include selfish interests.

By examining a few recent and significant legislative and special interest actions, it's easier to understand how special interests impact school budgets and why organizations like teachers and federal employee unions can't operate in a more businesslike manner. Through these examples, it's also easier to see why fitness and healthy lifestyle education isn't a priority or a core course requirement and why there'll never be any money for it. This makes no sense—especially when data shows childhood and adult obesity cases are increasing, along with related diseases. But neither the near epidemic childhood obesity problem nor disadvantaged and disabled children are a priority for them.

Remember sequestration? The automatic spending cuts began March 1, 2013, resulting from the Budget Control Act of 2011 as an austerity measure to get government spending under control. As a result, on October 1, 2013, the government temporarily shut down because of budget disputes over debt ceiling. Government function was then resumed on October 17, 2013. It shut down until an approximately $1.5 trillion budget deal was made to make spending cuts over a ten-year period. Who made these cuts and under what deals? Whose interests were served and whose weren't? Who will be harmed the most over the next decade? It doesn't appear these projected cuts were in the best interests of childhood development and education.

The Congressional Budget Office projected sequestration would put a number of programs at risk. Cuts to Title I programs that include special education and other large K–12 programs will impact more than four thousand schools and an estimated 1.8 million disadvantaged children, along with other support to 6.6 million children with disabilities if enacted. These cuts would impact services of more than fifteen thousand teachers and aides and would take effect in the fall of 2013 (Press Office 2012).

Who knows? President Trump may be able to bridge the projected Title I cuts by redirecting a $20 billion grant for a school choice voucher program. With it, schools could provide the common core standards and criteria necessary to ensure children receive a fit, healthy education. It may be the only way to squeeze it in through private school charters— because of the No Child Left Behind Act.

School budgets continue to cut comprehensive education programs, partially because of the No Child Left Behind Act President Bush signed into law on January 8, 2002. Whereas common core curriculum is K–12 educators' priority, the act provides federal grants to states who set standards based on common core criteria, and teacher unions want more control over these resources. They also don't want to compete with charter schools and for good reason.

If teacher unions had to compete with charter schools, they'd likely lose leverage in future labor negotiations, which equates to job security. School choice would also create a trickle-up effect in higher education curriculum and competition for student seats and tenured professor jobs. Government workers, elected officials, lobbyist, and collective bargaining positions would also be at stake.

According to one analysis:

> Data collected from 2008 to 2010 by the National Center for the Study of Collective Bargaining in Higher Education and the Professions show that about 440,000 faculty and graduate students are members of collective bargaining units, a 17% increase from five years ago ...
>
> According to a 2010 report from the Bureau of Labor and Statistics, the majority of the country's union members are government workers, rather than private-sector workers ... Moreover, the anti-corporate tone on many campuses and the left-leaning political views of college professors on campuses make them naturally more receptive to the union message ...
>
> Some observers worry that unions desire more than job protection ... Peter Kirsanow, a former member of the National Labor Relations Board, has noted that unions "want to get into curricula, class schedules, grading norms, etc." (Riley 2011)

Collective bargaining laws throughout the country vary from state to state and within local cities and municipalities but are similar in the way politicians and unions negotiate contracts to get the best deal possible for both sides. These deals are negotiated without competition or public input and behind closed doors. One side represents the taxpayer, and the other side agrees to provide educational services regulated by a plethora of complicated union, federal, and state education and employee laws that appear to put other interests first.

For instance, the Fair Labor Laws and Standards protect both private and public employee worker rights, wages, and benefits. "The department of labor (DOL) administers and enforces more than 180 federal laws ... The Fair Labor Standards Act (FLSA) prescribes standards for wages and overtime pay, which affect most private and public employment" (US DOL 2018).

What do sequestration, the No Child Left Behind Act, collective bargaining, FLSA, affordable health care, and the FDA have to do with fit, healthy childhood development education? And why can't these interests shift priorities to put our children's needs first?

It's partially about the special interests negotiated behind closed doors that continue to drive costs upward at the expense of our children's health. "The yearly cost of wages, health coverage, pensions, step increases, cost-of-living raises and other state employee benefits is no longer decided through public hearings in the normal legislative process. These operating costs are now decided in a series of secret collective bargaining meetings between union representatives and executive branch officials" (Guppy 2011). How can our children's best interests be represented and served when union wages, benefits, and jobs discussions are not part of a public process?

Public servants and collective bargaining interests are not representing our children's best interests by putting their needs first. Government and union interests don't stop with our educational resource shortfalls. They also are major players in the health care industry who are responsible for driving up unsustainable costs. For instance, just take a look at the projected 2001 to 2013 health care cost increases that have caused wages to stall while growing bigger union and governmental control over our lives and wallets.

Health care costs are escalating with no end in sight. "The cost to cover the typical family of four under an employer plan is expected to top $20,000 on health care this year, up more than 7% from last year, according to early projections by independent actuarial and health care consulting firm Milliman Inc. In 2002, the cost was just $9,235, the firm said" (Dickler 2012). So much for affordable health care and keeping your doctor.

"Health insurance premiums for employer-sponsored insurance nearly doubled over the past decade, with total premiums (employers' and workers' shares) increasing from an average of $7,601 per year in 2001 to $15,073 in 2011 for family coverage. Rising premiums contributed to a rise in the proportion of people without health insurance" (Komisar 2013).

The IRS expects both families of four and families of five "to pay a minimum of $20,000 per year for a bronze plan" (Cover 2013).

These consumer cost trajectories have proved to be true, and the increases don't appear to be over. However, with the insurgence of Trump promising to repeal Obamacare, it is possible these costs could come down as the marketplace becomes more competitive in the health care industry over the next decade. But there are no guarantees.

Heavy-handed and growing public agencies show us how their interests continue to benefit them and not our children's growth and development. They continue to create expensive, ineffective, and unnecessary bureaucracies that manufacture nothing, grow bureaucracies, and have a tax spending appetite that can't be satisfied.

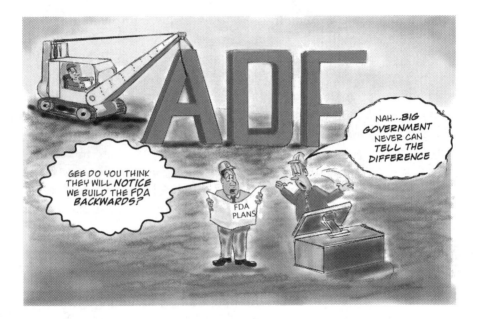

Consumers looking to live healthier lifestyles also need to know the Federal Drug Administration (FDA) is another huge bureaucracy involved in consumer food and drug safety and a health cost driver.

I'll be the first to admit the FDA has a huge consumer safety job to tackle, and it needs to be done. But would it be better to privatize parts of this business, as with other government agencies, to make it more competitive and efficient and to lessen the tax burden on hardworking families?

For example, in the case of "off-label" prescriptions, these relabeled products are approved by the FDA to repurpose drugs for different treatment use than originally intended. This information is especially important to know if working on a fitness plan where exercise activity is programmed around treatment that may make you drowsy or not feel well or create other health risks. For adults working through physical adversity, this is important health literacy knowledge relative to fitness programming.

"Since off-label prescribing is sometimes the standard of care, defending off-label cases takes the perspective of patient harm versus patient benefit." Other issues to consider are "whether physicians or the FDA have been misled in any serious way" (Policy and Medicine 2010). And if the off-label process were to be put to a halt, many patients may lose their life. On the flip side, many lose their lives due to secondary health complications.

Another point I want to make obvious—and most would agree—is that, when it comes to government service and access to government programs, customer service experience and the ability to actually reach a government employee by phone is not the same compared to access and service in the private sector. Simply recall any experience you had in a large public service agency, like a school, a city permits building, the DMV, the Veterans Benefits Administration, Social Security Disability Administration (SSDA), the post office, and Medicare to name a few.

The experience is often less satisfying, less efficient, and more costly to operate because government doesn't have to compete with a shareholder mandate to produce a profit. Therefore, no incentives or performance accountability are required to produce a better public service. Those inefficiencies in operations come at greater cost to the taxpayer. Now you begin to understand how taxpayer interests and wealth redistribution are controlled by industry and government interests. So how good of a job are these agencies and organizations doing spending your tax dollars?

If the government and educational institutions were doing such a great job at protecting consumers and educating our youth to be healthy producers of American products, why are there now more chemically and genetically engineered, modified foods with hyperpalatable ingredients that are addictive to consumers and known to cause obesity, diabetes, congestive heart disease, and cancer? If government and marketplace interests cared about our health and our children, these numbers would be going down, not up.

Another consumer truth that must be realized during early childhood development revolves around a balanced, whole foods diet. Without this knowledge, achieving a sustainable and natural fit healthy lifestyle is less likely, and future generations will need more health care services at the expense of taxpayers (chapter 14, "Processed vs. Organic Food").

Until you read chapter 14, I leave you the following quote to ponder: "For the last 100 years we have been witnessing dramatic advances in the scientific understanding and engineering techniques that increase agricultural production and allow for the commercial-scale production of countless processed foods. Through the concerted efforts of chemical engineers and others, the yields and quality of farm crops have increased exponentially, and the industry producing and packaging foods and beverages has evolved to a business worth many hundreds of billions of dollars" (Rodowicz 2009). And the plethora of chemicals used to produce those billions is now inside us—and taking a toll on the health of our people.

Finding a way to inclusively and comprehensively provide our kids ill-health prevention and fitness and health literacy education is one thing. Holding government and food industries accountable for chemicals that make us sick at the expense of hard-earned tax dollars is something else. These things are all connected by way of our culture. Unless we teach our children about unhealthy interests that drive cultural interests, the increasing ill-health trajectory in this nation won't change.

I've often thought about this unchanging trajectory or status quo and how it could be reversed through early education. I believe the answer is in a specialized educational module titled, e.g., Fit Healthy Lifestyle for Life," based on the principles in this book. And I believe the dissemination of this model should be funded by the Department of Education and implemented as soon as possible.

I have no other better solution on how to begin reversing these cultural interests. Until something like this is implemented on a national scale, it is important for parents and their children to understand that our marketplace is full of unhealthy interests, more than I could possibly cover.

Regardless, you must take matters into your own hands for the sake of good health and well-being. Being aware of such things opens the mind to discovery of other unhealthy interests. You may want to think twice before buying into a system, service, or program—be it political, social, or economic—that favors the marketplace and the bottom line over consumer health.

Personal Fitness Challenge: "Life Adversities"

Throughout my youth, I recall parents working together to raise money for school projects, extracurricular activities, and weekend social events where educators, community, and families worked together for the benefit of children. It seemed I grew up in a time when government stayed out of people's lives for the most part. Taxes didn't compromise a family's ability to provide recreational activities for kids. And foods weren't loaded with chemicals that harm health.

Even if a child was not one's own, parents understood all children needed a well-rounded education, balanced meals, and a safe place to play. Families also socialized, bonded, and developed healthy relationships. This was just part of a wholesome and well-rounded upbringing I experienced during childhood. As a point of reflection, I can tell you that seeing an obese child at that time was rare.

Although I experienced a balanced mix of schooling, recreational, and social activities, that balance provided no guarantee I wouldn't face a serious physical challenge later on in life. However, recalling the well-rounded education I received, along with the ample recreational opportunities and experiences during my youth contributed to multiple physical, mental, and spiritual healing events as an adult.

As you read through each "Personal Fitness Challenge" story, the importance and necessity of a fit, healthy lifestyle and of ill-health prevention and health literacy education becomes more obvious. It becomes ever clearer that such education could benefit this generation and the next and save a nation in pain.

Nursing my way back to health was not easy. Physical rehabilitation was one of the hardest challenges I've ever faced. Like others, I've experienced life adversities where bouncing back was not easy. But when I experienced serious physical injury and disease simultaneously, it was a devastating blow to me in every imaginable way.

The physical limitations during the healing process had a very powerful effect on the way I viewed life and prioritized daily activities and how I saw myself in the mirror.

My once athletic and agile, muscular frame, which knew no physical limitations, was reduced to a pile of rubble within a very short period of time after the destruction of one hip and a disease that threatened to destroy the other. These things complicated an already chronic back problem I'd suffered over the years from a head-on car collision caused by a drunk driver.

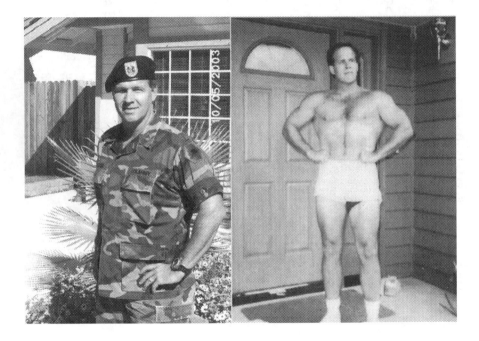

I went through all the phases of loss—you know, denial, anger, depression, and acceptance. Then it started all over again on multiple occasions, while I was dealing with never-ending nerve pain throughout my body.

Never before had I put so much planning and effort into developing and applying a rehabilitative fitness program for any client as I did for myself. And a big part of this challenge included scrutiny of foods, pharmaceuticals, and medical referrals and therapeutic and exercise choices.

I certainly didn't need unnecessary toxins and excess body weight while on the mend. Nor did I need to complicate a bone disease that could possibly spread elsewhere. So I left no stone unturned to heal and get on with life.

Should you experience disease and/or physical adversity, I'm confident that, after you read these chapters, including my "Personal Fitness Challenge" stories to conclusion, you'll have the tools necessary to reach a better state of mind, body, and spirit; to heal what ails you; and to live life to the fullest.

Chapter 3

Muscles' Fuel Preference during Exercise

> Working muscle metabolism prefers specific fuel
> mixtures to optimize fitness results.
>
> —MirrorAthlete Principled Fitness and
> Healthy Lifestyle Philosophy

When you perform work or exercise, you're going to burn calories at a faster rate than when you're at rest and then need to replace them. For some, exercise overstimulates appetite and causes weight gain. I recollect reading a *Times* article on this topic many years ago; a particular statement caught my eye. The statement read, "I get hungry after I exercise, so I often eat more on the days I work out than on the days I don't. Could exercise actually be keeping me from losing weight?" John Cloud coined this the "compensation effect" (Cloud 2009).

Do I personally believe in the compensation effect? Absolutely. Both eating and activity habits have a cause and effect on the body, behavior, and habits. For a percentage of you, hunger is a challenge that requires behavioral change around diet and exercise to offset the compensation effect.

I consulted a thirty-eight-year-old woman who wanted to lose weight and tone her body. Kelli had been participating in a high-impact aerobics dance program for at least six weeks before she sought my fitness consulting services. She stated that she was eating healthfully, but her body weight had increased, and her tone hadn't appeared to change. Her body fat per simple BMI (body mass index) calculation (chapter 5, "Caloric Exchange: A Balancing Act") put her at around 32 percent body fat weight.

As a side note, it is important to understand that BMI does not measure body fat directly. Research shows BMI is moderately correlated with more direct measures of body fat from skin fold thickness measurements, bioelectrical impedance, densitometry (underwater weighing), dual energy x-ray absorptiometry (DXA), and other methods. Furthermore, BMI appears to be strongly correlated with various metabolic and disease outcomes consistent with these more direct measures of body fatness (CDC 2012).

In our consult, Kelli mentioned feeling hungry, especially after each aerobics session. I asked her if her goal was to lose body fat or work towards sustaining high-cardio and muscular endurance activity. During our discussion, she seemed confused on how exercise, muscle metabolism, diet and weight gain/weight loss were connected. So I helped redirect her focus to achieve a desired weight-loss goal through a modified fitness program plan.

I explained that, when you work out intensely during aerobic exercise, working muscle will prefer burning carbohydrates before fats. And when total calories consumed are not burned daily they're stored as fat.

Next, I'm going to break down these concepts by getting into exercise activity intensity effort required to burn more body fat versus performing exercise at high levels of intensity and then refueling those calories.

Intensity of training effort determines the fuel source preferred during exercise. For example, "Carbohydrate is the main nutrient that fuels exercise of a moderate to high intensity, while fat can fuel low-intensity exercise for long periods of time. Proteins are generally used to maintain and repair body tissues and are not normally used to power muscle activity" (Quinn 2018a).

It is shown through various exercise physiology studies that the more intensely the body works, the greater the demand for carbohydrate fuel after digestion breaks it down into glucose. Excess glucose in the body is then stored in the liver and muscle glycogen. After those stores are full, it accumulates and stores as fat (Daussin et al. 2008).

Glycogen is sometimes called "animal starch" because of its resemblance to starch found in plants. "In the liver this conversion is regulated by the hormone glucagon. Under certain conditions, between meals for instance, liver glycogen is an important source of blood glucose ... Glycogen is the primary glucose (energy) storage mechanism" (Orthomolecular 2013).

For those who wish to lose weight, compensation effect can be a challenge to overcome—especially when the quick energy stores deplete and the brain's hunger center senses it's low on blood sugar and needs refueling. When this happens, a blood sugar level indicator signals the brain to crave and want carbohydrate foods to satisfy hunger through a quick blood glucose fix. To avoid overeating habits, behavior has to change; one must stay out of starvation mode by managing the compensation effect.

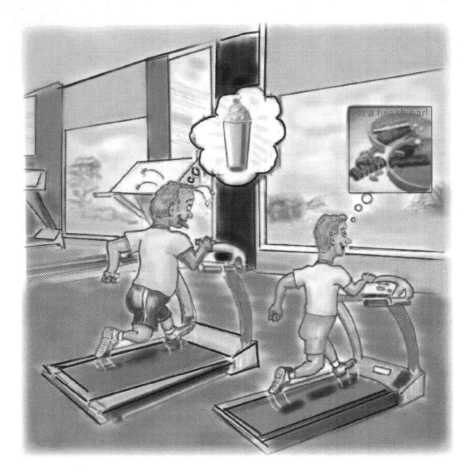

Like Kelli, if you're fitness goal is to lose body fat, you'll want to program yourself to do more low-medium aerobics activities of longer duration and modify food habits. Why? Because lower-intensity aerobics exercise "optimizes" the use of oxygen to burn body fat. Low-intensity aerobics centers on endurance activities like walking, jogging, swimming, biking, and the like. In addition, a healthy snack strategy between meals will mitigate the sensation in the brain's hunger center that blood sugar levels are low throughout the day.

To better understand how people gain weight through improper exercise and diet, it is necessary to define, relate, and expand on the muscle fuel preference, exercise intensity, and duration. No worries, I'll make this as painless as possible while showing how this information can be applied by anyone who wants to lose weight naturally and safely to get fit and stay healthy.

During aerobic exercise, "oxygen is used to burn fats and glucose in order to produce adenosine triphosphate, the basic energy carrier for all cells. Initially during aerobic exercise, glycogen is broken down to produce glucose, but in its absence, fat metabolism is initiated instead" (Science Daily 2013a).

"The anaerobic energy pathway, or glycolysis creates ATP (adenosine triphosphate) exclusively from carbohydrates, with lactic acid being a by-product. Anaerobic glycolysis provides energy by the (partial) breakdown of glucose without the need for oxygen. Anaerobic metabolism produces energy for short, high-intensity bursts of activity lasting no more than several minutes before the lactic acid build-up reaches a threshold known as the lactate threshold and muscle pain, burning and fatigue make it difficult to maintain such intensity" (Quinn 2018). Athletes refer to this muscular burn out phase as hitting the wall.

When the body runs low on blood glucose and/or stored muscle glycogen during high-intensity training, the next available energy source is provided from stored body fat. During this time, muscles' natural response is to rest or slow down once the fast-burning fuel glucose and then glycogen is expended. When glycogen fuel tanks are empty and blood glucose levels are low, aerobic exercise can continue at a slower pace by burning fat fuel and then speed up once the quick fuel sources are replenished.

The liver and muscle storage fuel tank replenishment helper is glucagon. When the pancreas releases the peptide hormone glucagon, it signals the brain's hunger center that fuel tanks are low and need replenishment. Once hunger is satisfied, then glucose, glycogen, and fat storage tanks are refueled. This fuel cycling occurs throughout the day as we eat and move about. To learn more about metabolic exchange rate, refer to chapter 5, "Caloric Exchange: A Balancing Act."

Anaerobic metabolism, unlike aerobic metabolism, occurs during high-intensity exercise activity and burns very little body fat to perform the task. Anaerobic exercise metabolism engages when maximum speed, strength, and power are needed for a short duration of time. The muscles' cellular energy during 100 percent anaerobic training effort is "able to take place where free oxygen is not present" (US Environmental Protection Agency 2009).

Kelli was working out hard with intensities of 90 to 95 percent aerobic-anaerobic effort and was overloading on carbs daily. Also by the time she went home after exercise, she was extremely tired and famished. Satisfying hunger through a high-carb diet caused her to consume more total calories in a day. Hence, the compensation effect occurred. Here are the four adjustments I recommended within her exercise program:

1. Don't wait to eat until famished.
2. Focus on medium-intensity aerobic exercise.
3. Cut back on total carbohydrates.
4. Consume more protein.

Achieving a desired body weight and muscular tone is a balancing act that requires some dietary and exercise planning and discipline. This includes drinking more water throughout the day and possibly applying a minimeal and/or food-drink snack plan to keep blood sugar levels elevated and a feeling of satiety.

Knowledgeable fitness buffs avoid the compensation effect by adding a protein or carbohydrate supplement powder to a water bottle and consuming it while training and between meals. They also carry around a gallon of water to stay hydrated. These refueling techniques have been used by weight lifters and competitive sports players throughout the years as hydration, satiety, and quick energy fuel training strategies to minimize hunger spikes and keep blood sugar levels elevated.

Why is water so important? Water replenishes bodily fluids and energizes the metabolism to endure more exercise activity. Proper water hydration also reduces risk of tendon, ligament, joint, and muscle injury.

How does water do all of this? Water helps to cushion and lubricate joints and also keep muscles working properly. As the body performs exercise and while at rest, it requires hydration to dispose of waste products, perform chemical functions at a cellular level, and support efficient metabolism.

The body's chemical functions rely on hydration to transport nutrients and oxygen to every cell in the body. Also, the elderly are at higher risk for developing arthritic conditions when adequate water is not incorporated into the daily diet. Water is the cellular filler that nourishes our body to keep us healthy (European Hydration Institute 2015). Today, I, like many others, use similar hydration practices during exercise and eat healthy snacks throughout the day to offset hunger.

The dietary and exercise weight-loss strategies discussed in this chapter should not be used in a limited or restrictive way to lose weight. If the concepts in this chapter are incorrectly or abusively applied, they then become restrictive and harmful to the body's metabolism and fitness goals, as you'll soon discover.

Many years ago during my military career, I trained as an amateur bodybuilder. During that time, I learned the value of applying safe refueling techniques to maintain body weight while sustaining high-performance bodybuilding exercise. I recalled packing empty water bottles with supplemental powders in them. I carried them in my backpack to the places I trained.

I'd typically take three to four 12-ounce bottles. Two of these bottles would have electrolyte powder and one to two others would contain a fiber-protein powder supplement. It was a convenient energy and hunger suppression fix. Just add water, shake, and drink. Decades later, the marketplace caught on to a similar product ideal and began selling premade powered drink bottles ready to be reconstituted with water. I still prefer an empty water bottle and buying the powder to add when needed. In the long run, you save money and you mix the drink you want. You're not limited to product selection.

The practice of carrying nutritious drink supplements in a ready-to-mix water bottle or meal replacement bar has not changed much from the days when I trained hard. However, there are a lot better fiber and whey proteins and carbohydrate products in the marketplace. My advice on selection is to look for natural meal replacement powders and/or bars that pack at least three to five grams of fiber, six to eight grams of whey protein, and 40 to 60 percent carbohydrates per serving.

If using the empty water bottle filled with powder, get into the habit of preparing for the next day. Simply rinse and stand your empty bottles at an angle to air out overnight. Then use a small funnel to add power to dry bottles and restock energy bars to go. If you don't prepare, you won't continue the habit of carrying these supplemental nutrients to elevate blood sugar levels when needed. And this may lead to compensation effect when hunger strikes. The beauty of a refueling strategy like this is that unconstituted drinks can be carried around indefinitely.

I can't emphasize enough about underhydration because of its connection to weight gain. It's not commonly known that, when the brain's hunger center tells you it's hungry, it's often not related to low blood glucose levels. Instead, the body is craving water, not food—which is a contributor to compensation effect, causing one to overeat or snack.

So make frequent hydration a common practice throughout the day and especially when you work out. "Many weight loss experts recommend drinking a glass of water before eating a meal or snack. If that satisfies you, then it was thirst. According to ADA (American Dietetic Association), recognizing 'real' hunger for many people sends them searching for food, often before they need to eat. Feeling hungry at the start of a meal is good, but knowing when you could wait longer is also important" (Little 2007).

If you're still hungry between meals after implementing these changes, try incorporating a minimeal diet strategy. For example, consume six to nine smaller meals a day. The ideal is to eat smaller meals throughout the day to suppress hunger and provide the body the energy it needs while balancing total calorie intake. Dietary concepts like this are further discussed in chapter 10, "Choose Favorite Foods to Lose Weight," and chapter 14, "Processed vs. Organic Food."

I've personally never use a minimeal diet strategy. I know it works for some and not others. I prefer a traditional meal strategy that allows me to eat three main meals (breakfast, lunch, and early dinner). Then have the option to eat two to three snacks before and after workouts.

I typically don't get severely hungry between meals unless I work out intensely.

My snack choices mostly consist of fruits, vegetables, nuts, protein-fiber drinks, and power bars. Since I love homemade chocolate chip cookies, I might substitute one instead of drinking a protein drink or meal replacement bar. Depending on the cookie size and calories, I may eat more than one. My bad?

Many weight-loss promoters sell weight-loss programs that limit or restrict favorite foods or macronutrients from the daily diet. Many of these I consider to be weight-loss fads and gimmicks that, in the long run, don't work and harm health. Safe and natural weight loss does not require intense training effort or using the latest weight-loss product or gimmick. It's more about dietary balance related to daily tasks, work, or exercise goals.

Muscle Fiber Fuel Preference and Fuel Mix during Exercise Effort

It has been well documented and established through scientific studies that muscle metabolism requires a mix of basically two fuel sources used during physical activity. During low-intensity aerobic exercise, muscle fiber prefers to metabolize stored body fat. During high-intensity anaerobic exercise, it prefers carbohydrate (CHO) fuel.

Ross Tucker, PhD, explains that during low-intensity activities, such as walking or cycling slowly, about 80 percent of your energy comes from fat, while only 20 percent comes from carbohydrates. "As the exercise intensity rises, the relative contribution of fat falls while CHO rises" (Tucker 2010).

Tucker's study shows that, with moderate exercise (60 percent intensity effort), working muscles burn around 50 percent CHO and 50 percent fat fuels. With high-intensity exercise effort, working muscles burn around 80 to 90 percent CHO and 10 to 20 percent fat fuel.

George Brooks, a very famous exercise physiologist, calls the point at which the contribution from CHO becomes greater than that from fat "the crossover point." "When carbohydrate stores are depleted it is equivalent to hitting the wall" (Tucker 2010). Hitting the wall occurs when an intense pace cannot be sustained for lack of oxygen, and glycogen muscle fuel needs replenishment.

For example, during a two-hour marathon race, muscle glycogen stores become depleted and fat burn conversion ramps up to continue producing blood glucose to fuel muscle fiber innervation at a slower rate of speed. The slowing of running speed to finish the race is not by choice when the crossover effect, or hitting the wall metabolically, occurs within working muscle.

Exercise studies also confirm muscle fiber types play an important metabolic role in burning fat during aerobic exercise. Take low- to moderate-aerobic exercise that uses large muscles within the legs and buttocks. These muscles have higher concentrations of slow-twitch muscle fiber, shown to prefer fat oxidation during prolonged aerobic endurance activity. On the other hand, with fast-twitch muscle fibers "in the particular situation where subjects regularly train at high exercise intensity, there seems to be some mitochondrial adaptations favoring the CHO pathway over the lipid pathway" (Daussin et al. 2008).

A related concept I'd like to share at this time is target heart rate (THR) monitoring, as THR is connected with muscle fuel burn preference during exercise. I believe this insight can provide a pretty good indicator of what fuel source is being used during low-, moderate-, or high-intensity aerobic to anaerobic exercise effort. For example, when THR reaches 60 percent, then an approximate fuel ratio can be assumed. For instance, 60 percent THR may approximately equal 60 percent moderate exercise effort or perceived exertion.

Therefore, it can be approximately measured that you're burning 50 percent CHO and 50 percent fat fuel at 60 percent THR, or intensity of aerobic exercise effort.

Muscle fiber fuel preferences based on exercise activity are not intuitively easy to understand. However, providing a different way to relate to this information can help. Thus, the concept is illustrated through personal experiences, tables and charts, and client examples throughout the book. More examples of intensity of exercise effort, fat fuel ratios, muscle fiber fuel preference, and THR are comprehensively covered in chapter 18, "Customized Fitness Programming."

I recall working out with Dan and Tom many years ago. Dan was mainly a high-intensity, anaerobic, free weight power lifter. Tom, on the other hand, was a high-intensity, aerobic jogger/runner. Tom's aerobic activities included using three different stationary pieces of aerobic equipment daily and running for a total of five to eight hours a week. Both trained at approximately 80 to 90 percent effort, or (as explained below) 8 to 9 perceived intensity of effort on average.

A perceived exercise exertion chart would have a range of 1 to 10. A client would point to a number on the chart as a perceived measure of how hard the client felt he or she had exercised. The perceived exercise effort chart was as simple as the following illustration:

1–4 = low-intensity effort
4 –7 = medium-intensity effort
7–10 = high-intensity effort

My eating and exercise habits have not changed much from the days I trained with Tom and Dan. What has changed for all three of us? We don't train on average at 80 to 90 percent intensity of exercise effort any more. Last I heard from the other two, their fitness routines (other than intensity of effort) had not changed much either over the last thirty years. So what did change?

Dan is about sixty pounds over what's considered a healthy weight but has sustained muscle mass and is strong as an ox, with no apparent health problems. Tom is extremely well conditioned to run marathons and still very lean. But he suffers from hip and knee joint pain. I still cross-train in a way that's aerobically and anaerobically balanced and don't jog or run anymore because of hip and back pain. And I can always stand to lose a little more weight, as is the case with most people my age.

Dan still prefers a high-protein diet, while Tom continues to favor carbs. I make a conscientious effort not to favor any macronutrient over the other. However, I do prefer proteins over carbohydrates. But I do make a conscious effort to boost my macronutrient intake depending on my fitness goal.

What does boosting macronutrient intake mean? When intensity of a fitness goal changes, so does my intake. In the case, for example, where aerobic exercise drops below 60 percent of perceived or measured exercise intensity effort, I cut back on carbohydrates and fats and consume more proteins to sustain my desired body weight.

But if I'm above this perceived aerobic effort, I'm going to consume more carbohydrates so that I can perform at higher levels of exercise intensity. In addition, I'm mindful of the total calories I consume if the goal is to lose more body fat.

Jason R. Karp, PhD, is a nationally known speaker and writer, an exercise physiologist, and an Olympic coach. I think Dr. Karp summed up my point nicely by stating, "Fat and weight loss is about burning lots of calories and cutting back on the number of calories consumed. For the purpose of losing weight, it matters little whether the calories burned during exercise come from fat or carbohydrates… You use both fat and carbohydrates for energy during exercise, with these two fuels providing that energy on a sliding scale. During exercise at a very low intensity (e.g., walking), fat accounts for most of the energy expenditure" (IDEA 2010).

Personally, my favorite fat-burning activity today is medium-intensity aerobic walking exercise at 60 to 70 percent intensity of aerobic effort six days a week and mid- to high-anaerobic intensity strength training two to three days a week at 80 to 85 percent intensity of effort. On days of rest, I consume fewer total calories relative, more or less, to what I prefer to eat (versus what my fitness goals would prefer I choose). I don't gain any weight on these days.

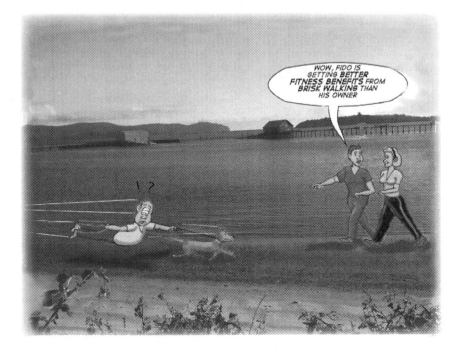

As you continue to read and learn more on how to plan, develop, and customize a fitness program, the following instruction will get you well on your way to achieving a desired weight-loss, fitness, or well-being goal prior to consuming the contents of this book.

You don't have to finish reading to begin losing weight and feeling well right now. I challenge you, as of this moment, to make a commitment to walk daily. Simply walk as far as you can at an easy, comfortable pace each day as you read on.

Although you won't feel the benefits at first, your internal metabolism will. I'm simply asking you to take a leap of faith by committing to a low-intensity aerobic exercise activity that only involves walking or riding a bike. Either of these activities can be performed on a stationary piece of equipment if you're mobility challenged.

Another thing I'd ask of you is to record your body weight now. Then put that recorded weight into a drawer and don't look at it again or weigh yourself until you've finished reading the book.

Also, each day, strive to walk or ride a little farther at a comfortable pace. Think of an aerobic walk or biking effort or pace as a pace that allows you to talk to someone without struggling to catch your breath. If you can speak comfortably while walking with purpose, you'll be well within a 2 to 4 perceived exercise exertion effort, or 20 to 40 percent intensity of aerobic walk/bike effort and will begin to burn more body fat and lose weight within a week's time.

After reading the book, compare the beginning body weight and walk times and distance results, and you'll note that one or all of these measurements have changed significantly. But most important, if you apply consistent walking effort daily, you'll notice significant weight loss, your clothes will fit more loosely, and you'll feel great!

Once these hard-to-find, life-changing truths are further revealed and as you become addicted to low-impact aerobic exercise and see the effortless results, it doesn't take much willpower to stay the course.

I'm not asking you to change anything within your daily diet or other habits or behavior. After reading the book, any further fitness or lifestyle changes are entirely up to you.

If you do choose to take the daily low-impact aerobics challenge now, I highly recommend you also prepare the feet for the task at hand—especially if you're overweight and/or have weight-bearing joint pain.

"People who are obese—classified as having a body mass index (BMI) of 25 or above—should pay more attention when selecting footwear, [Dr.] Tsai [Yung-Hu] states … Because of their body weight, overweight people may be susceptible to greater physical harm with a higher chance of injuring their tendons if walking in flats or uncomfortable shoes" (Hsu 2012)." To learn more about BMI, refer to chapter 5.

I walk many miles a week as my low-impact aerobic exercise of choice. Thus, my shoes wear quickly, and weight-bearing pain increases the longer I wait to replace them when needed. The first place I begin feeling pain is in the neck, back, hips, knees, and midfoot area. Since I literally have no foot arch and suffer from weight-bearing joint pain, replacement of walking shoes occurs on average every three to four months, and insole replacement is necessary annually. When I start feeling more weight-bearing pain sensation, I don't ignore it. Otherwise, I begin limping, and walking distances decrease.

The body will tell you when you're experiencing postural mal-alignment, which is the cause of musculoskeletal stress and radiating joint pain. Prior to feeling significant pain, I replace my insoles and/or shoes. Immediately after doing so, the limp and pain vanishes, and walking distances increase.

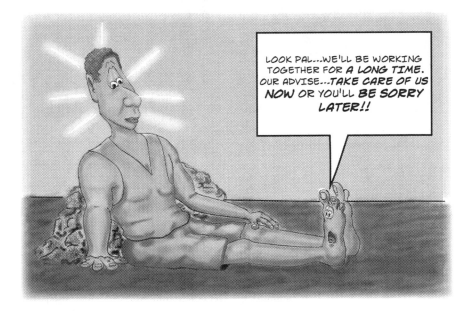

Your greatest expense as an avid walker will be your shoes. But this is a small price to pay for the fitness and health benefits you'll receive. Since I'm passionate about the walking habit, I average from fifty to sixty miles per week. I put a lot of wear and tear on my shoes and insoles. I'm not asking you to walk those miles. But one day, you may be motivated to do it—as you'll soon learn, for the same reasons I am.

If you take nothing else away from this book but a commitment to walk daily, your quality of life, health, and well-being will improve in ways you have yet to experience. And once you do make the commitment, you'll not turn back to old sedentary habits—especially once you see how easy and enjoyable it is to sustain the activity and once you see and feel the results.

Personal Fitness Challenge: "Lifestyle Change"

I must say, living a healthy lifestyle wasn't new to me prior to the time of disease and injury. Not until I was challenged with mobility loss did I focus harder than ever on finding new ways to customize a fit, healthy lifestyle program based on fitness goals.

During my downtime, I understood how the body's metabolism would change when mobility effort declined and food habits didn't change. If a person has an understanding of how working muscle metabolism and macronutrient foods are connected to health and fitness levels, then during physical adversity, this knowledge can serve as an advantage to enable him or her to heal sooner than later.

Prior to limited mobility, I could eat almost anything in the quantities I wanted without gaining weight. But once I became sedentary for lack of mobility, I knew I'd have to change habits to reduce a creeping weight gain.

Immediately, I cut my total daily calories and consumed a higher percentage of protein. I also began low-impact mobility exercise with walking aids and made use of deep-breathing exercises. If I didn't do these three things at a minimum, I'd slowly gain weight each day. Then I'd be at risk for other ill-health complications, while slowing the healing and mobility progress.

When the body's metabolism is not able to perform mobility exercises, no matter the macronutrient mix, if you can't burn it off, it will be stored as fat.

Why did I lean more toward a high-protein diet at this time? High-protein diets have been widely used as a weight-loss strategy because of their satiety effectiveness. But a diet high in protein is a dangerous strategy if it becomes a restrictive diet choice, is applied incorrectly, or is sustained for too long (chapter 5, "Caloric Exchange: A Balancing Act").

I was somewhat desperate at times to manage my body weight. However, I didn't cut out carbohydrates completely. I just reduced them and was very selective about what I ate. I went with a macronutrient balance of approximately 40 percent protein, 40 percent carbohydrates, and 20 percent fats. The carbs I left off the plate were mostly dessert, candy, baked and processed foods, sodas, sugar, and so on. I replaced them with complex carbohydrates—fibrous grains, cereals, rice, beans, fruits, vegetables, and the like.

The bottom line is that walking and other low- to moderate-aerobic activities are considered the best fat-burning exercise one could participate in to safely and naturally remove stubborn body fat. It is also easy on weight-bearing joints and good for overall health, and almost everyone can do it.

Regardless of mobility ability, include a deep-breathing exercise routine. Why? Because deep breathing supports weight loss, posture, and health and boosts the immune system, enabling you to heal more quickly. See chapter 16, "Don't Take Breathing for Granted."

Chapter 4

Fitness, Diet, and Antiaging Gimmicks Are Profitable

Due diligence on unnatural consumer products reduces health risk.

—MirrorAthlete Principled Fitness and
Healthy Lifestyle Philosophy

The fitness, diet, nutrition, and health industries offer services and products that may or may not work and could be unsafe. Learning to recognize the sales pitch hype and distinguish it from reality requires due diligence. And that's something you must do if you hope to optimize fitness results and sustain good health long-term. This line of reasoning also allows me to understand why fitness and health literacy education is not a Common Core State Standard (CCSS) and taught within our children's classrooms. The biggest reason is this: Fitness, diet, and antiaging gimmicks are too profitable to too many special interest groups.

It isn't my intention to say that every person who works within the fitness, health, and antiaging industry lacks integrity and doesn't have your best interests at heart. To the contrary, there are many reputable people who offer safe, quality goods and services within these industries. I'd like to think I've been one of those people to past clients.

But it's knowing what's safe for each individual's fitness, health, and lifestyle goals that's important. For example, is applying a quick weight-loss program repeatedly that only can be sustained on a short-term basis a healthy long-term strategy? Or what about participating in a high-intensity exercise program designed for someone in his or her twenties at age fifty? And regardless of age, is it good for someone who is overweight and out of shape or who has a medical condition to participate in any diet or exercise program?

Often we see fitness celebrities appearing on infomercials making a testimonial sales pitch proclaiming unbelievable physical results in a short period of time. Truth be told, quick weight-loss, antiaging, and physical performance-boosting and muscle-bulking products have health risks and don't always work. And if they do, the results are short-lived.

For example, a high-protein diet seems harmless enough, right? Well, what do we know about these types of diets? The marketplace sells high-protein supplement products to help suppress appetite and repair and build muscle. But how healthy is consuming more protein than a body needs?

And like a high-protein diet, is a high-carbohydrate diet any better?

"It appears that consumption of ~20-25 g ... of rapidly absorbed protein may serve to maximally stimulate MPS [muscle protein synthesis] after resistance exercise in young healthy individuals. Ideal candidates to fulfill such criteria appear to be whey or bovine milk ... For the elderly, consumption of high quality leucine-rich proteins, such as whey, may be of primary importance to maximize MPS" (Churchward-Venne, Burd, and Phillips 2012).

If the goal is increased muscle mass and strength, then the quality and quantity of protein may support the anabolic muscle growth fitness goal. Also protein is not normally used to power muscle activity like carbohydrates and fats. Protein, carbohydrates, and fats also represent calories. What the body doesn't burn it stores as fat and excretes from the body. And as you'll soon learn, both overconsumption and underconsumption of protein can cause illness and disease.

A question clients often ask is, When is the best time to consume protein to repair muscle and stimulate anabolic growth? And is protein effective for all types of exercise activity? A cyclist study on muscle protein synthesis (MPS) provides a pretty good answer to these questions.

Twelve cyclists were put through a two-hour cycling test at 55 percent peak workload (intensity of effort) in order to study the effects of co-ingestion of protein and carbohydrate on MPS. Researchers collected blood and muscle biopsies to evaluate whether the protein boosted rates of MPS during endurance activity.

The findings showed, "Protein co-ingestion does not further augment muscle protein synthesis during continuous endurance type exercise." The study concluded, "Also if the goal is muscle bulk and strength training at high anaerobic intensities, consume a rapidly absorbed protein after exercise" (Beelen et al. 2011). The study further shows that muscle is stimulated and energized by co-ingestion during continuous endurance activity and in between resistive training sets with no significant increase in MPS. Regardless of whether or not a supplement is taken, muscle protein synthesis is stimulated naturally by performing high-anaerobic strength exercises.

Why is this important information relevant to a muscle-bulking strength goal? Because there are specialized drinks sold in the marketplace as anabolic, or muscle-bulking protein drinks. But when you look at the co-ingestion mix (or carbohydrate-to-protein ratio), it would be better to consume this product to provide the energy needed to power through endurance exercise or between meals to alleviate hunger.

The bottom line, why waste money on a product that doesn't support a fitness goal or consume more than you need if it can't be used by the body and may increase health risk?

I remember during the late eighties when bodybuilding was at its peak and aerobic dance was becoming very popular. Back then, protein drinks were popular before, during, and after exercise. There was no reason not to overconsume protein. We simply believed the more we drank, the bigger the muscle and strength gains. We also added raw eggs to boost protein concentration as recommended by trainers, muscle mags, and celebrities.

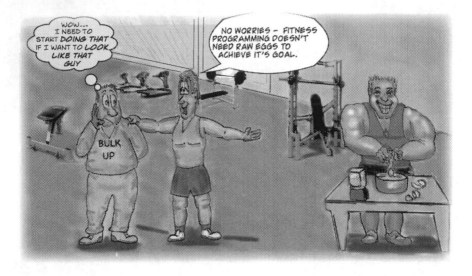

It seemed high-protein powder formulas and raw eggs were the breakfast of champions of the time. Today, the very same products under different labels and brands are used for the same purpose—to include being used as meal replacement liquid diets to lose weight fast.

But as you'll continue to learn, an excess of protein or carbohydrates or fats in the diet is not healthy for us. I call this *macronutrient ingestion imbalance*. Soon you'll learn how some of the most popular diet products are causing illness and disease.

Why Do Marketers Target the Boomers to Sell Self-Image Hype?

With approximately seventy million boomers strong and growing, there's big money to be made in the weight-loss and antiaging industries! Some of the most popular diet and fountain-of-youth products appear to offer positive results for the aging. But how healthy are they for long-term use?

"*Dr. Atkins' Diet Revolution*, first published in 1972 and reissued 20 years later as *Dr. Atkins' New Diet Revolution*, sold 12 million copies, making it the bestselling diet book in history" (Lenzer 2003). The Atkins diet is probably the most famous weight-loss program, as well as one of the most controversial. The latter is because the weight loss is dependent on consuming large amounts of protein. What is the health risk exactly?

High-protein and high–fat diets like the ever popular Atkins and Ketogenic "KETO" diets (respectively) cause the body to go into an unhealthy metabolic state called ketosis, since your body burns fat instead of readily reduced carbohydrate blood glucose for energy. Too many ketones produced by ketosis can cause gout, kidney stones, or kidney failure. Diets that are high in protein and low in carbohydrates have been linked to high cholesterol, heart disease, cancer, and kidney damage. "Any diet that advises against consuming whole grains and legumes is focused less on your health and more on selling books" (Cherny 2012).

On the flip side, science shows that, like eating too much protein, excessively high-carbohydrate intake is unhealthy, only it presents different health risks. "Because they pass through your intestinal wall so easily and quickly, simple carbohydrates trigger a more rapid increase in your blood glucose levels. Such foods are said to have a high glycemic index. According to a March 2011 review in *Nutrition Journal*, the routine consumption of high-glycemic-index foods is associated with an increased risk for diabetes and heart disease. Conversely, consuming more complex carbohydrates—those with a low glycemic index— confers a protective effect" (Christensen 2015).

In addition, "Older people who load up their plates with carbohydrates have nearly four times the risk of developing mild cognitive impairment … Sugars also played a role in the development of MCI, often a precursor to Alzheimer's disease, according to the report in the *Journal of Alzheimer's Disease*. Eating more proteins and fats offer some protection from MCI" (Lloyd 2012).

To sustain good health and feel well daily appears to be highly correlated with balanced macronutrient and eating habits and less emphasis on high protein or carbohydrate intake. "The American Heart Association, the National Cholesterol Education Program, and the American Cancer Society all recommend a diet in which a smaller percentage of calories come from protein" (Smith 2015).

However, a balanced diet, in accordance with the 2010 Dietary Guideline from the US Department of Health and Human Services, includes 45 to 65 percent of your calories coming from carbohydrates, 10 to 35 percent from protein, and 25 to 35 percent from fat. These guidelines represent the approximate macronutrient percentages the adult body needs to sustain healthy body weight, good health, and well-being. To ensure you likely fall within these percentages, consume more whole foods of variety.

Commercialization of Fitness Products and Services Is Big Business

As a former fitness trainer who owned a supplement business and customized fitness programs for clients, I can tell you a one-fit-for-all dietary or exercise product that guarantees similar results for all (or claims to be healthy for everyone) is less than honest. If anyone should try to sell you on this logic, it's a sham. Yet this type of sales tactic is just as prominent today as it was decades ago.

Do you recall watching fitness infomercials or reading magazine advertisements where exercise gadgets, intense aerobic dance, and weight-loss products promised great results in a short period of time? If so, you likely recall the plethora of aerobic workouts on VHS and now DVD discs and streaming video. How about the thigh and abs flex and other home-use exercise products promising pounds and inches would melt off in ten to thirty days or your money back guaranteed? Well, if you bought into these things, how did it work out for you?

After all, the models that use the product appear very fit. So the product must work, right? The first question in my mind as a former trainer is how would I know if or when these perfect specimens used the products they peddle? Did they use them at all? And if not, were their results achieved naturally and through a healthy or unhealthy process? I believe the following insight provides the answers too many consumers are oblivious to.

Fitness models and celebrities sell a lot of things that don't work and are flat-out dangerous. "What most people don't know about the fitness models and bodybuilders who are promoting the next pill, powder or potion is that these models are scheduled for photo shoots immediately after competitions. This is to ensure the model is in extreme shape after months of dieting, intense training (oftentimes with the use of steroids and growth hormone), tanning, posing practice, using diuretics, and other photo-enhancing products and tricks" (Del Monte 2015).

Some products do cause weight to come off quickly but in unhealthy ways. "Miracle diets, pills and potions are mere shortcuts that will lead you to a dead end. If a healthy body is aimed, you have to work for it. You have to earn it … The fat cannot just come off on its own by just using a gadget. Genetics has to do with it. Diet has to do with it. Lifestyle has to do with it" (Hubot 2012).

I know celebrities and marketers use trickery to enrich themselves at the expense of others' health. However, the peddlers will never agree with this premise. And if they do, why would they tell you? Their bank accounts are busting at the seams.

For example, Jillian Michaels, the Kardashians, and even Ronnie Ortiz-Magro from *Jersey Shore* all want you to burn calories, flush fat, and cleanse your system with their endorsed weight-loss products. 'The cleanse is going to have a lot more diuretic products in them and laxative effects, whereas the weight loss has more appetite suppressants and things that can actually cause anxiety and heart palpitations because you feel like you're on speed, basically, DeFazio a registered dietitian said. 'Ask yourself, am I doing what Kim is doing? Is my medical history the same as her and her family?' dietitian Ashley Koff said" (Corbin 2011).

Any one of my past client cases could be used as an example to make a lessons learned point relative to a diet fad or fast weight-loss gimmick. This is especially true for those who partook in one without my knowledge during fitness programming.

I recall working with Pam, a forty-eight-year-old woman who stood five foot five. She had a weight problem all her life and was grossly obese at around three hundred pounds. I knew through profiling and medical history that she was prone to knee, hip, and lower back injury; took insulin shots for diabetes; and had been diagnosed with early symptoms of heart disease. She also disclosed being treated for a thyroid problem, which caused a slower than normal metabolism.

After taking her vitals—heart rate and blood pressure—and in consideration of the entire fitness assessment profile, it was obvious she was at high risk for circulatory problems and weight-bearing injuries during exercise.

The only safe exercise program I would prescribe at the time included warm-up and cooldown stretching and low-aerobic stationary biking or walking, combined with guidelines for a reduction of calorie intake to begin losing weight slowly.

I did tell her this would be a slow weight-loss process and that achieving the fitness goal safely would require medical services. I recommended she consult a doctor for advisement prior to exercise. She also asked which diets were the best ones to lose weight quickly. This is a common question with overweight clients. I recommended that, to avoid unhealthy weight loss, she get a referral from her doctor to see a behavioral therapist; she needed help with a compulsive eating disorder she'd had since childhood.

At this point, I didn't think she took me seriously based on her behavior. In the long run, my hunch would prove to be correct.

Weeks later, I saw Pam in the fitness center riding an aerobics bike. I also noted that she had lost a lot of weight in a short period of time. I was concerned after I asked her how she was doing and she replied, "Your program is working great."

Unfortunately, I knew that was a lie. Natural fitness and weight-loss results don't work that fast. At least mine don't. What could I do about it? Nothing. It's simply a fact that many people don't want to change habits and behavior and don't want to take the time to achieve the desired results naturally.

Despite the fact that two-thirds of Americans say they are on a diet to improve their health, very few are actually decreasing in size. "Dieting is a skill, much like riding a bicycle, and requires practice and good instruction," says Dr. Bartfield. "You're going to fall over and feel frustrated, but eventually you will succeed and it will get easier" (Loyola University Health System 2013).

Later, I found out through the grapevine Pam fell ill. She had been consuming a liquid diet of eight hundred to a thousand calories daily and taking appetite-suppression pills. Fortunately, she had a complete recovery after starving herself and getting sick. Unfortunately, she regained all her weight back and then some.

In the world of weight-loss hype, a large segment of consumers buy into unknown health risks to achieve quick results—similar to an athlete who wants to enhance physical performance at any cost. And it's not just the young who take the bait to improve appearance or physical performance. Active adults (seniors) want similar results and buy into unhealthy antiaging products in hopes of reliving their youth.

Instead of wasting your money on gimmicks that won't work long-term, if at all, and risking your health, consider a mind-set shift. There are qualified fitness trainers who can help you achieve the desired antiaging and weight-loss results naturally.

If you do take this advice, know what to look for in a qualified fitness trainer or healthy lifestyle coach or consultant. Many fitness trainers do not make use of fitness profiling and dietary assessments and medical history screening to evaluate clients prior to exercise and weight-loss programming.

My advice, if you're now grossly obese and out of shape, look for trainers with a degree in exercise science or exercise physiology with specialized certification in fitness assessments, health profiling, and programming. When certified fitness profilers are used, client success stories are more often the result.

For example, Sally, at the time of her consult, was a thirty-two-year-old female interested in losing weight and gaining muscle strength. She also mentioned she was lacking energy to exercise and wanted help in this area. After a fitness assessment, medical history, and review of her recent exercise log, I noted she was using a restrictive diet plan referred to her by a previous trainer.

Sally mentioned she felt hungry all the time, didn't feel well, and didn't want to continue her strength-training routine. Posted on her workout log, a declining trend in exercise effort was obvious.

She was into this diet program for five weeks before she sought my advice. The plan required eating mostly carbohydrates, totaling around 1,400 calories daily. During this time she struggled to lose weight because of the compensation effect. She'd go on frequent binging episodes after workouts and especially over the weekends.

When I asked for the details of the plan, I found out it was a popular high-carbohydrate, low-fat and protein program. I considered it to be a minimeal diet plan and not compatible with her current fitness goals.

I asked her, "Did you have any follow-up consults with the previous fitness trainer who sold the product and developed the fitness program for you?"

Sally told me she didn't because she felt his advice would not help her. This makes the point. When fitness and diet programming is not compatible or related to encompassing a person's needs, failure often ensues. The total calories in her diet were a bit low, and the macronutrient balance was off. The protein and fat intake were too low. Hence, satiety was short-lived after a meal or exercise, and compensation effect overwhelmed her ability to stay the dietary and strength-training course.

My diet change recommendations for Sally were that she consume three balanced meals that included 30 percent protein, cut back on carbohydrates, get as much fiber in the diet as possible, and drink more water. I didn't limit her food choices but impressed upon her that, when you're working out intensely, you're going to feel hungrier, especially if you're consuming mostly carbohydrate foods. I also talked about protein and carbohydrate co-ingestion snacks that satisfy hunger and provide energy between workouts. I also asked her to remain mindful of total calories consumed in a day.

During our discussion, she understood that, as muscle mass increased, so too would total body weight. Muscle mass weight per pound is greater than equivalent body fat in weight.

During exercise, muscle fiber is conditioned to grow and increases muscle density weight. Muscle growth typically outpaces body fat weight loss at first. I also explained that, when balancing aerobic and anaerobic exercise, weight loss would occur naturally but take longer to achieve. However, once muscle density peaked, total body weight would drop more rapidly. Of course the rate of muscle growth and body weight results are going to vary dependent on metabolism, dietary consistency, genetics, and exercise effort.

I tweaked her strength-training program by adding fat-burning aerobic exercise at 60 to 70 percent effort of intensity (or 6 to 7 on the scale of perceived effort) for thirty to sixty minutes per session, three days per week. These exercise modifications seemed to suit her (chapter 18, "Customized Fitness Programming").

Sally's results: Within four weeks, she comfortably lost five pounds. I asked her if she was satisfied with the results. Although she wanted to lose weight more quickly, she understood the value of a safe and natural weight-loss program. I asked how she felt physically. She stated her body felt good and strong and that she had plenty of energy and didn't feel hungry all the time. Plus, she was motivated to continue the program. She never came back for further programming advice. Sally continued to lose more weight following the plan modification I provided. Months later, she appeared to have reached her set weight-loss and strength goals.

Do you think the marketers know a thing or two about about Sally's behaviors, habits, and personal fitness goals? You know they do. It's their job to target consumers and fix whatever needs fixing. But without a basic understanding of fitness and healthy lifestyle programming skill sets, marketplace gimmicks can put anyone into a hurt locker.

Let's check to see if you or a friend has been bitten by a fitness celebrity sales pitch. Simply look around your house or the homes of friends and family members; see if you notice fitness equipment, supplements, diet books, or workout videos. Have they been used, barely touched, or not used at all?

Why purchase this stuff and let it collect dust if the intent is to lose weight and get fit? I believe it's because people don't have a solid foundation in fitness and health literacy. So they'll fork over hundreds of dollars to find the right solution to get the results they desire based on visuals and a good sales pitch.

What I find fascinating about product relics collecting dust is that most had a thirty- to ninety-day return policy; no questions asked. But as I discovered, very few clients returned these products, even when barely used or not used at all or when the client wasn't satisfied with the results after use.

If the product didn't produce the results you wanted or you lost interest after the first use or didn't use it at all, why keep it? Regardless of the reason, the product is sitting in your home as a conversation piece and likely serves as a reminder of a failed fitness goal attempt. Again, why keep things around that don't work? For me, the answer is clear. It's about trying the latest fad or gimmick and hoping it will work at some point in time. If not today, there's always tomorrow. But tomorrow never comes.

If you're a person who needs to lose weight or change your appearance rapidly, you're a perfect prospect for marketers to target. They are also experts in predicting young adult behavior and shopping habits. A study revealed, "Young adults appear to place a greater emphasis on appearance, social factors, and physical activity and less emphasis on their health and the use of formal programs." Whereas younger older adults are mostly motivated by an emotional trigger, a medical or health trigger is more often the motivation for older adults (LaRose et al. 2013).

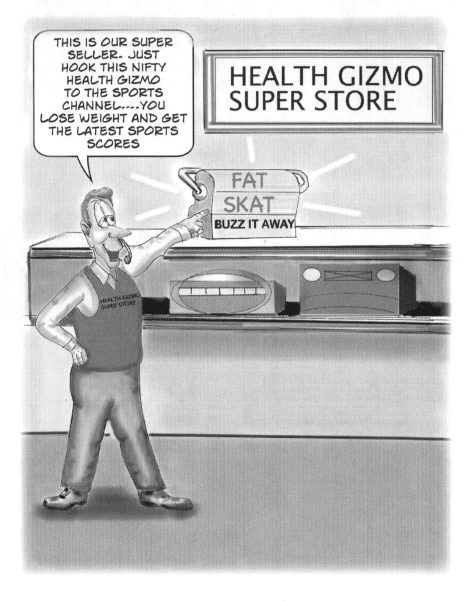

When consumers don't understand promoter interests and motivations, they become prey to deceitful sales pitches. If it sounds too good to be true, believe me, it is. And wanting these things to be true as opposed to understanding the reality of the marketplace is what's putting our youth into a state of obesity and ill health at near-epidemic proportions.

Physical performance is just as important to young athletes and professional sports athletes as weight loss is to a young lady who only sees a fat person or someone who wants to be young again. And so are a youthful appearance and youthful physicality equally important to someone who wants to be young again.

What do these groups have in common for a marketer? These people need something now and the marketplace has the next "fix-it" product to give them what they want.

A product that can give athletes what they want now—and at huge risk to health—is steroids.

I recall writing a paper on what motivated professional football players to use steroids. A scientific study questionnaire given to a group of retired players between the ages of twenty-eight and thirty-eight years old provided the answers I sought. Their answers shed light on why fix-it products work.

Two questions immediately caught my eye. The first asked, If given a chance to play again, would you use steroids to remain competitive? The answers were quite clear; a good percentage of those retired players would use steroids to relive their glory days if given a chance to play again. They were also asked, Would you do it if you knew you'd die within five years? More than half of those retired NFL players stated they'd take the deal.

I've shared a portion of this study to illustrate how motivating factors drive self-image and behavior from a very young age, as young people watch and listen to those who they admire and aspire to be. Children learn motivational triggers that influence behavior by watching their favorite athletes and celebrities. Our youth, like adults, learn through example to value riches and reward and quick results over anything else. In many cases, the takeaway is simple—live for today and don't worry about the consequences of tomorrow. People don't care about (or want to know or think about) health risks associated with fitness, diet, and antiaging product use. In the case of an athletic steroid user, it's not about self-image, physical appearance, or health. It's more about achieving fame, popularity, power, and lucrative money deals. These things are the motivators that often drive unhealthy behavior and increase health risk for far too many youth involved in sports.

Media pressure and societal expectations of sports is that their players are to win games. And if you're not winning, you're yesterday's news. "The media puts undue pressure on these guys to perform at the highest levels at all times. The pressure cooker that is our society has to be tough to deal with. So I don't blame athletes for using PEDs (performance-enhancing drugs). If I could take a pill or a shot to be better at my job and make a ton more money, I would do it in a heartbeat" (Abbamonte 2013). I rest my case.

I've found this study to be enlightening and disturbing at the same time. I have also experienced firsthand what some will do to recapture their glory days, including disregarding health risks. Like retired football players, each client I've worked with wants to look younger, feel well, and participate in youthful activities. And many are willing to risk their health like an athlete who wants performance-enhancement drugs or an overweight person desperate to lose weight or a thin person who only sees a fat person or someone who wants to be young again.

The reality of our culture is that quick-result gimmicks that promise to fix us sell. And these products are just as addictive and tough to quit for some as a tobacco, drug, or alcohol habit is for others. It's important to understanding that use increases health risk, and damage caused may not be reversed.

For these consumer industries to support any form of fitness and health literacy education in an open and honest way would be the equivalent of profit share suicide—and the end of the quick-fix gimmick game. For these reasons the industries fight consumer safety advocates and spend a lot of money to defeat legislative action that would overly regulate them or stand in their way of making windfall profits. You are their cash cows, and they'll fight to the death to sustain the marketplace status quo.

Personal Fitness Challenge: "Black Cloud"

Through the rehabilitative process, I gained more weight, took more pain pills, and became more depressed for a period of time.

For me, working through the healing process after injury and surgeries caused a lot of radiating pain throughout the body—the brain said, "This is painful. Stop moving!" On more days than I care to recall, exercise was trumped by pain. And a new habit of sedentary behavior and unhealthy food habits began to take its toll.

Severe injury and recovery is certainly a different pain experience, as opposed to the willpower necessary to stop eating unhealthy crap and start exercising daily. Physical and mental pain often compromise healthy body weight and mobility if the pain is not managed correctly, which was what happened in my case.

Eventually I had to learn to embrace a certain amount of pain during recovery in order to heal and become more mobile. Learning to embrace a dark cloud within the mind's eye is not something we're taught or trained to do in school. It's more or less something forced upon us at a most inconvenient time. And to remove that cloud is more easily said than done—especially if you find yourself in a limited mobility situation, in pain, and overweight.

Sometimes, I had to remind myself in the moment when things seemed at their worst to simply focus on getting through the next minute, hour, and day. I never allowed myself to think in terms of days, weeks, months, or years to heal. To do so would have been mentally defeating. And I knew there were no quick-fix solutions in the marketplace that could repair me quickly or were healthy for me. Although I was tempted to buy hunger-suppression supplements and drink alcohol to kill the pain, I didn't go there.

If I got antsy during bed rest and wanted to take my mind off the time, I'd do some deep breathing and physical therapy exercise in bed. Or I'd take more steps that day with a walker. Or I would propel myself in a wheelchair around the house or outside of it.

In the long run, you must believe things will get better. But you have to have a plan in place to challenge yourself to take small, positive steps each day to give yourself something to look forward to. Realize, though, that certain adversity challenges are not going to come easy. To keep things in perspective, I had to retain a focused and positive mind-set in order to get through each day. This was a disciplined mind-set I had learned while serving in the army.

I had many challenging experiences during military training that led me to coin a phrase in 1997 during a come-to-Jesus moment: *Don't stop until your mind tells you to stop.* For me, this meant the body is able to endure more physical pain upon exertion before the mind tells it to stop due to physical discomfort or disabling pain. Here's another way to view this oxymoronic mentality that would drive me forward through physical adversity: For what reason should I allow the brain to shut down my body's ability to physically and safely move forward absent disabling pain? This is especially applicable when the alternative "to stop" is not in the best interest of self-preservation, well-being, health, mobility, or lifestyle.

This simply meant I resolved I would never give up on myself, even when I was at my lowest point. I believe everyone, at some point in life, is challenged by God to find purpose during good and bad times. For better or worse and for whatever reason, it was my time to experience pain, discomfort, and immobility for a lengthy time. And when that mission was over, I'd be ready to tackle the next challenge and new life purpose God had in store for me.

I believe today as I believed during my Roman Catholic upbringing that, when the physical body dies, the spiritual soul ascends to greater purpose. So unless I have physically expired, there's no reason to quit living life to the fullest. Otherwise, what's the purpose of being?

If you don't have faith, it would serve you well to believe in something. Religion, spiritualism, and other universal and earth energy come in many forms and can serve to provide the willpower and motivation to heal yourself once a dark cloud envelopes you.

I never allowed the physical and mental pain of depression to completely take me hostage for long periods of time. Nor did I accept a disabled mind-set. I also understood that I needed to repurpose and retool my life for whatever reason. I knew it was time to take that challenge in earnest and share it at some point in time with others in ways and for purposes I couldn't understand.

Faith and belief are powerful spiritual motivators that provide healing of the entire physical mind and body to retool perspective and purpose. Hence, my new motto—don't stop until your mind tells you to stop—was born. I knew I had further purpose per God's design. And no matter how painful the mission, I'd move forward and never quit on myself or others who depended on me.

I often doubted myself during periods of chronic pain and depression while recovering from multiple surgeries; and I'd never been overweight before. Losing thirty pounds and walking well again appeared to be a monumental task, as getting there was a long-term ordeal, without any guarantees of optimal mobility results.

Living inside my head during this time was the most challenging ordeal. And there was nothing out there to fix me quickly. I had to remain mindful daily not to succumb to the feel-good, quick-fix demons in the marketplace.

My advice to anyone who hasn't worked out for years, has medical challenges or injuries, and/or is in a sedentary condition, seek a doctor's consult prior to participating in exercise or going on a restrictive diet plan. And when you do begin exercise, seek the advice of a credible fitness consultant to help you achieve your fitness and mobility goals naturally and safely.

Chapter 5

Caloric Exchange: A Balancing Act

Balanced food nutrients support optimum health and fitness levels.

—MirrorAthlete Principled Fitness and
Healthy Lifestyle Philosophy

It is beneficial to know how the body spends food calories during rest, work, and daily exercise. And it's important to understand how sedentary habits and poor food choices affect the metabolism and can increase body weight and health risk. To make these connections, basic caloric exchange and metabolic terms must be introduced—beginning with a food calorie.

"A calorie is the amount of energy, or heat, it takes to raise the temperature of 1 gram of water 1 degree Celsius (1.8 degrees Fahrenheit) … It turns out that the calories on a food package are actually kilocalories (1,000 calories = 1 kilocalorie)" (Layton 2015).

"Calories are just a measurement tool, like inches or ounces. They measure the energy a food or beverage provides … When choosing what to eat and drink, it's important to get the right mix—enough nutrients, but not too many calories" (USDA 2015).

Foods come in various energy and nutrient densities. "Energy density is the number of calories (energy) in a specific amount of food. High energy density means that there are a lot of calories in a little food. Low energy density means there are fewer calories in a lot of foods" (Mayo Clinic 2017). You can think about it this way. One tablespoon of butter or oil can have nearly the same calorie count as two cups of cut green beans or Brussels sprouts. What is more filling and satisfying? It's really a no-brainer.

I know counting calories can be a drag. However, I believe it's a tool that will help some of you achieve healthy weight loss.

To be honest, I don't count the calories I consume. I used to, but now I can just look at food and come close to an approximate calorie count if I'm mindful of it or want to do it. Actually, it's not difficult to tally food calories to determine a net weight gain or loss once you know how.

The bottom line is, if you consume more than you burn, you gain weight. If you reduce calories, you lose weight. And if you don't consume enough high-nutrient foods daily, it may have a negative effect on health and physical performance goals.

It is true that many dieters can determine how successful a weight-loss program is simply by stepping on a scale or how the clothes feel and fit around the waistline. Although this is a good gauge of success, it's more important to learn how caloric exchange, daily activity, and marketplace influence affect body composition, health, and lifestyle choices.

I learned the value of consuming a balanced diet and daily exercise early on in life. Many of the basic diet and physical activity principles were taught in health, home economics, team sport, and physical education courses throughout my formative years. In addition, back then our foods were mostly purchased from farms and local mom-and-pop grocery stores. This was an era when big-box stores and fast food places didn't rule the marketplace. So it's fairly easy for those of my generation with a similar upbringing to relate to organic whole foods versus processed ones and the value of daily exercise.

The world has changed a lot in the last fifty years. Our K–12 schools don't provide the basic dietary, health, and exercise terms, concepts, and practices, I learned in the classroom, which I, like many, others value as adults.

This is why it's so important for the next generation to be able to relate to, at a minimum, the dietary guidelines by the US Department of Agriculture (USDA), which includes daily exercise activity. In relating to these healthy habit guidelines, it is also easier to digest and make use of the balanced caloric exchange concept to set, achieve, and sustain good health, fitness, and well-being goals.

The USDA "Dietary Guidelines recommendations encompass two over-arching concepts: Maintain calorie balance over time to achieve and sustain a healthy weight ... Focus on consuming nutrient-dense foods and beverages" (HHS 2010).

So what do these dietary guidelines truly represent? They represent the ideal and importance of knowing what percentage of food nutrients and calories our bodies need to stay fit, happy, healthy, and well. When mindful of these dietary guidelines, it is also true that natural weight loss is easier to achieve when these guidelines are applied with consistency.

Breaking down these guidelines a little further, it is also important to make the following relationship with respect to the percentage of total macronutrient calories consumed daily:

> The Institute of Medicine has established ranges for the percentage of calories in the diet that should come from carbohydrate, protein, and fat. These acceptable macronutrient distribution ranges (AMDR) to follow take into account essential nutrients known to decrease chronic disease risk:

1) Young children (1–3 years): Carbohydrates 45–65%, Proteins 5–20%, Fats 30–40%.
2) Older children and adolescents (4–18 years): Carbohydrates 45–65%, Proteins 10–30%, Fats 25–35%.
3) Adults (19 years and older): Carbohydrates 45–65%, Proteins 10–35%, Fats 20–35%. (USDA and USDHHS 2010)

I currently consume an approximate macronutrient balance of 45 percent carbohydrates, 30 percent protein, and 25 percent fats within the day's diet. And these percentages fall within the AMDR for my age. I consume mostly meat, chicken, fish, potatoes, rice, and vegetables. It's what I grew up on, and my body feels good and performs better with this food choice balance.

For the following exercise, refer to table 5.1, "Estimated Caloric Intake Requirement per Day, Age, and Activity." It will be easier to learn and relate to how calorie intake fuels daily work and how exercise activity burns those calories.

Table 5.1. "Estimated Caloric Intake Requirement Per Day, Age, and Activity"

Physical activity level				
Gender	Age (years)	Sedentary	Moderately active	Active
Child (female/ male)	2–3	1,000–1,200	1,000–1,400	1,000–1,400
Female	4–8	1,200–1,400	1,400–1,600	1,400–1,800
	9–13	1,400–1,600	1,600–2,000	1,800–2,200
	14–18	1,800	2,000	2,400
	19–30	1,800–2,000	2,000–2,200	2400
	31–50	1,800	2000	2200
	51+	1600	1800	2000–2200
Male	4–8	1,200–1,400	1,400–1,600	1,600–2,000
	9–13	1,600–2,000	1,800–2,200	2,000–2,600
	14–18	2,000–2,400	2,400–2,800	2,800–3,200
	19–30	2,400–2,600	2,600–2,800	3,000
	31–50	2,200–2,400	2,400–2,600	2,800–3,000
	51+	2,000–2,200	2,200–2,400	2,400–2,800

Information from chapter 2, page 14 of the Dietary Guidelines for Americans, 2010 (USDA and USDHHS 2010). Institute of Medicine. Dietary Reference Intakes for Energy, Carbohydrate, Fiber, Fat, Fatty Acids, Cholesterol, Protein, and Amino Acids. Washington (DC): The National Academies Press; 2002. http://health.gov/dietaryguidelines/dga2010/DietaryGuidelines2010.pdf

Although table 5.1 is a good illustration of how calories are used during activity, the data represent an average requirement per age group and, therefore, not an exact measurement. There are many free calculators online to conveniently approximate energy expenditure, as well as calories needed to gain or lose weight. HealthStatus.com has a good variety of easy-to-use calculators if you're interested in an online source to approximate health risk assessment and BMI (body mass index) (HealthStatus 2018).

You can also access the Centers for Disease Control and Prevention (CDC)'s BMI calculator (CDC 2015) to forgo the need of performing long, manual calculations as illustrated below to estimate body fat percentage. Regardless, I'll show you an example of how this is typically done longhand.

The following client example shows how to manually calculate caloric intake and expenditure if you want to do the math.

Marvin, at the time of consult, was a sixty-two-year-old man who weighed 175 pounds, stood five foot eleven, and was very physically active. He trained all his life to compete in marathon races and had retired from competitive runs. He planned to maintain his cardio-muscular endurance condition by jogging two hours daily at about six miles per hour, as opposed to his past flat road, marathon run pace average of about seven miles per hour.

He said he had retired from marathon events and wanted to continue training at a moderate effort of intensity (about 70 percent aerobic effort). After nutrition and activity analysis, it was determined his total caloric requirement to fuel his daily activities, including both the runs and other activities, was approximately 4,220 calories per day. I calculated Marvin's caloric needs by breaking down hourly activity tasks within a twenty-four-hour period to determine an approximate energy requirement needed to sustain daily metabolism. (Williams 1988)

I know, some of you are wondering how Marvin wouldn't gain weight with a daily calorie intake of 4,220—especially when you observe the caloric requirement per activity task listed in table 5.1. It shows a man his age does not need more than 2,800 calories to sustain a daily "active" lifestyle. That's the problem with averaged tables.

The caloric requirements in Marvin's case show how people use three different metabolic burn rates per day. Once you get this connection, it is easier to understand how daily exercise makes it possible for a sixty-two-year-old man to compete with someone decades younger.

Think about it this way. How many sixty-two-year-olds, let alone forty-year-olds do you know who jog or run twelve miles a day, seven days per week at an average rate of six to seven miles per hour? And how do his rest cycles and work habits influence caloric need?

His six-mile-per-hour jog/run, or task-specific exercise, when performed at current intensity and rate of speed requires approximately 1,356 calories. How do I know it will take approximately 1,356 energy calories to accomplish this two-hour activity? Because science has already shown, through controlled studies, that caloric expenditures based on age, weight, activity type, intensity, and time duration burn an approximate and measureable amount of calories. See Table 5.2, "Caloric Energy Cost per Activity per Minute" (USDA and USDHHS 2005). The table is presented within a few pages after the three metabolic rates are defined and calculated.

Marvin also has a diet that falls within the recommended food group balance (carbohydrates at 45 to 65 percent, protein at 10 to 35 percent, and fats at 20 to 35 percent). He does not have a restrictive diet that would deprive him of the calories and nutrients necessary to fuel his daily activities and keep him healthy.

Next, you'll see and relate to how caloric intake and expenditure, when in balance, is the sum of balanced caloric exchange daily.

In order to approximate Marvin's energy requirements for a twenty-four-hour period, I need to account for three types of metabolic rates that can be summed to more accurately reflect his daily caloric need.

Those three metabolic rates are as follows:

1) Basal metabolic rate (BMR), which is needed to sustain life function (for example, breathing, organ function, and respiration) twenty-four hours a day. During sleep, there is no activity and no extra calorie requirements other than to satisfy BMR function. The BMR rate also varies with weight, height, sex, age, and environment.
2) Resting metabolic rate (RMR), which is higher than BMR because it requires a little more energy to digest food and perform sedentary activities, such as sitting and standing.
3) Exercise metabolic rate (EMR), which calculates the calories needed during exercise, work, or physical task.

A more accurate formula to calculate caloric need requires summing the three metabolic rates of basal, rest, and exercise function and activities within a twenty-four-hour period. Therefore, the summation of BMR+RMR+EMR calorie expenditure can approximate the daily caloric intake need to perform a physical task efficiently.

To calculate daily caloric need, convert body weight from pounds to kilograms (divide body weight by 2.2 and convert to kilograms).

Then use a BMR factor of 1.0 kilocalorie (expressed as thousands of calories or kcalories) per kilogram of body weight for men, or 0.9

for women. Men typically have more muscle mass than women and receive the higher caloric factor. While working through Marvin's total metabolic calorie expenditure, refer to forms 5.1 "Marvin's calculated daily metabolic and caloric energy requirement" and his "Simple Body Mass Index (BMI) Calculations," form 5.3 (see appendix)

For example, let's find Marvin's BMR per hour:

1. Change Marvin's weight in pounds to kilograms (pounds/2.2 = k). 175 lb./2.2 = 79.55 kg
2. Multiply weight in kilograms by the BMR "male" caloric factor. 79.55 kg × 1.0 kcal/kg/hr. = 79.55 kcal/hr.
3. Multiply the BMR kcalories used in one hour by hours in a day. 79.55 kcal/hr. × 24 hr./day = 1,910 kcal/day

The energy required to sustain Marvin's basic life functions twenty-four hours per day requires 1,910 calories.

Marvin's second metabolic rate occurs during digestion, standing, and sitting still. The third occurs during increased daily activities and exercise. After comparing lifestyle notes with Marvin, it appears these three metabolic rates break down daily in the following manner:

> BMR (includes sleep time of about eight hours per day) plus RMR (Marvin sits, comfortably moves about with ease, and stands for about fourteen hours per day, which includes about eight hours a day working in an office) plus EMR (jogging for two hours at a about six miles per hour). Now let's look at these metabolic rates in greater detail and sum the caloric macronutrient requirement for total energy expenditure requirement for one day:

Again, Marvin's basal requirements are found using the formula, 79.55 kg × 1.0 kcal/kg/hr. = 79.55 kcal/hr.:

Marvin's BMR: 79.55 kcal/hr. × 8 hr. = ~636 kcal/8 hr. of sleep.

I calculate Marvin's RMR for approximately fourteen hours of light-duty activity by increasing his energy cost one additional calorie over BMR (refer to table 5.2 below "Caloric Energy Cost per Activity per Minute").

> *Marvin's RMR*: 79.55 kcals/hr. × 14 hr. × 2.0 cal/min = 2,227.4 kcal/14 hr. (This increased energy cost includes his BMR energy requirement.)

Next up is Marvin's EMR, which relates to his daily jog and requires 11.3 calories per minute:

> *Marvin's EMR*: 11.3 cal/min × 120 min. = 1,356 kcal/2 hr. to jog/run 12 miles at an average rate of 6 mph.

So, the sum of caloric exchange to sustain Marvin's daily lifestyle is:
BMR = 636 calories (8 hours sleep)
RMR = 2,227 (14 hours light activity)
EMR = 1,356 calories (2 hours for 6 mph jog/run)

Marvin's total calorie requirement to sustain daily activities without losing or gaining is approximately 4,220 calories per day (Williams 1988).

Table 5.2. Caloric Energy Cost per Activity per Minute

Rest, Work, or Exercise Activity	Caloric Energy per Minute
Basal metabolic rate	1.0
Sitting and writing	2.0
Walking (2 mph)	3.3
Walking (3 mph)	4.2
Jogging/running (5 mph)	9.4
Jogging/running (6 mph) (extrapolated @ 1.88 cal/min.)	11.3

Note: Table 5.2 Calories/hour/minute were based on a 154-pound person. Marvin's caloric requirements and table examples are for illustration purposes only. His caloric expenditure would have been slightly higher by approximately 12 percent or an additional 400 calories based on a 175-pound body weight. This adjustment is not reflected in these calculations and examples.

Form 5.1 gives an example of a "Daily Caloric Expenditure Worksheet," showing how Marvin calculated his caloric expenditure and approximate requirements. Form 5.2, "Daily Caloric Expenditure Worksheet" is a blank form you can copy to make your own calculations. (see appendix)

The next thing to estimate is Marvin's BMI (body mass index). I've used BMI with clients to approximate whether they are overweight for their age and height. This information is also useful in tracking weight-loss goal success. (Refer to table 5.3, "Body Mass Index Standards" after calculating Marvin's Body fat %. Then use form 5.3 "Simple BMI Worksheet" (see appendix) to find your body fat % for your height and weight.

Looking at Marvin, it was my opinion he was not overweight. Regardless, I used a BMI to establish a body mass baseline for the record. I did offer skin fold and impedance testing at additional cost to get a more accurate body fat percentage, which he turned down. The Simple BMI calculations are based on height and weight and one of the least accurate methods to determine body fat. If you wish to get a more accurate body fat calculation, it will cost extra for the assessment.

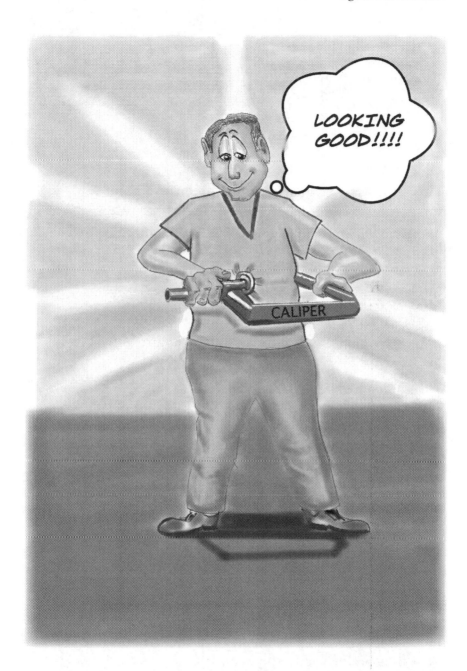

To calculate Marvin's BMI, I used the following methodology and plotted results on form 5.3, "Simple BMI Worksheet" (see appendix). I divided his weight in pounds by height in inches squared and then multiplied that number by 703. The BMI standard formula is:

Weight in pounds/height in inches × 703

So for Marvin, who weighs 175 pounds and is five foot ten (70 inches), the calculation is:

175 lb./(70" × 70" = 4,900) = .0357 × 703 = 25.10 % body fat

Use table 5.3 to determine whether Marvin falls within the body fat percentages for his height and weight (NIH 2015).

Table 5.3. BMI (Body Mass Index Standards)

BMI below 18.5 is considered underweight.
BMI between 18.5 and 24.9 is normal weight.
BMI between 25.0 and 29.9 is overweight.
BMI of 30.0 and above are considered obese.
BMI of 40.0 + extremely high obesity.

Marvin's 25.1 percent BMI falls mostly toward normal weight per BMI standards.

It is noteworthy to point out, "Those who have a waist size of more than 40 inches for men, or 35 inches for women, have a higher risk for obesity related health problems such as diabetes, high blood pressure, and heart disease" (Scott 2014). Marvin's waist size was approximately 36 inches.

Copy and use blank form 5.4, "Simple BMI Calculation and Body Mass Index" (see appendix) to copy and record a BMI baseline.

Marvin did not feel he was carrying too much body fat. And to tell you the truth, he looked lean and muscular for his age. He didn't want to restrict his calories and didn't think he'd gain any significant body fat within the next year, provided his activities and diet remained the same.

Do balanced nutrition and the types of food we eat really matter relative to fitness, well-being, and healthy lifestyle goals?

I believe this question can best be answered by illustrating how bad eating habits and restrictive diets can be harmful to fat-burning metabolism, health, and fitness goals.

Since one of my favorite foods is a cheeseburger, I want to show how a person could lose or gain weight eating cheeseburgers. I also want to show you how, if you do eat a favorite food consistently to lose or control body weight, this practice could destroy the fat-burning metabolism and result in obesity and related disease. Why am I emphasizing unhealthy favorite food habits? Because weight-loss marketers formulate favorite food plans based on unhealthy and addictive food habits.

I also want to emphasize that there is a healthy way to lose weight eating favorite foods, provided your diet consists of a healthy balance of macronutrients and variety in terms of food group as further covered in chapter 10.

To make this point, let's look at an example of an unhealthy favorite food strategy for weight loss—this one including only cheeseburgers. A cheeseburger diet alone cannot provide the balanced macronutrients needed to sustain healthy body weight over the long term. Here's why (I know you hate the math, but stay with me; I'm sure you'll appreciate the end game on this one):

- *Cheeseburger macronutrient totals by gram and calorie*: One quarter-pound burger with cheese has about 30 grams of fat (at 9 calories per gram), so 270 calories; 28 grams of carbohydrate (at 4 calories per gram), 152 calories; and 27 grams of protein (at 4 calories per gram), 108 calories.
- *Cheeseburger total calories*: 270 + 152 + 108 = 530 calories
- *Cheeseburger macronutrient percentages*: 270 calories/530 total calories = 51% fat content, 152 calories/530 total calories = 28.5% carbohydrate content, and 108 calories/530 total calories = 20% protein content.

Our cheeseburger has 270 fat calories (51 percent). The AMDR requirement shows us that adults should strive for a daily balance of 20 to 35 percent fats in our diet.

The USDA (United States Department of Agriculture), ADA (American Dietetic Association), WHO (World Health Organization), and Institute of Medicine, who established the acceptable macronutrient distribution ranges (AMDR), would not agree that 51 percent fat intake at each meal is healthy for anyone on a consistent basis.

Regardless, I bet you're curious to know whether you *can* eat a favorite food like a quarter-pound cheeseburger to lose weight. Is there any such diet plan on the market? I don't know if there is a cheeseburger weight-loss diet plan out there. But anyone could lose weight eating only cheeseburgers or sandwiches if you restricted how many calories you consumed in a day. And no, I don't recommend an *only* cheeseburger or sub sandwich diet to lose weight. That's a restrictive weight-loss ideology and, in my professional opinion, unhealthy for the body and an unnatural and unsustainable habit in the long run.

I'm showing you this example because some people do eat only one type of food or a few favorite foods or chose a restrictive fad diet to lose weight. But if you're considering such a course, it's important to understand that unbalanced macronutrient intake and diets that don't have flexibility in terms of food choice result in increased health risk and broken metabolism.

To continue this illustration, let's hypothetically put Marvin, our marathon runner, on this cheeseburger diet plan (which I'd never recommend to him). Then we'll examine the results.

Marvin does like cheeseburgers but would not be interested in restricting his diet to one kind of favorite food to lose weight if that was his goal. However, in our hypothetical situation where he does do this, we can use his previous daily caloric requirement to see how a cheeseburger diet would pencil out. Would he gain or lose weight eating six quarter pounders a day? Let's do the math.

Recall—Marvin's daily caloric expenditure is 4,220 calories a day to sustain daily activities and body weight.

If Marvin ate six quarter pounders with cheese per day (at 530 calories each) and drank only water, his food calories would equal 3,180 per day. If his activities stayed the same for thirty days (at 4,220 calories expended daily), Marvin would have a net caloric loss (4,220 calorie expenditure − 3,180 calorie intake daily = 1,040-calorie net loss/day). The caloric loss may actually be greater. Recall that I didn't factor in the additional 12 percent of calories required for a 175-pound man. Regardless, we'll stick with the 1,040-calorie net loss per day.

Let's look at the math that will help us determine how that calorie loss converts to weight loss:

- Calorie-to-body weight conversion – *3,500 food calories = 1 lb. of body weight*
- Calories lost per month – 1,040 calorie loss/day × 30 days = 31,200 calories lost/month
- Pounds lost per month – 31,200 calories loss/3,500 = 8.9

In other words, since Marvin would lose 31,200 calories during the month, he would also lose approximately nine pounds.

But is this a safe and balanced energy exchange that could be sustained on a long-term basis? And would his health be at risk as a result of eating six cheeseburgers a day?

You could lose weight safely this way, right? Not!

Oh, I know some of you are thinking, *Perfect. I'll just eat quarter pounders with cheese throughout the day because Marc demonstrated that this favorite food plan could help me lose weight.* Although that may be technically true, I never said this was a healthy or sustainable way to lose weight.

The lack of balanced macro and micronutrients—derived from eating a variety of foods from various food groups—would eventually starve Marvin's metabolism of the nutrients required to sustain his active lifestyle. Favorite food habits can also cause unhealthy weight gain for those who are living a sedentary lifestyle.

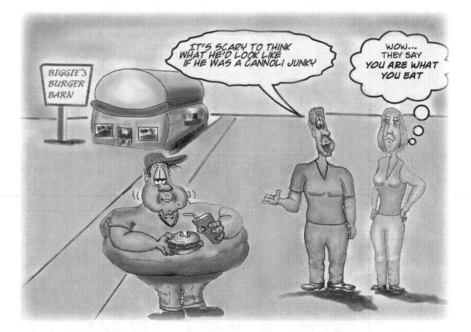

Do you recall the documentary *Super Size Me* by Morgan Spurlock? The object of Spurlock's experiment (thirty days of eating only McDonald's food) was not to lose weight but, in fact, to show

how eating fast foods daily was bad for your health. This experiment made national news and brought unwanted notoriety to a popular hamburger chain. In the long run, it provided consumers with an important lesson. If calorie intake far exceeds exercise output and an imbalance of macronutrients is consumed for long periods of time, health can and does become compromised, increasing health risk.

For his experiment, Spurlock ate three McDonald's meals a day every day for one month. After his first supersized meal, he threw up. At the end of the experiment, "He only felt well after eating junk food. These are sure signs of addiction" (Hyman 2011).

Here's what *Wikipedia* noted about the film:

> As a result, the then-32-year-old Spurlock gained 11.1 kilograms (24 lbs.) a 13% body mass increase and increased his cholesterol to 230 mg/dl. He also experienced mood swings, sexual dysfunction, and fat accumulation in his liver …
>
> Critics of the film, including McDonald's, argue that the author intentionally consumed an average of 5,000 calories per day and did not exercise, and that the results would have been the same regardless of the source of overeating…
>
> One reviewer pointed out, he's telling us something everyone already knows: "Fast food is bad for you" (Wikipedia 2015).

What about the popular Atkins diet? It appears to be no exception when considering the potential harm macronutrient imbalances or high protein intake can have on health and well-being.

Robert H. Eckel, MD, director of the general clinical research center at the University of Colorado Health Sciences Center in Denver expresses concerns over whether the Atkins diet "is a healthy diet for preventing heart disease, stroke, and cancer." Other concerns Eckel notes include "possible bone loss and liver and kidney problems resulting from high protein levels." This diet has also been criticized regarding overconsumption of fats. "The American Heart Association recommends a maximum of 30% of fat in a person's daily diet" (Admin 2011).

"The American Dietetic Association also has concerns about the Atkins diet. Gail Frank, PhD, former spokeswoman for the organization and professor of nutrition at California State University in Long Beach, says, 'The body needs a minimum of carbohydrates for efficient and healthy functioning—about 150 grams daily.' Below that, normal metabolic activity is disrupted" (WebMD 2015).

The other less obvious restrictive weight-loss diet plan, which surfaced in the marketplace not long ago, is the caveman diet, commonly referred to as the paleo diet. As with all innovators of the latest and greatest diet plans, its creators always disagree with their critics.

"The paleo diet is a very healthy diet," says Loren Cordain, PhD, Colorado State University professor and author of *The Paleo Diet*.

This diet is based on eating plants and animals; it includes meat, fish, shellfish, eggs, tree nuts, vegetables, roots, fruits, and berries. It does not include dairy, grains, sugar, potatoes, processed oils, legumes or any other foods grown after agriculture started. The plan also calls for exercise activity daily.

However, I believe the pro-paleo diet argument crumbles based on a preagricultural fact—cavemen didn't have a variety of high-nutrient and balanced macronutrient choices compared to the organic foods found in today's marketplace. Also, early man's way of life was one of survival—very stressful and short-lived. So I don't know how one could qualify or quantify the paleo diet as a superior diet in today's whole foods marketplace relative to overall fitness levels, health, well-being, and longevity.

"'People who eat diets high in whole grains, beans and low-fat dairy tend to be healthier due to the high nutrient values in these foods,' says Keith Ayoob, EDd, RD, an assistant professor at New York's Albert Einstein School of Medicine. Heather Manigieri, MS, RD, says, 'The diet has some great aspects, but the limitations make it another diet that people can't sustain for long for lack of food group variety and potential nutrient inadequacies'" (Mustang CrossFit 2018).

On the surface, innovative weight-loss diet fads may look and sound good. But they always fall short of providing organic whole foods and/or a balance of nutrient variety as recommended by nutritional guidelines.

High-carbohydrate diets are just as unhealthy as high-protein diets. They are known to cause obesity, often resulting in diabetes and other ill-health consequences.

If you're a carbohydrate lover, did you know that all carbohydrates are not equal? For example, refined sugars or simple carbohydrates should not be a daily overindulgence, especially for those who are diabetic or want to lose weight.

Unfortunately, refined carbs are not only bad for you but also the tastiest and most habit forming. "Anything with added sugar, or made from refined (white) flour is likely to lack the fiber to balance out the sugar, and has little nutritional value to make it worthwhile" (WeightLossForAll 2018).

When too many refined carbohydrates are consumed, the brain's hunger center is triggered more often, making it harder to control over eating.

The more complex and less refined (processed) the carbohydrate, the longer it takes to digest. Thus, the body gets its fuel slowly and steadily, which is healthier for you. Your metabolism will be able to process the energy more efficiently and won't overload the body with energy, and you will feel hungry less often. On the other hand, "simple carbohydrates are good when quick energy conversion is needed fast, especially during a pick-me-up during exercise activity" (Elements Database 2015).

There are good reasons to make complex carbohydrates the bulk of the required AMDR carbohydrate choice. A healthy balance of complex carbohydrates (whole grain breads and starchy vegetables like beans, corn, potatoes, peas, lentils, and so on) in the body works quite a bit differently with the fat-burning metabolism than do simple carbohydrates—and in a way that is much healthier.

The USDA, DHHS (Department for Health and Human Services), and CDC (Center for Disease Control and Prevention) have years of scientific studies to show that daily macronutrient intake, attained with a balance of vegetables, fruits, grains, dairy, and protein, is necessary to lower disease risk and keep us healthy (Nutrition.gov 2015). So why do so many consumers disregard the scientific studies and dietary truths? I believe this question can be best answered by sharing a past personal experience from another client case.

Kyle, a client at first, eventually became a good friend. In late fall 2006, he tried to sell me on the merits of the Atkins diet. During this time, I was working through my own rehabilitation and fitness challenge, which included weight loss. So of course I was interested in other diet plans that could help reduce weight safely.

He provided firsthand knowledge of the Atkins diet, and I witnessed his results over a course of six months.

At the one-month mark, I noted Kyle was losing weight really quickly (about ten pounds already). I had to admit I was impressed. But I was also concerned about this aggressive weight-loss approach, as Kyle's macronutrient consumption was imbalanced.

I wondered what impact it would have on his long-term health should he continue the course. Although I was tempted to start the Atkins diet, I never did. I'm more of a wait-and-see type of guy. I need to evaluate risk versus reward before I apply a strategy. In the case of Kyle, I determined quickly that the risk of ill health far outweighed the quick weight-loss results.

I hadn't seen him for three months after that first visit. As life has it, we all get busy. But when I did meet up with him, I was shocked. I almost didn't recognize the person sitting in the chair as I entered the house.

He'd lost a lot of weight and did not look well. I thought he looked ten years older and was genuinely concerned for his health. He appeared to have lost forty pounds and actually looked like an AIDS patient or as if he'd gone through chemotherapy. But in his mind's eye and mirror image, he saw uncontroversial weight-loss success. I agreed he'd experienced dramatic weight loss, and I was genuinely stunned by it. But I disagreed that it was the result of a healthy weight-loss process, and I let him know how I felt about it.

I didn't immediately tell him I was concerned about his health. Instead, I wanted more information about what he was eating daily. I found out that, like an anorexic obsession, he had taken the Atkins diet to a new level. From what I gathered, what he was doing was a self-modified version of the plan, not the plan specified by Atkins instruction.

For instance, I asked him what he was eating daily. He confirmed he had been eating mostly peanuts and peanut butter and only animal products like lunch meat, eggs, bacon, cheese, and beef jerky. In addition, he was drinking low-carb beers. He claimed he was drinking at least a liter of water daily. But I never saw him drink any water.

During this visit, his wife made pizza for lunch.

What appeared sacrilegious to me was the fact that both he and his wife only ate the toppings off the pizza and threw away the dough. I wondered why his wife, who also was on the diet, didn't share the same dramatic weight-loss results. It soon became apparent she was cheating. She confided in me she was still consuming carbohydrates throughout the day, just not in front of her husband. Of course, like me, he didn't understand why she wasn't having the same weight-loss results. I left this issue alone.

At first I didn't let on I was worried about Kyle's health. But eventually I did tell him my concerns about putting the body in a state of ketosis for long periods of time.

Ketosis in the body occurs when an excessive breakdown of fatty acids is metabolized due to lack of or inadequate use of carbohydrates. Ketosis is known to cause kidney failure, including the formation of kidney stones and a whole list of other diseases including cancer. Untreated ketosis can progress to a ketoacidosis condition. That condition's worst-case scenario can lead to coma and death.

Kyle thanked me for my concerns and said he would add more carbs into his diet. I took that to mean he would get the carbs by drinking more beer.

The next time I saw him, I was really concerned. After six months, his body weight had dropped from a starting weight of 235 pounds (on a six foot frame). He now weighed in at 175 pounds. Again, prior to leaving that day, I advised him to modify his diet plan for the sake of his health. I warned him that the path he was following was akin to starvation or a wasting away syndrome, and if he didn't change his food habits and behavior, he'd fall ill, or worse.

Two months after this conversation, I received a call from his wife. Kyle was in the hospital and very sick with kidney stones.

Luckily, Kyle came out of this health scare okay. After his return from the hospital, he went off the Atkins diet and gained back all his weight, including an additional ten pounds.

So a question comes to mind. Why do so many people disregard the signs, symptoms, and risk factors of unhealthy eating habits, which include long-term fad dieting? There are many possible answers. But the decision to embrace an unhealthy dietary course has much to do with a belief that the marketplace can provide a safe and fast weight-loss product without increasing the user's health risk. You know the answer to this: No, it can't.

Is Our Genetic Code Influenced by Food Choice?

The data shows us chemicals found within our environment and food chain can be just as harmful to our DNA as a restrictive diet plan is to metabolism. This insight should scream out loud to fad dieters. In terms of genetic expression, what is the consequence of frequent macronutrient imbalance, restrictions on food group variety, and foods with too many chemicals?

An individual may not be born with a disease but may be at high risk of acquiring it. The World Health Organization's Noncommunicable Diseases and Mental Health Cluster (NMH) has done extensive work on major diseases, such as cancer, diabetes, cardiovascular disease, asthma, and some mental illnesses.

Some of us, to varying degrees, may be genetically compromised, or predisposed—meaning that we lack the ability to tolerate or defend against certain environmental toxins and chemicals. Regardless of this assumption, genetics may progress disease no matter the lifestyle, environment, or cultural engagement. "Diseases can occur due to a defect in a single gene or in a set of genes. According to the degree of gene mutation, diseases categorized …" (WHO 2018a).

Twenty-two thousand chemicals have been introduced into commerce since 1976. "Chemical manufacturers have provided little or no information to the EPA regarding their potential health or environmental impacts." It is now commonly understood that some toxic chemicals persist in the environment, sometimes for decades, and build up in the food chain and in our bodies. It is now well-recognized that some chemicals are able to disturb our hormonal, reproductive, and immune systems and that multiple chemicals can act in concert to harm health (NRDC 2015).

The following statement was alarming when it was made and even more concerning now. "The growth in the use of food additives has increased enormously … now over 200,000 tons per year … Each person is now consuming an average 8–10 lbs. of food additives per year, with some possibly eating considerably more … There also has emerged considerable scientific data linking food additive intolerance with various physical and mental disorders, particularly with childhood hyperactivity (Tuormaa 1994). As you'll continue to see and learn, both the amounts of chemicals in foods and food intolerances among consumers have continued to rise within the twenty-first-century marketplace. This is especially true when it comes to the connection between food chemicals and childhood obesity and related diseases that are plaguing our nation.

"Recent cumulating evidence suggests that obesity may represent an adverse health consequence of exposure during the critical developmental windows to environmental chemicals disrupting endocrine function. Moreover, exposure to these chemicals seems to play a key role in the development of obesity-related metabolic and cardiovascular diseases" (Latini, Gallo, and Iughetti 2010).

"Because the obesity epidemic occurred relatively quickly, it has been suggested that environmental causes instead of genetic factors may be largely responsible" (Baillie-Hamilton 2002). Baillie-Hamilton's paper hypothesizes that "the current level of human exposure to these chemicals may have damaged many of the body's natural weight-control mechanisms" (2002).

These environmental and cultural realities highlight the importance of balanced diet, healthy food choice, and daily activity to achieve the caloric exchange balance necessary to sustain a healthy body weight, healthy fitness levels, good health, and well-being for a life time.

Personal Fitness Challenge: "Therapeutic Cooking to Expedite Recovery"

The injuries, surgery, and rehabilitative episodes in my life caused my body to balloon from 195 pounds to 225 pounds. My muscle had left the building; my body fat had increased and my muscle mass had decreased. After spending ten months lying around too much, I felt lousy. I knew I needed to come up with an in-house and outdoor activity plan to get my broken body moving.

It occurred to me more than once that I'd have to change certain food choices and come up with a plan to become more progressively mobile so that I could heal sooner rather than later.

Although I had been consuming a decent balance of calories prior to injury and recovery, I knew too many of those calories came from convenient processed foods with too much salt, sugar, trans fats, and other unhealthy chemicals. If I wanted to lose weight and increase my energy levels, the processed foods had to go.

These changes also required a greater balance of organic whole foods, which included plenty of fruits, vegetables, and nuts and water to help curb hunger between meals.

I rarely felt hungry or craved processed foods after the first week of dietary change. I credit much of my successful recovery and weight loss to a balance of favorite meals made of fresh whole foods. My wife made many trips to the store to purchase and then cook those healthy wholesome recipes at home. I eventually helped with meals as I became more mobile. During this period of time, I referred to this activity task as "therapeutic cooking to expedite recovery."

The activity task called for food prep and cooking in the kitchen. I used a wheelchair, in combination with crutches, to gather ingredients to make dinner. I recall standing on one leg in the kitchen as long as I could tolerate it to accumulate other things from drawers and cabinets and then moving the ingredients and pots and pans to a seated area.

This daily dinner ritual was both a mobility exercise and a lesson in how to cook healthier foods. Although it took me three times as long to cook and serve dinner as it did my wife, it was therapeutic and gave me purpose. This provided a very low-impact aerobic activity that gave me something therapeutic to do for three hours a day. I knew the meal was to be served at 6:00 p.m. So I began prepping in the kitchen at 3:00 p.m. each day.

This activity was important for me to achieve the next exercise activity task above and beyond cooking a daily meal and attending physical therapy sessions. Cooking in the kitchen forced me to move more and also provided an opportunity for me to learn how to tolerate a certain level of pain. My goal was to eventually venture out and exercise outdoors.

Through better whole food and recipe choices, you can remove a large amount of the man-made processed chemicals. Be aware of what to look for in order to achieve a better balance of caloric energy exchange in order to stay healthy and heal sooner. Chapter 14, "Processed vs. Organic Foods," dives deeper into the dietary differences between various processed foods and organic whole foods and their respective effects on health.

Chapter 6

Consumer Trust at What Cost?

> Consumer needs and wants determine the marketplace supply and demand.
>
> —MirrorAthlete Principled Fitness and
> Healthy Lifestyle Philosophy

I've worked with many clients throughout the years who are desperate to lose weight. They share similar stories about weight loss and the latest services and products to battle the bulge and reverse the hands of time—to become forever ageless.

The particular clients I'm talking about subjected themselves to risky and unnecessary surgeries, prescriptions, and herbal or supplement products in hopes of achieving quick improvements to appearance or physical performance or rapid weight loss. These types of people are not easily persuaded to change unhealthy habits and behaviors.

They also look to persuade others—similar to marketers promoting the next weight-loss fad and hoping others will jump aboard the bandwagon. The cycle this creates—including professional testimonials and actual physical results—affirms they've made good decisions. Seeing is believing, right? In this case, it is. In a world of cure-all, "natural" products that appear to work quickly, there is nothing more powerful than personal testimonies with before and after shots. These quick-fix products and services are big business for the fitness, antiaging, physical enhancement, and weight-loss entrepreneurs.

I've never fully understood or realized all the different ways you could cheat, tricking the body into weight loss, improved physical performance, increased muscle mass, and changed appearance—harming it in the process. If I didn't have the client fitness consulting experiences I had offered for many years, I wouldn't have known about many unsafe and epic failure products and the related disease truths the industries promoting these products don't want divulged.

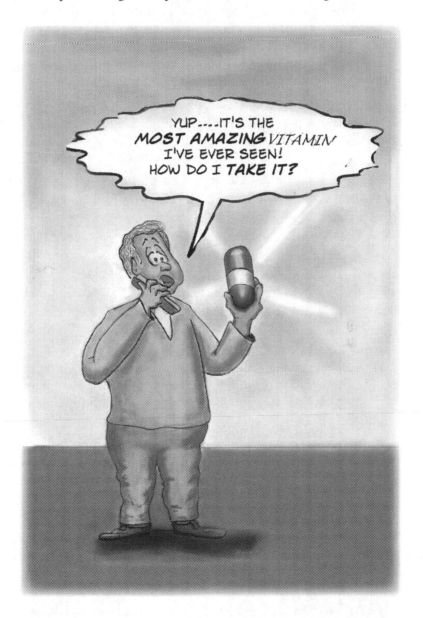

Since the general public is unaware of many of these truths, the quick-fix product advertisements aren't going away anytime soon either. If anything, consumer exposure to them is greater than ever. They now appear on smartphones, along with streaming internet and cable TV advertisements, with greater consumer reach than ever before. How many times have you seen personal testimonies and infomercials selling quick-fix everything to cure all that ails you? I'd bet you see them every day if you're connected to the internet. Many infomercials or advertisements start out harmless enough but grab your attention immediately. Testimonials often include beginning and ending photo shots and statements like "I know this gal who's taken this diet product and dropped fifteen to twenty-five pounds in ten days." Or the advertisement will say something like, "Just take these pills, and you won't be hungry anymore and weight will melt away like butter." Another typical promise states that by using a particular supplement, pill, or natural cure, you'll gain ten to twenty pounds of muscle in twenty-one days.

These testimonials and ads are very powerful persuaders to buy products and services. However, before making that purchase, consider the following truths.

Did you know dietary supplements don't undergo FDA review for safety and effectiveness like medical drugs? Medical doctors warn, "Be skeptical about anecdotal information from personal 'testimonials' about incredible benefits or results obtained from using a product" (FDA 2010). Check with your doctor before using any form of supplement that does not state "FDA approved."

The marketplace influences our habits and behaviors at a very young age. The food, fashion, diet, and antiaging industries often tell us what we need and sell a lifestyle, fad, and mirror image visual, along with Band-Aid cures to solve a problem that may temporarily make us feel better. But if we're not educated on the other half-truths, the snake venom is powerful enough to cause irreversible disease.

Pure and simple, marketers target and condition consumers by providing products to increase muscle mass, sports play, rapid weight loss, and sexual performance. Men have to be especially cautious when it comes to performance-enhancement products.

"American men have a mania for pills and potions that can add muscle or stiffen their sex lives. Shady drug labs supply the demand by dosing 'natural' nostrums with illegal meds and hidden health threats." These products are then sold by "sellers who want to grab a share of a $27 billion market by touting a pill that really delivers" (Beil 2011). Beil's article also notes, "Products most likely to be spiked are weight loss, bodybuilding and 'sexual enhancement'—categories pitched largely to men" (2011).

As a cautionary note, it is wise for men to seek advisement from a doctor before experimenting with the body's hormone-metabolic system (chapter 15, "Antiaging and Physical Performance-Enhancement Truths").

It's not just the antiaging, physical enhancement, and fitness industries that consumers need to pay attention to. A plethora of chemicals is used to grow genetically modified (GM) food crops. Many unknowingly consume these chemicals through whole and processed foods, weight-loss and muscle-building products, and so on. There are three things to pay attention to here: 1) GM seeds farmed in a lab, 2) chemicals used to grow the crop seeds, and 3) the processing of crops into foods after harvest.

In 2007, consumer data showed a heavily processed food market. And I've not even begun to discuss GM food crops and chemicals used to grow them. "Over 12,000 chemicals are used in the production of our food. Many are used intentionally as 'direct' additives, but some are 'indirect' contaminants or used accidentally. As of 1995, complete health risk assessments were available for only 5% of food additives. The food industry uses about 3,000 different food additives in various packaged and preserved foods. These include preservatives, emulsifiers, buffers, natural and artificial colorings and flavorings" (Lipman 2010).

Be very skeptical of special diet foods and supplements that claim to be organic in nature and safe for use but don't have an FDA stamp of approval. There is enough scientific evidence to support strong correlations showing processed and refined foods, including genetically modified foods in concert with food chemicals leading to obesity, diabetes, and other related disease.

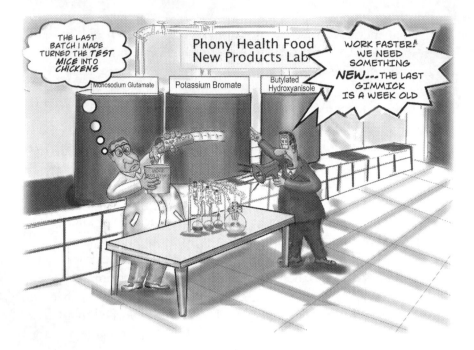

Over a decade ago, childhood obesity had crept to epidemic proportions and is on target to continue that trajectory. "Worldwide obesity has nearly tripled since 1975. In 2016, more than 1.9 billion adults, 18 years and older, were overweight. Of these over 650 million were obese … Forty one million children under the age of 5 were overweight or obese in 2016. Over 340 million children and adolescents aged 5-19 were overweight or obese in 2016" (WHO 2018b). Childhood obesity is increasing at a near epidemic rate, even among preschool children, and causing related health problems.

"Prevention should be the primary goal and, if successful, will help reduce adult obesity. Accordingly, we will have the greatest chance to successfully reverse the obesity epidemic if we consider it a crisis, make it a funded government and public health priority, and join forces across disciplines to mount an effective public health campaign in the prevention and early treatment" (Deckelbaum and Williams 2001, 239S–43S).

The early childhood obesity forecasts are disturbing. "Over the past four decades, obesity rates in the United States have more than quadrupled among children ages 6 to 11, more than tripled among adolescents ages 12 to 19, and more than doubled among children ages

2 to 5. Today, more than 23.5 million US children and adolescents—nearly one in three young people—are either overweight or obese" (Robert Wood Johnson Foundation 2018). It is becoming more apparent than ever that there is an obesity connection between engineered foods and food chemicals as key contributors to obesity and related ill-health conditions.

Approximately 70 percent or greater of our processed foods are now genetically engineered. Of course, these numbers do vary depending on the source. Consumers are becoming more aware that our nation has a dependency on hyperpalatable, addictive foods made from GM crop foods and food chemicals. Consumer advocacy groups increasingly demand that manufacturers identify the unhealthy chemicals, including GMOs, in food product labels. However, it will take some time to advance these efforts because of opposing commercial interests.

States like Oregon, Colorado, Washington, and California put to a vote on November 4, 2014, a consumer right to know ballot measure that would have required companies like Monsanto, a biotechnology company, to disclose GMO products in foods had it passed. Although these western states did not pass GMO ballot measures at that time, there is a consumer movement that demands to know what ingredients are in our foods. And this issue is not going away anytime soon.

This is only the beginning of a consumer push toward right to know legistlative actions. The Vermont legislature approved a labeling bill that's set to take effect. This initiates a state precedence and shows the serious nature of how humankind's meddling with the food chain has caused a consumer and voter backlash that demands to know if GMOs and other man-made ingredients are used in processed foods. Maine and Connecticut legislatures also passed GMO labeling bills. "Similar legislation has been introduced in about 30 states, according to the National Conference of State Legislatures" (Wilson 2014).

However the Protect Interstate Commerce Act (PICA), introduced by Representative Steve King (R-IA) in 2015 is intended to protect big food and big pharma and could undermine hard-won state GMO labeling bills should they pass. "It would allow states that do not have labeling laws to freely sell their unlabeled products in states that *do* have labeling laws" (ANH-USA 2017). Unfortunately, consumers will continue to draw the short straw for some time as deep-pocketed interests oppose the growing consumer right to know movement.

On the positive side, the marketplace may ultimately adjust to change as more state legistlators feel the pressure of voters' desire that unsafe ingredients be listed on food labels.

For your information—if you don't already know—the most common genetically modified foods found in Western marketplaces today are fresh corn, corn syrup, soy lecithin, sugar, other vegetables and fruits, and cottonseed oil, to name a few.

Some of you may wonder, what exactly are GMOs and how did they get here? Let's look at the short of it.

GMOs are crop seed organisims, in which the DNA has been genetically altered and farmed in a lab. Thereafter, these superseeds are sown in farm fields, and chemical sprays are applied to prevent crop disease—resulting in high-quality crop yields with low spoilage. The crops are sold at lower costs in comparison to organic crop foods.

For example, "herbicide-tolerant (HT) crops are genetically engineered to survive direct application of one or more herbicides during the growing season, chemicals that would otherwise kill, or severely stunt a crop. There are also pest control [pesticides] and fungus resistant [fungicide] crop seeds that manage plant disease" (Benbrook 2009).

"If you want to avoid obesity, then avoid eating genetically engineered (GE) corn, corn based products and animals that are fed a diet of GE grain" (Samsel 2012). Organic and processed food differences and related weight gain and disease are further covered in chapter 14.

"Despite the recognition of the severe health and psychosocial damage done by childhood obesity, it remains low on the public agenda of important issues facing policy makers. Perhaps this is because the most serious health effects of obesity in today's children will not be seen for several decades. Action must be taken now to stem the epidemic of childhood obesity" (Hill and Trowbridge 1998, 570–74). Consumer right to know advocates and state labeling laws and health literacy education is slowly gaining traction in consumer health and educational advocacy circles.

But as noted, the impact on health will be paid at the expense of future generations, as prophetically observed by Hill and Trowbridge in 1998. In my opinion, the obesity epidemic will unfortunately get worse before it gets better.

Why are these issues so difficult for consumers to act upon even when they know the truths about the connection between dietary choices and obesity? "Why is it so hard for them to lose weight despite the realization of health consequences such as high blood pressure, diabetes, heart disease, arthritis, and even cancer even though they have an intense desire to lose weight? It is not because they *want* to be fat. It is because certain types of food are addictive" (Hyman 2014).

You'll never hear the food industries admit their lab-farmed and chemically manufactured products contribute to obesity and related disease. This is because GE foods processed with addictive chemicals are too profitable to stop supplying to the marketplace. It should be no surprise to anyone that addictive products sell and make a lot of money for industries and shareholders.

I believe to date, there are approximately eight major marketplace dynamics that contribute to obesity and other related health problems. And until these things change, childhood obesity and related illness and disease will not be reversed anytime soon. The eight dynamics are as follows:

1) Food and agricultural industries harm health by injecting unnecessary chemicals into the food chain and environment.
2) Americans simply consume too many engineered foods sprayed with pesticide and fungicide toxins.
3) Children are not educated to become fitness and health literate and conscious of unhealthy lifestyle habits.
4) Consumers value fix-all solutions.
5) Too many people are addicted to certain foods and don't want to stop eating them.
6) Unhealthy foods are too profitable.
7) Processed foods are cheaper than organic foods.
8) Powerful consumer lobbyists, special interest groups, unions, and large conglomerates influence political and marketplace interests.

People are consuming processed foods at greater frequency and quantities and at younger ages than any other generation before us. The damaging health effect of toxic and chemically processed foods, like those of pharmaceuticals, lie within chemical toxin potency, along with frequency and duration of use.

Fortunately, the FDA does require that pharmaceutical companies identify health risks on labels of approved drugs. In addition, food labels must identify things like amounts of trans fats or recombinant bovine growth hormone (rBGH) steroids in certain dairy products.

How hard would it be to change Western culture to a healthier one? I'd say it's a monumental but not impossible task—especially if there was a national push to provide fit, healthy lifestyle development and obesity literacy education in our K–12 schools. Then the next generation would learn to value the things necessary to change our culture in a big way.

It is my opinion that there is no one government agency, industry, or group to blame for the childhood obesity problem we now face in this nation. Instead politicians, educators, parents, special interests, and voters must all be held accountable for our growing obesity epidemic. And we must work together to find resolutions if we hope to reverse childhood obesity anytime soon and, thus, lower related health care costs so the next generation doesn't have to bear its overwhelming burden. But what instrument or gauge or process will be used to combat biased research that is less than honest with consumers?

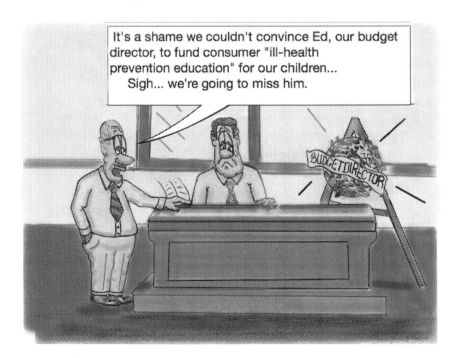

Pharmaceutical Research Bias and
Class Action Lawsuits

Consumer safety takes on a different meaning when you understand that the approval of many drugs and their introduction into the marketplace have been based on biased studies influenced by billions of research and development (R&D) dollars!

Past class action lawsuits claimed biased R&D harmed consumer health. Since 2010, it appears that recent class action lawsuits are in decline. So does this mean R&D bias is on the decline? Not necessarily.

For example, according to *Rx Compliance Report*, "Federal prosecutors are reporting that the pace of new *qui tam* filings (whistle blower cases for pharmaceutical and device companies) has slowed considerably and the alleged illegalities cited in new suits are less egregious than in years past" (Policymed 2010).

Although this statement on the surface appears to look out for the little guy, looks can be deceiving. "One reason for this slowing is due to pharma companies working to stop the steady flow of qui tam suits alleging drug marketing fraud over the past decade, and according to several federal prosecutors, these efforts are now paying off" (Sullivan 2010).

Biased prescribing of FDA-approved drugs requires consumer awareness and scrutiny. Why? Have you ever wondered why some doctors prescribe certain brands over others or prescribe medications *not* lab tested or approved by the FDA as an alternate form of treatment for a medical condition? Here's why:

"Approximately 90 percent of the $21 billion marketing budget of the pharmaceutical industry continues to be directed at physicians, despite a dramatic increase in direct-to-consumer advertising ... The purpose behind such industry contacts with physicians is unmistakable: drug companies are attempting to promote the use of their products ... Does physician disclosure ensure that patients are getting a doctor who is not 'under the influence' of pharmaceutical company marketing practices?" (Shomon 2015).

This is simply an example of how a free marketplace can influence sales of biased prescriptions to patients. Since our marketplace is an imperfect one, my advice is to remain mindful of biased prescriptions and consider a habit of due diligence research to determine what's not in your best health interest.

How safe and beneficial is an FDA-approved drug compared to a hyperpalatable food chemical that addicts us to it? Well, in both cases, depending on dose and frequency of use and duration, there is a potential for health risk.

For example, do consumers realize certain drug treatments are designed in similar ways to unhealthy processed foods? Here's a good analogy. Food made of sugar, fat, and salt can be addictive, especially when combined in secret ways the food industry will not share or make public. According to Mark Hyman, MD, "We are biologically wired to crave these foods and eat as much of them as possible." Adds Hyman, "We all know about cravings, but what does the science tell us about food and addiction and what are the legal and policy implications if certain food are, in fact, addictive?" (2014).

Let's take this line of reasoning one step further. When an FDA drug or a chemical ingredient farmed in a lab is approved after it passes clinical animal and human trials, does this mean it is safe for adult consumption and nonaddictive? And how safe is it for children?

Many are surprised to learn the exception for human drug testing is that it does not include children. After all, how many would volunteer children to be guinea pigs prior to an approved drug or food chemical ingredient entering the marketplace? However, adults volunteer all the time to test new drugs, and some receive payment to participate.

So what does it mean when humans and animals are used during clinical studies and the drugs or chemicals are approved by the FDA? Are they safe for both children and adult use?

Let's digest this another way to answer this question fully. How many FDA-approved pharmaceuticals have you been prescribed where there is *no* risk to health per warning label? None exist that I'm aware of. All FDA-approved drugs have health risk statements on their warning labels.

Although animal studies will continue to advance new drugs and ensure they are approved for consumption on the market, it is wise to understand that animals don't have the same DNA or metabolism as humans. Did you know drug manufacturers only have to meet the minimum acceptable health risk criteria based on animal studies prior to approval of a product's entrance into the marketplace? Many drugs, like pediatric medications for children, have only been tested on animals before FDA approval. For children, the health risks appear higher because animal DNA is so different than that of humans.

Regardless, patients need to accept some risk when using an FDA-approved drug to improve an ill-health condition. But aren't food and diet products entirely different matters? Shouldn't parents, as well as children have the right to know what product ingredients are the cause of rapid weight loss? Shouldn't we know what addictive qualities, behavioral changes, and health risks may result?

A five-year study of 2,500 female teenagers in St. Paul, Minnesota, found the use of diet pills among high school age girls nearly doubled from 7.5 percent to 14.2 percent. Specifically, "21.9% of teenage females used very unhealthy behaviors to achieve their fitness results that also included laxatives, vomiting or skipped meals as a weight control modality ... Of the 2,500 males in the study, their rates were half the females. 'We have found that teenage females who diet and use unhealthy weight control behaviors are at three times the risk of being overweight,' said Neumark-Sztainer. '... Parents can play a key role in helping their children to build a positive body image and engage in healthy eating and physical activity behaviors'" (University of Minnesota 2006).

At a minimum, our kids shouldn't get sick consuming diet, meal-replacement, and weight-loss products found in the marketplace. And when unhealthy dietary behavior and addictive habits occur, they should be recognized by parents and educators and treated accordingly.

Since the food, drug, and educational institutions are not likely to change anytime soon, the best parents can do is set a positive, healthy lifestyle example for their children. In addition, parents must educate children on how the marketplace is mostly interested in their wallet and not their long-term health interest.

Personal Fitness Challenge: "Guilty as Charged"

The depression hit hard when my orthopedic surgeon told me I might likely be dependent on a wheelchair and canes to get around for life because of my hip disease, prior broken back, and pain complications.

These things weighed heavily on my psyche in a way that was tough to shake initially.

I know from personal experience that depression can be temporarily relieved through food, drink, and prescription drug use. These things do provide a false sense of comfort. Yes, guilty as charged.

At certain points, I was consuming more calories and drugs than my body needed, while experiencing more physical and mental pain over long periods of time. I had never imagined or seen myself in a situation like this. But it became my reality.

There were days I couldn't have cared less if I lived or died. The mental and physical pain often trumped common sense, reasoning, and a plan to move forward and get excited about life again. Reflecting back, there was someone else in my head, and I didn't like it.

If any of you have experienced physical and mental pain and limited mobility for years, you know what I'm talking about. Imagine acute radiating neural pain throughout the body that could easily become chronic at any time. This is a recipe for out-of-control pain and depression.

I ultimately accepted the "physiatrist and psychiatric diagnosis of substantiated injuries related to psychosomatic pain-depression." Being treated for the symptoms required a daily pain management program to alleviate both mental and physical pain. Once I fully understood the diagnosis, I was able to minimize the depression triggers through medical consultation and applicable treatment. Then I began moving forward with a coordinated, customized fitness and pain management program. Unbeknownst to me at the time, it would take over five years to heal mentally, physically, and spiritually and get back on track.

Physical pain is one thing, and mental pain and anguish is something entirely different. Managing the two is very challenging but possible with the right medical support and resources. You have to learn to take small steps each day. Recall what I said earlier—each minute and each hour counts. No matter how small or insignificant the progress may seem, don't quit trying to improve a bad situation and make it better. It does take time for the body to heal naturally.

If you need someone to talk to, swallow your pride and seek medical consultation as soon as possible. I know this is extremely hard for most men. But keep in mind an expression known by all veterans: "No man has to go it alone."

Do not depend on family members, friends, or mind-numbing vices to fill this void. Untrained individuals can't begin to relate to or understand what you're experiencing. And drug dependency will not help move you forward. I guarantee that pain management and mental health professionals will make a huge difference by providing the tools you need to help maintain a positive self-image while working your way through depression and physical challenges.

Another physical issue I faced was correcting a severe limp that stayed with me for years. The limp left an emotional scar in my head. Self-image afflictions are often caused by poor health, immobility, and general appearance. Mine was the appearance of being less capable or weak. Either way, I needed to improve upon this mental and physical affliction to strengthen my ego and how I saw myself in the mirror.

I knew by walking daily I could strengthen muscle tone, tendons, and ligaments and overall body posture while losing weight naturally. However, it was understood there were no guarantees I would completely remove the limp or be completely free of walking aids.

The reason I tell my personal adversity story is to provide hope for those who want to increase mobility efficiency and fitness levels and overall health while alleviating pain. I'm also here to tell you that all hope is not lost. It is possible to change an adversity situation. But it does take some effort to get better and move forward.

My personal fitness and health literacy education, including physical challenges and doctor referrals, gave me the tools I needed to turn adversity into personal triumph.

But I'm also going to be realistic and truthful in saying we're all emotionally motivated to find purpose and move forward differently. What helped me muster up the willpower to move forward was the belief my life had purpose. And that purpose was to take care of family.

As you can imagine, I'm happy I made the decisions I did back then. I now have the ability to walk on average ten to twelve miles per day or more, and I walk religiously, as if my mobility independence and life depended on it.

Thinking about and planning a lifestyle change strategy that would enable me to heal sooner rather than later was easier said than done. And I used no fast-track products or services to do it. I simply applied the natural and truthful information found in this book, which provided a purpose—to share the knowledge with you.

I inherently knew that if I didn't change or try to improve my situation, I'd be trapped in an overweight and pain-ridden body that would be a drain on me, my family, and society. My present health, fitness levels, and life purpose may have been completely different had I chosen to ignore what I knew was true.

When you hold these hard-to-find truths in the palm of your hand, I believe that, should adversity strike, you will make an informed plan to move forward. That plan will serve to guide you, provide hope, and enable you to repurpose what it means to live life to the fullest. While you continue to gain purposeful healing, remain strong in your resolve to attain self-improvement. And take comfort in knowing you're not alone on this journey.

Chapter 7

Substitute Addictive Habits

Removing a bad habit may require a substitute practice
to achieve the goal.

—MirrorAthlete Principled Fitness and
Healthy Lifestyle Philosophy

Lifestyle change becomes especially challenging after sedentary habits
and weight gain have settled in. To help reverse, moderate, or stop an
unhealthy weight-gain habit, I'm presenting an unconventional ideology
about changing habits as a tool that will be useful for some. It's a
different way to think about food and, ultimately, achieve your fitness
goal.

However, I'm also realistic about hyperpalatable, addictive cravings.
I understand that, as with most addictions, going cold turkey won't
work well as a solid weight-loss strategy that'll last long-term. That's
why I'm sharing a substitution food practice that may allow you to have
your cake and eat it too.

However, there are caveats to food or drink substitute practices as
you pursue weight loss. This strategy is in no way perfect. But for some,
it offers hope to help moderate unhealthy eating habits. At best, it may
enable you to abstain from the hard-to-quit food and drink habits that
are currently putting your health at risk.

Think of a food substitute practice like a smoker's patch. You can
still get the "nicotine" while eliminating the bulk of the toxic garbage
entering your body. In time, the smoker's habit may or may not resolve.

Regardless, you have a substitute strategy that may be the silver bullet to help you change a bad habit and get closer to your healthy living goals.

It is my experience after client consultations that there are unhealthy food chemicals people crave and that cause weight gain and unhealthy, sedentary habits. And those addictive cravings, to a large degree, are caused by chemical sweeteners, alcohol, and caffeine that also end up in unhealthy concoctions, including energy and coffee drinks, diet supplements, and the like.

I created the healthy food substitute practice while working with a particular client who craved drinking too much beer and artificial sweeteners in coffee. This client's goal was weight loss. If your goal is to lose weight, moderation of these things won't rock your world. But when combined and consumed frequently, they can increase your health risk.

The analogy I used to discuss a healthy food substitute practice for this client began in the following manner. During the consult, I likened a beer in calories to a pork chop. Why a pork chop? Because I *first* needed to make a relative point and in a way that would show him how liquid calories, like food calories, contributed to weight gain. That would then lead to a discussion on hyperpalatable food addiction.

For instance, twelve ounces of beer have the calorie equivalent of a fried pork chop. There are approximately 165 calories in one small or thinly cut fried, breaded, or floured pork chop. Or think of the previous chapter's example, where we learned there are around 530 calories in a quarter-pound cheeseburger. So when you drink three beers with around 150 calories each, you've just about consumed those burger calories in the drinks. The connection here is this—if you're serious about losing weight, you must plan how you're going to consume those calories.

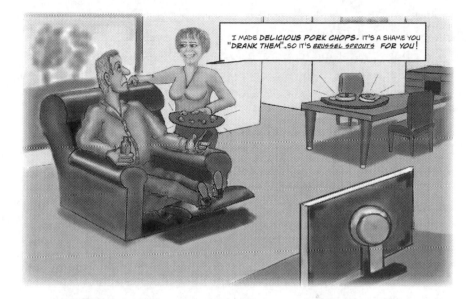

What if you could relate each drink to a food item? You'd begin to think, I wouldn't typically eat four pork chops for dinner or drink away the equivalent calories of a quarter-pound burger with cheese. So in essence, you begin to realize you've drunk your calories for dinner and haven't satisfied the solid food hunger mechanism in the brain. When you add food after drinks, that's additional calories your body will store as fat.

This is a mindful practice that can be used to limit portions of addictive and unhealthy food and drink choices enjoyed a little too much. In this case, a few beers could be substituted for a healthy food choice. I'm not going to tell anyone to stop drinking or stop eating hyperpalatable foods. Instead, I find providing examples of how to moderate unhealthy food habits through a healthier balance of food calories, which can help people achieve their goals.

Will substituting a bad food or drink habit work for everyone? The answer is no. But compromise does help some achieve the weight loss goal while moderating a bad food or drink habit.

Recall Kyle's story from chapter 5. Kyle was the client who tried to sell me on the merits of the Atkins diet plan. Not only did he become obsessed with a high-protein diet; he also substituted carbohydrate food choices for low-carbohydrate beers. Ultimately, he ended up in the hospital with kidney stones. Only after inpatient treatment did he make drastic lifestyle changes. He stopped drinking altogether, swapped those beers for healthy foods, and began drinking more water (which is good). But without moderation, he ate too many food calories without adequate exercise activity and caused excess body fat weight gain.

Many consumers know the absence of alcohol in the diet is better for overall health. But a daily glass or two of red wine appears to be the exception. For those who don't know, resveratrol from red wine is considered heart healthy per multiple scientific studies. However, there are limits on how much one should consume.

"The alcohol and certain substances in red wine called antioxidants may help prevent heart disease by increasing levels of 'good' cholesterol and protecting against artery damage" (Mayo Clinic 2014). However, in the same breath, many doctors won't recommend you start drinking any type of alcohol to improve your overall health condition. So it appears wine drank in moderation may be a healthy habit for some.

Nevertheless, when one vice ends, often another that can be just as addictive and dangerous begins.

Did you know that "emergency room visits related to energy drinks doubled from 10,000 to 20,000 visits between 2007 and 2011, often due to heart problems linked to a caffeine overdose?" That's likely because these drinks "contain unknown and unregulated amounts of caffeine and other stimulants that raise the risk of heart palpitations, insomnia, and dehydration" (Kotz 2013). "Colorful packaging, appetizing pictures, and nutrition claims hide the truth: unhealthy chemicals are lurking in many these seemingly harmless foods" (McCarthy 2009).

Regardless of the type of calories consumed, it is wise to consider a quality antioxidant supplement to minimize the effects of addictive, hyperpalatable foods on the organic body. Not only do we human beings contaminate our air and water; humankind also contaminates almost every food product, including those that appear to be healthy diet foods and supplements.

How does this happen?

Chemical additives and preservatives are in all of our consumables because they come from our crops and livestock and other lab-farmed foods and are absorbed at a cellular level. "Contaminants get into our food in a variety of ways," concluded Irva Hertz-Picciotto, principal investigator of a study on contaminants and professor and chief of the Division of Environmental and Occupational Health at UC Davis.

"They can be chemicals that have nothing to do with the food or byproducts from processing. We wanted to understand the dietary pathway pesticides, metals and other toxins take to get into the body" (2012).

When clients asked how to assure their bodies receive adequate and safe antioxidant nutrients to protect them from toxic foods and stressful environment, I said, "Nothing is 100 percent guaranteed." However, for an added layer of environmental and consumer safety protective insurance, I recommend a good *absorbable* daily vitamin and mineral supplement at a minimum—especially for those who don't get enough fresh fruits and vegetables daily for whatever reason.

Absorbable means the supplement can be easily broken down by the digestive system and used by the body. In this way, you can ensure a layer of some antioxidant protection, as detailed throughout chapter 14.

"For best results, look for multivitamins and all other supplement products that are free of binders, fillers, artificial colorings, preservatives, yeast, sugar, starch, hydrogenated oils or other additives" (Turner 2012). If you have food allergies, Turner notes it's important to stay mindful that, in multivitamins, "lactose, corn starch, various sugars, soy and yeast can be used as fillers, and may cause digestive disturbances in sensitive individuals" (2012).

Many essential nutrients, such as vitamins B and C, are water-soluble and are used by our bodies daily. So they need to be replaced for optimum health, energy levels, and cellular repair each day. Very few of us get four to five servings of fruits and vegetables a day, yet our bodies crave them whether we know it or not. I've advised clients for years on the importance of fresh fruits and vegetables, "supplemental insurance" (absorbable vitamins and mineral supplements), and healthy food substitute practices that avoid unhealthy food choices.

Do our bodies use all the nutrients consumed from foods and supplements? My answer is a simple no. Am I throwing away some money on "supplemental insurance"? Many say yes, and I'd agree in part. And just because a supplement is labeled "all natural" doesn't mean it's safe—or effective. "The FDA does regulate dietary supplements; however, it treats them like foods rather than medications. Unlike drug manufacturers, the makers of supplements don't have to show their products are safe or effective before selling them on the market" (WebMD n.d.).

The peace of mind that comes with ensuring a level of protection against environmental toxins while substituting addictive food habits is worth the cost of high-quality antioxidant supplements. However, "Some supplements are riskier than others … And if you have a health condition, check with your doctor before you take supplements. He can tell you if they have side effects or interfere with other medicines you use" (WebMD 2013). Report any side effects to your doctor, and to the FDA, as soon as possible. You can reach the FDA at (800) FDA-1088, or go to www.fda.gov/medwatch to report a problem (MedWatch 2018).

Get into the habit of having a bowl of fruit and a bag of mixed vegetables in the kitchen. Substitute these foods regularly to help curb hunger and sweet addictions throughout the day. After practicing this habit repeatedly, you begin to crave these high-nutrient foods. A natural sweets addiction is a good substitution for a craving for artificial sweeteners. These substitutes will provide the energy and nutrients needed to move the body more while providing cellular health protection and a feeling of well-being.

"'The safest route to a long life is to eliminate all processed and synthesized foods from your diet,' illuminates Dr. Messerlian. 'It's just that simple.' … 'Drinking soda each day, even diet soda, dramatically increases your chance of type 2 diabetes and weight gain; it's not good for you.' … For example, in the 1970s the artificial sweetener Saccharin was shown to cause the formation of bladder tumors in rats, especially in male rats … 'The issue is that if your body grows used to absorbing these products, and if you actually do eat a fruit or something good for you, your brain remains hungry because it's not satisfied'" (West 2013).

The information that follows reminds us all that sweets are not created equal. If you're diabetic, it is wise to pay attention to sugar alcohol content within the total carb count. You may or may not have noticed sugar alcohols on food labels as the low-carb craze began at the turn of the century. Now the FDA requires a nutrition label's total carb to include the full amount of grams from sugar alcohols and fiber.

Why are sugar alcohols important information? Sugar alcohol "carbs have less impact on blood glucose than others because they are only partially converted to glucose, or not at all, by the body. Some food companies started using the term 'net carbs' and defined it to mean the total grams of carbohydrate minus the grams of sugar alcohols, fiber, and glycerin. This equation is not entirely accurate, because some of the sugar alcohols and fiber are absorbed by the body. In fact, about half of the grams of sugar alcohols are metabolized to glucose" (Wheeler 2015).

If you're on an intensive insulin management program, be sure to consult with your physician to determine whether you need to be concerned with sugar alcohols and carbohydrate ratios in food substitutes to control diabetes and manage weight loss. This is important why? When these ratios are considered within balance, blood glucose or blood sugar count may be better controlled.

Important Facts Found on Aspartame and Shocking Health Risks

Aspartame continues to be a huge topic of concern about consumer health risk. It has long been argued that the sweetener is a health risk because of its chemical properties. Inadequate distribution centers and high-temperature environments during transit and storage are partially to blame. There is a health risk multiplier when the chemical sweetener in sodas is aspartame (United States Congressional Senate 1985).

"When the temperature of this sweetener exceeds 86 degrees F, the wood alcohol in aspartame converts to formaldehyde and then to formic acid, which in turn causes metabolic acidosis. Formic acid is the poison found in the sting of fire ants. The methanol toxicity mimics, among other conditions, multiple sclerosis and systemic lupus" (Wilson 2009).

Aspartame appears to be a common artificial sweetener found in many popular brands, among them NutraSweet, Equal, and Spoonful. And consumer safety advocates and others claim it makes people sick and causes them to gain weight.

"Technically the chemical is called aspartame, and it was once on a Pentagon list of bio warfare chemicals submitted to Congress" (Mercola 2002). It was originally developed to have deadly consequences on human beings. But then it was chemically formulated so it could be added into the food chain. Aspartame has a very interesting history of research and other intended use before it found its way into the foods and drinks we consume.

Consumer safety advocates, including myself, believe everyone's health would be better off if we all substituted the aspartame chemical with a natural sugar drink and moderated the habit. Otherwise, weight gain and associated diseases are likely to become problematic as the habit continues.

If you are suffering from unexplained, acute, and symptomatic health problems and are a heavy consumer of aspartame products, try removing them from your diet. Then substitute that bad habit for a natural sweets habit. The symptoms may be greatly alleviated or simply go away when you remove aspartame from your diet. There also appears to be a significant weight-gain connection with aspartame. How ironic is it that manufacturers use aspartame to sweeten weight-loss diet foods?

"There is absolutely no reason to take this product. It is NOT A DIET PRODUCT!!! The Congressional record said, 'It makes you crave carbohydrates and will make you FAT.' Dr. Roberts stated that when he got patients off aspartame, their average weight loss was 19 pounds per person. The formaldehyde stores in the fat cells, particularly in the hips and thighs … All physicians know what wood alcohol will do to a diabetic … The aspartame keeps the blood sugar level out of control, causing many patients to go into a coma" (Emery 1999).

There are now more than six thousand products on the shelves containing aspartame and neotame (Equal and NutraSweet) (ANH-USA 2012). Are uninformed parents unknowingly poisoning their families? It doesn't help when the FDA does not agree that aspartame is harmful to health. Nor is it useful that the American Diabetes Association, the American Dietetic Association, and the Conference of the American College of Physicians are all part of the choir. But this is no surprise, given that they all depend on Monsanto funding and must endorse Monsanto to continue receiving a "piece of the aspartame pie." This was exposed in *The New York Times* (Wilson 2009).

It is important to understand and not forget that deep-pocketed industries, including many special interests, have a lot to lose should this product be removed from shelves. After all, we know aspartame is very profitable. For instance, let's look at the effect to a supplier's bottom line when a company's aspartame contract ends.

A Gaitherburg, Maryland, biotech company, Genex Corp., went from reporting $14.3 million in revenues in 1985 to $2.8 million in 1986 (New York Times 1987). Genex had been a main supplier of aspartame ingredient to G.D. Searle & Company (who merged with Monsanto in 1985). The cause of the revenue loss was a direct result of NutraSweet Company marketing the chemical itself. And a suit was filed by Genex Corp. against Searle & Co. for failing to disclose gearing up to "its own L-phenylalanine plant" in Augusta, Georgia. "In 1984, 58 percent of Genex's $34.8 million in revenue was from sales to Searle" (*LA Times* 1985).

Most consumers don't know phenylalanine represents about one-half the aspartame within foods and drinks that contain this chemical sweetener. Keep this in mind as you read through the aspartame portion of this chapter. Although phenylalanine is an essential amino acid, it should be consumed with other amino acids naturally occurring in whole foods. Too much consumption of processed phenylalanine in high concentrates is said to support cancer cells.

If data shows a chemical or processed additive is likely to be unhealthy, why do manufacturers adamantly defend its safe merits at all costs? Simply recall who has the most to lose should the marketplace remove a multibillion-dollar food chemical from the food chain.

"In 2007, a review study was published by a panel of experts, declaring aspartame to be 'very safe.' The panel was chosen by the Burdock Group, a consulting firm serving the food, dietary supplement, and cosmetics industries, which was in turn hired by Ajinomoto, the world's largest aspartame manufacturer. Michael F. Jacobson, executive director of the consumer group Center for Science in the Public Interest (CSPI), said that the study was 'totally unreliable' and that some members of the expert panel were longstanding industry consultants" (SourceWatch 2013).

Maybe the best way to impress upon you the importance of substituting an artificial sweetener with a natural one is to convince you by sharing a famous aspartame animal study. Then you decide whether or not to continue a particular sweets habit.

Victoria Inness-Brown went above and beyond the typical consumer search for the truth about aspartame. She was concerned that her children were consuming too many diet sodas and wanted to know more about the harmful effects of aspartame.

Concerned this chemical sweetener would one day lead to illness or death, Inness-Brown performed a unique aspartame experiment. Although she is not a credentialed researcher or food manufacturer, Inness-Brown's work was found to be a powerful motivational tool. It became the reason for Dr. Marcela (a world-renowned alternative medicine proponent who markets dietary supplements and the like and a critic of many aspects of standard medical practices) to quit consuming aspartame products.

Inness-Brown performed a famous scientific study starting with 108 rats that lasted for two and a half years. A group of 60 rats was fed aspartame doses that, adjusted per rat weight, were less than acceptable daily intake (ADI) levels set by the FDA. The FDA allows for "50 mg of aspartame per kg of body weight per day, which is equivalent to a 150-lb person drinking about 20 12-oz cans of diet soda." Controversial studies, however, suggest the safe ADI for aspartame ingestion should be less than one-eighth a can equivalent of diet soda or that aspartame should be cut out of the diet all together. The other 48 rats of mixed sex remained as the control group. Although some small tumors in a low percentage of the control rats were naturally occurring, tumor growth in this group was unremarkable compared to the group of rats that was fed aspartame.

The results—within the group of rats consuming aspartame 67 percent of the female rats "developed tumors the size of golf balls or greater." In addition, 23 percent of the male rats "developed visible tumors." The rats also "developed other apparent health issues, such as paralysis, difficulty walking, spasmodic torticollis (also called dystonia, where the neck is twisted and the head continually tilted to one side), infected and bleeding eyes, skin lesions, thinning and yellowing fur, and obesity—which is sad, because people often use aspartame to lose weight" (Inness-Brown 2008). If the rats get sick when consuming amounts of aspartame that are adjusted for their body weight and far under ADI, why wouldn't we?

The fact that aspartame is endorsed by the FDA as a safe product and recommended by many doctors as a sweet alternative to sugar and a healthy weight-loss option appears to defy common sense logic.

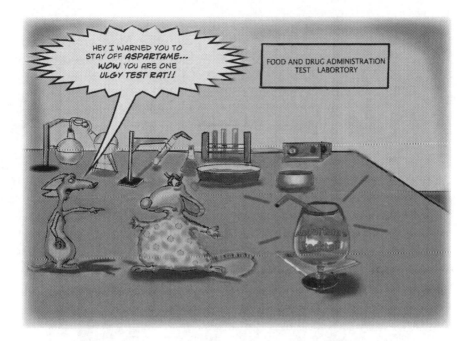

If you'd like to remove aspartame from your diet, popular brands to avoid when listed on ingredient labels include NutraSweet, Equal, Spoonful, Equal-Measure, and Canderel, to name a few. This artificial sweetener is found in diet sodas, beverage mixers, juice drinks, flavored waters, chewing gum, tabletop sweeteners, diet and diabetic foods, breakfast cereals such as Fiber One, fiber supplements like orange-flavored Metamucil, jams, and other sweets. Read your labels when you're looking to substitute sweet calories with healthier ones.

"According to Dr. Betty Martini, popular anti-aspartame advocate, the sweetener is an 'addictive, exitoneurotic, carcinogenic, genetically engineered drug and adjuvant that damages the mitochondria.' Moreover, Dr. Janet Hall, another famous advocate against aspartame, shares on her website that all artificial sweeteners create an artificial need for more sweetness" (Geib 2012).

Thus, the group of altered foods created by such sweeteners is a trap that causes people to become addicted to sweeter-tasting food with no nutritional value. "Recent studies have shown that aspartame is addictive because it affects the absorption of dopamine in the brain" (Geib 2012).

Changing addictive food habits requires removing as many chemical additives as possible from the diet to allow natural brain chemicals and functions to do their job through uninhibited dopamine absorption. When brain chemicals are affected, so is the balance of natural feel-good brain dopamine. "The major behaviors dopamine affects are movement, cognition, pleasure and motivation" (Siddiqui 2005). Since certain foods are known to release dopamine, if one knew which ones to substitute, then a more positive behavior would result, along with increased willpower to live a healthier lifestyle.

Substituting healthier foods and drink that don't obstruct but produce more naturally occurring dopamine may be a way to break an unhealthy food habit. "Load up on foods that contain vitamin B6 and phenylalanine [recall that a balance of natural amino acids is healthy] and tyrosine, the building blocks of dopamine. Good sources of all three nutrients include chicken, turkey, lean beef, eggs, salmon, tuna, shrimp, crab, tofu, dark-green leafy vegetables and reduced-fat dairy foods" (Dworkin-McDaniel 2012). The amino acid phenylalanine is not good for us when it is artificially isolated. However, when it occurs naturally in whole foods, it is very good for us.

When one neurotransmitter, such as dopamine, is not effectively doing its job, it has an effect on other chemicals that are naturally produced in the body, such as adrenaline. "Most people with addictions have weak adrenal glands. They essentially crave the euphoric feeling that goes with more active adrenals. They gravitate to substances, activities, habits, behaviors, relationships or other situations that stimulate, or perhaps nourish to a degree, the adrenal glands." These addictions may include "caffeine, sugar, cocaine, depressants, stimulants, anger, fear, sex, vigorous exercise, or job or marital drama. Furthermore, these stimulants eventually weaken the adrenals, causing a deepening of the addiction" (Wilson 2013).

When unnatural stimulation of brain-body neurotransmitter chemical exchange occurs on a daily basis, unhealthy habits tend to continue. And that chemical imbalance has much to do with how we feel and whether we sustain our fitness, health, and lifestyle goals.

Personal Fitness Challenge: "Diet and Autoimmune Connected"

I did then as I still do today have a preference toward high-protein foods. They make me feel full longer and, when mixed with green leafy and other assorted vegetables, support increased dopamine production. Increased dopamine production equates to increased willpower and motivation to perform daily exercise. More exercise also produces a healthy dose of adrenaline daily to support fitness goals.

Since dopamine is the brain's driving motivation to voluntarily push the body, the adrenal glands are the nitro boost that keeps the body in motion. Once the natural high from adrenalin is experienced during and after exercise activity, the craving to repeat it is reinforced daily.

I didn't severely restrict any macro or micronutrient food group or go on some strange diet regiment. Nor did I overly exert myself physically. I wanted to achieve a natural brain-body boost so I could lose weight naturally.

I took in roughly the same amount of calories daily but modified my food preference by substituting unhealthy addictive foods for more whole foods. My carbohydrate food preferences were multigrain breads and cereals, trail mix, potatoes, rice, noodles, and assorted fruits and vegetables and other wholesome favorite food choices (chapter 10, "Choose Favorite Foods to Lose Weight"). I also took a quality vitamin and mineral supplement to increase my energy levels, improve my mood, and ensure antioxidant cellular protection. These daily nutrients also provided the energy I needed to exercise daily.

For me it's not all about removing every bad food habit or vice. It's about balance, moderation, and quality of lifestyle experiences. However, during the healing and recovery period, I didn't consume any sodas, artificial sweeteners, or alcohol for five years. Giving up these things completely was not an easy ordeal, but it was necessary to heal and confirm whether or not I had lupus and/or fibromyalgia. I believe the painful fibromyalgia and autoimmune-like symptoms and false positive after positive lupus test results - resulted from overconsumption of artificial sweeteners. The range of joint pain, stiffness, and swelling I experienced before and after quitting aspartame was the difference between night and day.

The chronic pain disorder I was diagnosed with (and most of you will be familiar with) was fibromyalgia. At the time, I was being treated by an immunologist, as well as a physiatrist who recommended testing for lupus. Those tests were not consistent, often showing a false positive result. At the time, this led me to believe something in my diet may be a trigger to the musculoskeletal joint pain, fatigue, and swelling in multiple areas characteristic of lupus.

If I wouldn't have had these referred medical experiences, I couldn't have reasoned out a possible aspartame connection as suspect and/or the likely cause of my acute symptoms and revolving positive and false test results.

My medical records still reflect a diagnosis of fibromyalgia with medically substantiated service injuries. If I could change the details within the transcripts to be more precise, I'd add, an allergic reaction note reading, "Aspartame products trigger acute lupus-like and fibromyalgia symptoms in this patient." But that would never happen, because there's no medical study or evidence that validates this connection. At least, none exist that I'm aware of anyway.

A major point I want to make is that not one of those medical doctors connected the false positive test results and fibromyalgia symptoms to my diet. Nevertheless, to this day, I do my best to ensure I don't consume any aspartame of any form. Since I no longer drink or eat any artificially sweetened drinks or foods, I've not experience any lupus-like or fibromyalgia symptoms. Nor am I treated by a physiatrist or immunologist for total body pain any more.

Is it a coincidence that the physical pain is no longer present throughout my body to the same degree? Not as far as I'm concerned.

Why didn't I drink any alcohol for five years? No, I wasn't a reformed alcoholic who needed to sober up and get my life on track. I'd rather eat good food than drink those calories and not increase health risk while on the mend. Everyone knows alcohol mixed with almost any drug is not a good idea.

I'm a firm believer that, when the healing process is hampered with too many toxins and mind-altering substances, it can lead to sedentary and other addictive habits known to cause disease.

Chapter 8

All Fats Are Not Equal

Man adds hyperpalatable ingredients to foods that
addict us and harms health.

—MirrorAthlete Principled Fitness and
Healthy Lifestyle Philosophy

When choosing favorite food substitution strategies to lose weight, one
must consider hyperpalatable fats as part of the dietary equation. There
are animal models that show findings that suggest sugars and fats are
addictive and, when combined, can be just as addictive as a bad drug
habit and "result in increased body weight." These are key nutrients
and do play an important role in balanced diet. However too many
people tend to binge on them and consume too much (Avena, Rada,
and Hoebel 2009, 623–28).

It is not hard to understand how certain foods can be addictive and,
coincidently, cause obesity. For example, give kids a choice between a
fruit or vegetable and a bag of chips or cookies. Most of the time, they'll
prefer processed foods that have lots of sugar, fats, and salt in them.

What makes unnecessary additives especially bad is many foods
are processed in ways that make us want more. Consuming too many
hyperpalatable fats, sugars, and salt isn't healthy for us in general.
"Nothing about a natural additive makes it safer than a man-made
additive. An individual food additive consists of chemical elements
combined in a particular way. Whether grown in a garden or
manufactured in a laboratory, the chemical structure and composition
is the same" (Curtis, Meer, and Misner 2006).

However, lab-farmed ingredients like trans fats, although structurally similar appear to be malformed at the molecular level in comparison to natural trans fats. Since trans fats are abundant in our food chain, it's time to get better acquainted with them.

First, we must define and relate to trans fats as naturally occurring in animal products—for example, meat and dairy. Then we must realize that when engineered vegetable oils are partially or fully hydrogenated, it increases unhealthy trans fat intake.

A trans fat naturally exists in organic foods in small amounts. However, the process of adding more hydrogen atoms (hydrogenation) to vegetable oil(s) monounsaturated fat carbon chains changes the molecular composition. The vegetable oil then becomes a *partially hydrogenated* product with more unnatural trans fat composition.

When the vegetable oil's carbon chain molecules are *fully hydrogenated*, they become *saturated fats* or *"trans hard fats."* Vegetable oils are partially hardened to achieve "firm" soft spreads and vegetable shortenings with long shelf lives, great for baking and frying and known to cause health problems.

"Eating hydrogenated fats has been associated with some very serious diseases such as cancer, atherosclerosis (hardening of the arteries), diabetes, obesity, immune system dysfunction, decreased visual acuity (sharpness, clearness, keenness), sterility, difficulty with mothers lactating and problems with bones and tendons. These types of 'processed' oils are not healthy" (Vigil 2007).

"Trans fats, it turns out, take the place of healthy saturated fats throughout the body and effectively block things like nutrient absorption, waste elimination, and immune function—this is why they are so uniquely dangerous for your health. Though chemically identical to saturated fats, according to *GreenMedInfo.com*, trans fats are inherently malformed and unnatural" (Benson 2013).

In the long run, cubed butter and lard appear to be "more or less" better for health in moderation when compared to the hydrogenation of vegetable oils and margarine soft spreads. Why? Because saturated animal fats have carbon atom chains that are "naturally" filled with hydrogen atoms.

This does not mean overconsumption of saturated animal fats is good for us either. Looking at fats in general, too much of any kind can cause bad cholesterol to rise. This can increase blood pressure and, under worst-case scenarios, predispose one to heart disease and stroke.

Once you understand partial and full hydrogenation of oil fats are *nonessential* to the diet, you may then determine *certain* vegetable oils, butter, and lard to be healthier fat alternatives when used in moderation.

Today, trans fats are found in many processed foods, such as soups; chips and crackers; breakfast and dairy products; cookies and candies; and thousands of other convenient fried, baked, and frozen products. And a major source of trans fat calories is one of America's favorite fried foods—french fries. "To make vegetable oils suitable for deep frying, the oils are subjected to hydrogenation, which creates trans fats. Among the hazards of fast food, 'fries' are prime in purveying trans fats" (MedicineNet.com 2015).

"In the late 19th century, chemists discovered that they could add hydrogen atoms to unsaturated fats by bubbling hydrogen gas through vegetable oil in the presence of a nickel catalyst" (Harvard School of Public Health 2015). The trans fats frying oil industry, the long-standing investor interests behind it, and the frying oils themselves will not go away anytime soon.

The trans fats industry innovators have figured out ways to survive the consumer health backlash by reducing trans fats while leading people to believe that the trans fats are being removed altogether. Simply note that, on margarine containers and other processed food ingredient labels like frying oils, you see the words, "Trans Fat, 0 grams" along with something like "Partially Hydrogenated, Soybean Oil," for example.

What's most deceptive for consumers is that the "0" does not mean trans fats are not in a processed food product (a point that will soon be covered in greater detail). But what's most important to understand is that, when these vegetable oils become partially hydrogenated and intentionally mixed with other hyperpalatable additives, people become addicted to them.

"In his book *The End of Overeating*, David Kessler, M.D., the former head of the Food and Drug Administration, describes the science of how food is made into drugs by the creation of hyperpalatable foods that lead to neuro-chemical addiction" (Hyman 2011). And that neurochemical addiction can be identified in brain receptors.

"A new animal study looked at what happens to the brain when rats are fed these fast food oils—they became drug addicts! … What was really concerning was that the trans-fats and soybean oil changed the brain receptors to make the rats more susceptible to drug addiction. Yep, you read that right; these rats had withdrawal type symptoms when they weren't being given uppers (amphetamines). The upshot? Yikes! Are we fabricating a nation of drug addicts with mass manufactured food?" (Centeno 2014).

If you see the words *partially hydrogenated* before an oil ingredient you know it has hydrogen trans fats added to the oil's carbon chains. "Trans fat was originally added to foods to increase the shelf life. Trans fat does not stand for 'transformed fat,' but comes from the fact that the hydrogen atoms in the double bond are actually across from each other. This comes from the Latin meaning of trans, which is across" (theLabRat.com 2005).

I know many of you are health conscious when it comes to eating too many animal fats because you remove it from meat or ladle it from broth prior to serving. However, in the case of man-made or naturally occurring trans fats or partially hydrogenated fats, they can't be seen as they're blended into foods. In other words, as opposed to fats floating on top a broth or within a cooled frying pan, they're impossible to detect.

I believe Hyman and Centeno are on point regarding engineered foods that addict you to them. I recall working with a client who had a bad food habit that, in essence, resulted from hyperpalatable food choices.

At the time of consult, Kate was twenty-four years old, stood at five foot five. Kate was an attractive woman with inquisitive charm, very personable, and weighed in at a stout 210 pounds. I was interested in working with her because I knew she was a dedicated fitness buff, had good muscle mass, and was motivated to lose body fat weight. She simply needed a relevant fitness and nutrition plan that would work for her. But in order for Kate to be successful at weight loss, the exact cause of her weight gain had to be identified.

Her fitness goal was to lose the weight she'd gained over the previous year, and she had a goal of becoming a competitive bodybuilder. She needed a different fitness program strategy to achieve both goals.

After a nutritional assessment, it was clear she was consuming too many fats and sugar calories from convenience store coffees, processed cookies, muffins, and microwave popcorn. I calculated she consumed approximately four hundred calories per day more than her body burned. The excess food calories were being stored as body fat.

I explained to Kate how her weight had gotten out of control. Then I provided a simple BMI worksheet calculation (chapter 5, "Caloric Exchange: A Balancing Act" and BMI form 5.4).

To calculate Kate's BMI, I divide her weight in pounds by her height in inches squared and multiplied that by 703. The formula:

Kate's weight is 210 lb. / [height 5' 5" (65")] ^{2} × 703

210 lbs. / (65" × 65" = 4225) = .0497 × 703 = 34.94% body fat

Kate's BMI shows she is considered obese for her height and weight. Recall the BMI Standards:

BMI below 18.5 – underweight

BMI between 18.5 and 24.9 – normal weight

BMI between 25.0 and 29.9 – overweight

BMI of 30.0 and above – obese

Kate desired to drop her body fat (BF) from 35 percent to 25 percent. First, I needed to calculate her BF weight based on her 35 percent BMI calculation and then determine her lean body weight (LBW). Lean body weight is comprised of water, muscle, bone, organs, connective tissue, and blood.

Recall the difference between BF and LBW can be calculated through a simple formula for both men and women:

Total body weight (BW) × body fat (BF) % = fat weight (lb.)

Then total body weight – fat weight = LBW

Given Kate's current stats—210 pounds, five foot five, with a calculated BMI of about 35 percent BF—let's do the calculations:

Kate's approximate body weight composition

210 lb. × .35 BF = 73.5 lb. of BF

210 lb. – 73.5 lb. BF = 136.5 lb. LBW

Kate's desired body weight (DBW) at 25 percent body fat

210 lb. × .25 BF = 52.5 lb.

136.5 lb. LBW + 52.5 lb. = 189 lb. DBW

Current weight 210 – 189 DBW = 21 lb. weight-loss goal

To achieve her DBW and fat-loss goal, Kate must lose approximately twenty-one pounds.

The BMI is a convenient starting baseline tool to approximate unhealthy body weight; it's easy to use and costs nothing. But it is also the least accurate assessment method if you want to accurately measure body fat within an acceptable margin of error. "BMI is simply based on height and weight, and it fails to assess lean muscle mass or body fat percentage, and indicates most lean individuals are overweight simply by definition." It is often used as a baseline by fitness trainers and consultants because it's "simple, inexpensive and non-invasive" (Han, Ko, and Cho 2012, 791).

At the time I calculated Kate's BMI, I also cross-compared those results using a digital skin fold caliper, taking measurements at the back of the upper arm, abdomen, and thigh. Though taking measurements with calipers still has a low rate of accuracy, it is still a more accurate method than BMI. On the other hand, the gold standard, the hydrostatic body weight technique, falls within a couple percentage points of body fat accuracy (Katch and McArdle 1993, 233–58). This technique is more accurate than any other body fat measuring test in comparison. The BMI is least accurate in measuring body fat compared to other tests that account for body composition—or what our bodies actually comprise (in other words, measuring body fat less muscle density, bone, and other organic bodily matter).

After comparing Kate's caliper results to her BMI calculations, her body fat weight was around 40 percent. She needed to lose closer to thirty-two pounds, as opposed to twenty-one pounds, to meet her desired lean muscle mass and body fat weight.

Since the accuracy of caliper tests and especially hydrostatic body fat analysis services is dependent on repeatable technique, equipment, and cost, I'd typically offer the BMI service at no cost with initial programming services. Then I'd provide the calculation worksheets to clients for future self-assessment. This allowed them to easily update their initial body fat weight baselines through simple calculation. Clients could then save money, compare body fat baseline increases or decreases, and choose a more accurate way to measure body fat if desired.

Kate realized that she'd put on the forty pounds of excess weight over a year's time. But she didn't fully understand how it happened. After showing how her body needed approximately 2,200 calories per day to sustain her metabolic rate, exercise, and other daily activities, the following caloric calculations became more meaningful to her.

I calculated, she was consuming around 400 calories more a day then she was burning. The math worked out like this:

400 cal × 7 days = 2,800 cal/wk. × 4 wks. = 11,200 cal added (recall 3,500 cal = 1 lb.)

11,200 cal/month/by 3,500 cal = 3.2 lb. weight gain per month × 12 months = 38.4 lb. gained in one year

Once Kate was provided this information, she changed to healthier fitness activities and made other healthy lifestyle habit choices. She started a two- to four-mile walking program per day, alternating other aerobic exercise in the gym throughout the week. For instance, she'd walk or ride her bike to the gym and then use a stationary bike, stair-stepper, or rowing machine in her local fitness center for approximately thirty minutes prior to her forty-five-minute weight lifting routine.

It is also worth mentioning that, "among women consuming a usual diet, physical activity was associated with less weight gain only among women whose BMI was lower than 25. Women successful in maintaining normal weight and gaining fewer than 2.3 kg over 13 years averaged approximately 60 minutes a day of moderate-intensity activity throughout the study" (Lee et al. 2010 1,173–79).

What favorite food habits was Kate willing to substitute to lose forty pounds? She gave up microwave popcorn during the evening and a variation of baked snacks and other fast foods throughout the day. Not only was Kate eating too many trans fat snacks; the other additives in those foods contributed to her weight gain. Once she became mindful of healthy snack substitutes, she replaced most of her bad snack choices with fruits, vegetables, and other healthy products. She also went back to drinking regular coffee, more water and tea, and eating three balanced meals a day.

By changing her eating habits and adding more aerobic exercise activity, she began having weight-loss success. What really made a difference for Kate was when she learned how to balance calorie nutrients and identify addictive foods known to cause weight gain and harm health.

Our bodies need only about 20 grams of dietary fats daily (saturated and unsaturated). Kate's three serving bag of microwave popcorn had 13.5 grams of fat (13.5 g × 9 cal/g = 121.5 fat calories) and 19 grams of carbohydrate (57 g × 4 cal/g = 228 carbohydrate calories). Kate's total calorie intake when consuming a three-serving bag of microwave popcorn equaled approximately 350 calories.

The total calories in her sixteen-ounce white chocolate mocha with whipped cream were 510. By removing these two addictive foods, she reduced nearly 860 calories from her daily diet.

She instantly understood how many trans fats and other calories and percentages of macronutrients she was consuming after a five-day nutritional assessment, which was instrumental in her ability to change her lifestyle habits. Her transitional dietary and exercise habit changes resulted in her losing forty pounds of body weight in fourteen months.

For many, it is nearly impossible to relate to trans fats in hyperpalatable foods because they're impossible to detect unless you're mindful of such things. In addition, product labels don't tell the story of the connection between unhealthy weight gain and consuming too many unnatural, as well as natural, addictive ingredients. There are also diet and weight-loss foods promoted as low calorie and heart healthy with 0 grams of trans fats and partially hydrogenated oils listed on product labels. But does "0" actually mean zero?

What is not widely known by consumers is that trans fats were not banned from use. However, during early 2006, companies began removing the "really bad" trans fat hydrogenation processes from foods, once it had been determined these fully saturated fats increased the risk of heart disease and other ill-health conditions. After the effective date of January 1, 2006, the FDA required manufactures to request extension to use existing food labels. Thereafter, the FDA considered, upon request, whether the trans fat values should have a declared value of "0.5 g" per serving or less.

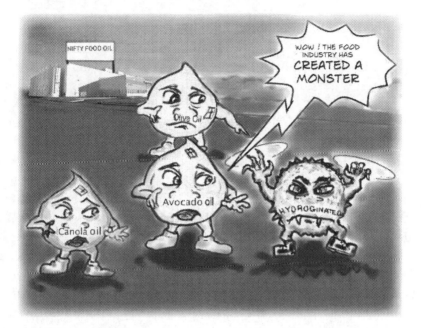

You'll see labels that list "0" trans fats in their products. The "0" reflects that food manufacturers replaced *most* of the saturated trans fats in products with partially hydrogenated vegetable oil(s). "Federal law allows manufacturers to report 0 g trans fats per serving as long as the product provides less than 0.5 g per serving. The American Heart Association recommends consuming no more than 1 percent of your total calories in the form of trans fats. For people following a 2,000-calorie diet, that means no more than 20 calories, or 2 g, trans fat" (Schuab 2015).

But have these actions quenched the trans fat health risk concerns completely? It appears the FDA's trans fat label laws address the identification of these unhealthy fats. It looks like consumers have won this battle. But have they? Also, some would say it's a guise making way for its replacement.

"In June 2015, the US Food and Drug Administration (FDA) announced it was phasing trans fats out of the food supply, finalizing a 2013 preliminary determination that partially-hydrogenated oils (PHOs) were no longer generally recognized as safe. Food companies will have three years to remove trans fats from their products. In the meantime, consumers should choose foods that have the lowest amounts of trans fats possible" (Public Health Law Center 2015).

However, "the timing and intent of the FDA's rule is suspect for three reasons. First, it was announced only after most companies had already eliminated trans fat—it's currently only in a handful of foods. Secondly, it was a quiet reaction to a lawsuit the FDA was sure to lose. And lastly, the ban will promote market demand for two new GMO soybeans by Monsanto and DuPont, which are engineered for trans fat-free oils" (ANH-USA 2013).

Even through the FDA recently determined trans fats are not safe for humans, the ban on these fats is not 100 percent. This is because naturally occurring PHOs are found in livestock and plants. Also none of the existing laws restrict trans fats in restaurants or in convenience and fast foods stores.

The good news is the ban on trans fats has made a significant difference in our children's school breakfast and lunch programs. The USDA supports rules for the national school breakfast and lunch programs. Meals will contain less than .5 g trans fats per serving or will be labeled "0" g trans fat under FDA regulation, mimicking the way other ingredients are currently labeled on food products. And the good news for consumers is that the FDA now requires food manufactures to follow more stringent trans fat label laws. For instance, if a food product has .5 g trans fats or more, that value has to be listed on the label (FDA 2017).

As previously stated, these actions will not remove all the trans fat from our children's diet because of the naturally occurring trans fats found in vegetables and animals. But it is a significant step in the right direction and a precedent set for restaurants, retail outlets, and convenience food producers to identify and/or remove unhealthy fats in foods.

Regardless, based on history, I wouldn't hold my breath on a 2018 removal or ban of all man-made trans fats. It is possible the FDA, in partnership with industry giants, will approve new PHO standards and continue unhealthy hydrogenated trans fats masquerading under a different guise as heart healthy.

Ultimately, the marketplace will determine the fate of trans fats and trans fat free oils. "Many food makers have realized that consumers, having the new information on the food label, would avoid products containing trans fat. Fearing lost sales, many companies have found ways to make their products without partially hydrogenated oils"

(Harvard School of Public Health 2015). Will this new process include Monsanto—will its genetically modified organisms be made with trans fats-free oil?

I can see a future without unhealthy saturated trans fat products, but not absent of GMOs; nor can I see the total elimination of a PHO fats additives. I believe food engineers will simply innovate another blend of hydrogenated vegetable oils processed using a new strain of genetic crop food and promoted free of trans fats and health risk. Then consumer health advocates in opposition to the new "industry oil substitute" will have to spend the next thirty to forty years proving why this new and addictive oil innovation is bad for our health.

In continuation of this topic, chapter 11, "The Impact of Cooking Oil on Health," thoroughly breaks down the good, bad, and ugly dietary fat choices.

Personal Fitness Challenge: "Weight-Bearing Pain"

To be honest, during the rehabilitative period in my life, I was not focused on unhealthy trans fats—not until I became aware of the labeling law requirements of 2006.

Fortunately, prior to this time I was mostly focused on how to reduce total fat calories from my daily diet. Simply by reducing fat calories, I was also reducing trans fats.

It was the thought of dealing with more weight-bearing pain that ultimately pushed me to lose body weight. I knew that, if I didn't have a plan to deal with weight-bearing pain, immobility coupled with more drugs and obesity would become a long-term reality.

Even though I cut down on portions of fatty foods and total daily calories, I wasn't losing weight. Since I don't believe in restrictive or starvation diets, I needed to further examine in detail what I was consuming from the kitchen and what I knew my metabolism needed, or didn't need, during a time of rehab or living a sedentary lifestyle. I knew that, in time, if I didn't get a handle on the weight gain, I was at high risk of secondary injury or other ill-health complications.

The food habit easiest for me to change involved removing all the processed and convenience foods from the fridge, freezer, and pantry. I did the things I had instructed past clients to do. I eventually removed products with trans fats, high fructose corn syrup (HFCS), and monosodium glutamate (MSG), as well as baked snacks and the like. Why? Because these things were unnecessary, addictive, and unhealthy foods that wouldn't help me lose weight.

Until I experienced personal adversity with mobility loss, I really never followed any dietary guidelines. Before this time, I was never overweight and in great shape. I suppose one of my dietary saving graces was that I have a craving and preference for natural whole foods.

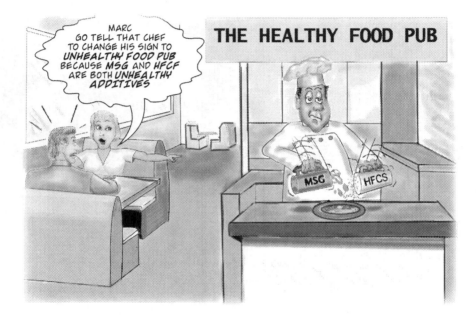

After I made the necessary changes in the kitchen and to my food habits, the weight began to come off and the weight-bearing pain was alleviated enough to allow increased walking distances while using crutches at first. Once out of the wheelchair, I never looked back.

What was amazing to my wife was how strong my upper body became and how fast I could move on crutches after I'd become conditioned to use them at one point in time.

I mean I could actually, at one point, keep up with a jogger using one leg and two crutches at a racehorse stride. But that was just me—and that very attitude has also been my reinjury and pain nemesis. I've always been competitive, and that mind-set didn't help one day on the job site. Ironically, I lost control of my wheelchair during an ADA parking and sidewalk safety inspection for my employer.

In short, I pushed myself too hard and nearly launched off and over a sidewalk curb. As I braked quickly with my hands on the wheels to prevent the launch, the stress in doing so permanently injured both of my shoulders.

Unfortunately, I tore both rotor cuffs. One was surgically repaired in 2012; the other is still pending. What can I say? Pacing oneself during recovery requires patience and self-control. I'd like to think I've learned something from this experience and can pass it on to others. That is, high-risk competitive behavior during recovery is just that—risky and not wise.

After I was no longer using a wheelchair, crutches, or a cane, I recall walking a couple of blocks with a painful and severe limp. At this time, my two-mile walk goal seemed impossible.

But I was determined and willing to put the effort in to increase my distances daily. If I didn't try to strengthen my weight-bearing walking posture and increase distances daily, I knew for certain the physical pain would worsen, immobility would follow, and sedentary habits would begin anew. This scared the hell out of me and was a key motivator that provided me the willpower to improve my walking distances, heal the best I could, and get on with my life.

Chapter 9

Health Risk Prediction and Prevention

Relating to lab results can influence lifestyle change and consumer choice.

—MirrorAthlete Principled Fitness and
Healthy Lifestyle Philosophy

I believe it is important to cover how blood test results can serve as predictive, preventative, and relatable health gauge indicators.

I've used blood test results shared by clients to educate them and help them plan dietary and exercise programs in coordination with their doctors. These discussions also ensured the client understood the various roles of a medical service provider, a nutritionist, a fitness trainer, and a healthy lifestyle consultant—and how this information could help them develop a better healthy lifestyle program.

A good example of a client relationship that involved medical coordination occurred while I was working with Tom to create a customized fitness program. Tom was thirty-four years old at the time. He appeared to be in good shape and had approximately 27 percent body fat, stood five foot ten, and weighed 204 pounds. Tom was muscular and didn't appear overweight. He had concerns about his blood fat test results and weight gain. His doctor gave him a brochure on healthy diet and daily exercise and recommended he consider a cholesterol-lowering medication (a statin).

Tom didn't want the medication. He preferred to lower his cholesterol and triglyceride levels through diet and exercise. He would then use future blood test results measured against a baseline to determine whether the lifestyle changes were successful. He would relate the baseline blood fat test results to tests taken after he'd applied healthier food choices and a modified exercise plan.

During the first part of our dietary consult, we defined the two types of fats circulating in the blood and stored in the body and the relationship between the two.

Defining Triglycerides and Cholesterol Fats

Triglyceride fats come from vegetables and their pressed oils and are also found in animal products. So how do triglycerides come from animal products? Since animals graze on vegetation, a portion of those vegetable oils gets stored in fat cells. Since plants don't produce cholesterol fat, it is the animal and human cells and liver that produce it. When consumers underconsume or overconsume fatty acids, it influences blood chemistry, body fat weight, and overall health.

The following three citations help define a triglyceride structure and its fatty acid composition, including the cholesterol fat count produced by the body and how that count changes when consuming animal products.

The triglyceride structure is a formation of an ester (organic compound), or glycerol's three fatty acids. "The word 'fat' generally refers to a chemical substance known as glycerides. These are the basic building blocks of glycerol, and there are as many as 3 units of fatty acids that would normally link to the glycerol backbone. Because of this type of attachment of the fatty acids to glycerol, fats are usually defined as triglycerides" (FitDay 2018).

"Fatty acids are arranged as chains. Each fatty acid from a triglyceride is classified as a saturated (SFA), a monounsaturated (MUFA) or a polyunsaturated (PUFA) fatty acid. Triglycerides are mixtures of the three different types of fatty acids. The proportion of each determines the characteristics of fats in food and their effect on human health" (Henley and Misner 1999).

"Solid fats usually consist of saturated fatty acids, whereas liquid oils are made largely of unsaturated acids, however this can be artificially manipulated to produce triglycerides with other desirable properties" (Blamire 2005). This is very similar to the conversion of vegetable oil to soft spread margarine or the fry oil hydrogenation process discussed in the previous chapter.

Although Tom was exercising daily, he was consuming a high-carbohydrate diet including too many fried fatty foods. There are known health risks associated with high-carbohydrate diets. "A high carbohydrate diet translates directly to high triglycerides in the blood and on the body" (Eberstein 2015). In Tom's case, both triglycerides and cholesterol blood fat levels were elevated.

The cholesterol our bodies produce and consume is the other fat type. It also circulates and stores in the body and is in the steroid family. It is essential for normal function and integrity of cellular structure and efficient nerve conduction. Cholesterol is a vital precursor to our body's manufacturing of other steroid hormones—cortical, progesterone, estrogen, and testosterone. It also functions as a precursor for critical biosynthesis (manufacturing) of required bile acids for our digestive system and vitamin D.

Through the consulting session, I provided Tom a brochure and a better understanding of cholesterol's role in the body. We discussed how too many fats in the diet increase the risk of diseases such as stroke, diabetes, heart disease, and atherosclerosis.

"Because triglycerides and cholesterol can't dissolve in blood, they circulate throughout your body with the help of proteins that transport the lipids" (Mayo Clinic 2015). And since removal of both fat types is dependent on a finite protein transport system, if too many remain in circulation, they can gum up and plug blood flow pathways.

According to the American Heart Association, the liver produces about 75 percent of the cholesterol needed by the body. This leaves 25 percent that should be supplemented through diet to sustain optimum health. But this amount is very small, approximately 200 mg. And too many Americans exceed this cholesterol level.

Let's use Tom's 255 total cholesterol serum count to relate to his blood fat results, which include the VLDL (very low density lipoprotein) cholesterol levels found in his triglyceride count of 150. Most people don't know that a small amount of VLDLs is found in the triglyceride count and is not singled out unless a doctor requests a specific lipid fat count panel. VLDLs are considered the worst type of cholesterol fat to remain circulating in the blood. In order to bring meaning to these numbers and the related health risks, we must further define them.

Tom had a triglyceride (TGL) level of 150 mg/dl. This level should be less than 150 mg/dl. So Tom is on the border of a high TGL level (150–199 mg/dl). He had a HDL (high density lipoprotein) level of 40 mg/dl and LDL (low density lipoprotein) level of 185 mg/dl. In 1972, William Friedewald, a medical doctor, derived a simple equation to estimate the VLDL (very low density lipoproteins) found in the triglyceride level. They represent one-fifth the total amount of cholesterol bound to triglyceride fats.

The equation below is still used to determine routine laboratory estimates of HDL and LDL cholesterol levels. Because of the consistency of cholesterol content in plasma triglycerides, when measuring VLDL within specific parameters, it is possible to derive an approximate VLDL cholesterol level by dividing total triglycerides by five:

TGL/5 = VLDL

Let's take a look at a couple other equations:

Total cholesterol = (HDL cholesterol) + (LDL cholesterol) + (VLDL cholesterol)

Rearranging this equation to solve for LDL gives us

LDL = total cholesterol – HLD – VLDL

When dividing the 150 triglyceride level by 5, we get a result of 30 mg/dl of VLDL. The sum of 40 (HDL), 185 (LDL), and 30 (VLDL) derives an approximate total serum cholesterol level of 255 mg/dl (Friedewald 2012).

"Friedewald knew that it was easy to measure total cholesterol and HDL but difficult to measure the others. His insight was that the triglyceride level if divided by five could give a close approximation of VLDL. In running his experiments, he also realized that this relationship held only if triglyceride levels were 400 mg/dl or under. If they were over this, all bets were off" (Eades 2009). If triglyceride levels are higher than 400 mg/dl, it is wise to get a referral for a specific blood panel that includes an accurate VLDL count.

Doctors recommend total cholesterol levels remain below 200. Tom's good cholesterol level, or HDL, was at 40 mg/dl (60 and above is considered good). His bad cholesterol, or LDL, was at 185 mg/dl (anything over 100–129 mg/dl is considered too high). Of his LDL level, approximately 30 mg/dl of VLDL was present. The test results indicated his cholesterol levels, like his triglyceride levels, were positively heading in the wrong direction.

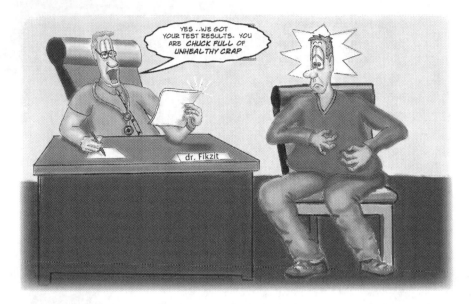

For ideal cholesterol level ratios, LDLs should be twice as high as HDLs. In Tom's case, the ratio was 185 LDLs to 40 HDLs, or a ratio of ~4.6:1—approximately two times over the unhealthy ratio. Tom was definitely pushing the health risk envelope. I told him the fat concentration circulating in the blood is important to pay attention to. Doctors and dieticians tell us to limit dietary fats for good reason.

But are all fats bad for us?

Fats are also categorized as essential and nonessential. Essential fats are considered those fats our bodies cannot manufacture on their own that must come from the diet.

"The only essential polyunsaturated fatty acids are linoleic acid [omega-6] and alpha-linolenic acid [omega-3]. The other fatty acids are not essential because you can survive without getting them from your diet" (Stein 2015). Nonessential fats, such as cholesterol, aren't necessary, as you learned earlier, because the cells and liver can manufacture them through *lipolysis* (the breakdown of stored body fat through hydrolysis). This cholesterol produced by the body is then converted to blood glucose for energy and other vital biosynthesis and cellular function.

Monounsaturated and polyunsaturated vegetable oils can have the opposite effect of saturated fats when used in moderation. For instance, "both oils have a blood-cholesterol lowering effect and can lower the risk of heart disease." Reducing total fat and replacing some saturated fat with unsaturated fats can help lower your risk of heart disease. Eating foods high in polyunsaturated oils can help lower blood cholesterol but may also lower HDL cholesterol, the "good" cholesterol (Henley and Misner 1999). During Tom's nutritional assessment it was important to identify the nonessential fat calories he consumed daily. Then he needed to cut back on them to improve future blood test results.

At breakfast Tom would typically eat pastries. Then for lunch he'd eat pastas and fried foods from the workplace cafeteria. His dinners were cooked by his wife and seemed more traditional and healthy, but it appeared he was also consuming too many baked snacks overall. By nutritional assessment, it appeared 75 percent of his daily calories came from carbohydrates. The 2010 Dietary Guidelines for Americans recommends average daily intake of 45 to 65 percent carbohydrates for both men and women.

For exercise, Tom worked out three days per week doing strength-training activities. He preferred using free weights and did not participate in any type of aerobic exercise.

I explained to Tom it was likely the high cholesterol and triglycerides counts were mostly due to poor food choice. His past and current medical and family history suggested no other cause for elevated blood fat serum levels. I emphasized that, at 27 percent body fat, a BMI between 25.0 and 29.9 is considered overweight to obese. Although he was not facing an immediate health risk, Tom realized it was a matter of time before an overweight condition could turn into gross obesity and disease if he didn't change his habits.

As a part of my fitness assessment services, I also sized up Tom's somatotype to determine a fitness plan relevant to his body type and fitness goals.

"Somatotype is a category to which people are assigned according to the extent to which their bodily physique conforms to a basic type (usually endomorphic, mesomorphic, or ectomorphic). An endomorphic body type is a person with a soft round body build and a high proportion of fat tissue. A mesomorphic body type is a person with a compact and muscular body build. An ectomorphic body type is a person with a lean and delicate body build" (Teachers Corner 2015).

Tom most definitely had the body type you'd associate and identify as a running back or defensive safety on a football team. As a matter of fact, during varsity high school football, Tom had been highly ranked in the state stats as an all-time yardage gainer and scoring fullback. "There is considerable corpus of evidence indicating that athletes succeeding in certain sports have distinctive body shapes that differ according to the demands of the type of sports and competitive level" (ShamseNajabadi, Dehkordi, and Ahdeno 2013).

After Tom's somatotype assessment, I determined he was approximately 50 percent mesomorph, 20 percent ectomorph, and 30 percent endomorph. These percentages were based on subjective viewing criteria of his body while in T-shirt and shorts. Assessment and classification of body type is important, especially when customizing a fitness program, for the following reasons. Somatotype analysis helps a fitness trainer discuss how realistic a client's goals and expectations may be in terms of whether or not they complement the client's body type, as well as customize a relevant fitness and nutrition program. In Tom's case, his metabolism and body type composition had an advantage in terms of its ability to burn more body fat than other somatotype combinations based on muscular density.

However, composition alone does not guarantee reduction of overall body fat and cholesterol levels. Other factors, such as genetics, metabolism, and environment, can significantly influence blood test results, regardless of someone in Tom's position putting his or her best foot forward. (See chapter 15, "Antiaging and Physical Performance-Enhancement Truths," and chapter 18, "Customized Fitness Programming.")

Tom was young and thought he could continue his current lifestyle for some time before running into any adverse health conditions. But he also understood and admitted it was the wrong type of thinking. He became very aware that if he didn't change his habits, ultimately, he could morph into an endomorphic body type with increased health risk. His lifestyle change decisions included removal of nonessential fats from his diet and a modification of his exercise routine that complimented his interests and goals.

Since Tom learned that excess cholesterol circulates and stores in the body and comes basically in two prominent densities (HDL and LDL), he had a better understanding of how HDLs in the blood are less involved in plaque formation and are more efficient at removing fats from the body. It is these high-density proteins that attach themselves to fat molecules and remove them from the body as opposed to storing them.

If you eat healthfully and exercise daily and your cholesterol levels remain high, it is wise to seek further follow-up and treatment by a medical specialist. There are people who have genetic predispositions with no family history of high cholesterol counts. When treated accordingly by a medical doctor, cholesterol levels can be controlled.

Although overproduction of cholesterol does not affect everyone, too many people get more than two hundred milligrams of it in their daily diet. In Tom's case, he was getting more than his fair share of carbohydrates and fat calories, which contributed to high blood fat levels and unwanted body weight.

"Elevated triglyceride can be caused by overweight and obesity, physical inactivity, cigarette smoking, excess alcohol consumption and a diet very high in carbohydrates (more than 60 percent of total calories). People with high triglycerides often have a high total cholesterol level, including a high LDL cholesterol (bad) level and a low HDL cholesterol (good) level" (American Heart Association 2014).

Once Tom thoroughly understood the cause and effect of elevated blood fats, he was motivated to modify exercise and food choice. Through these changes, he lost eight pounds in a few months. This decreased his body fat by approximately 3 percent. Although this may not seem like a huge improvement to some, I assure you this was a significant milestone for Tom.

Most importantly, his personal physician no longer recommended medications after comparing his most recent blood fat levels; recall that the recommendation for a medication was what had brought Tom to me in the first place.

Personal Fitness Challenge: "Weight-Loss Fad Half-Truths"

If I wanted to lose the weight while on the mend, I had to change my eating habits. That included removal of unnecessary fat calories and maintaining a balance of food nutrients.

However, it is important to understand, as I explained to both Kate and Tom, that "macronutrients, commonly referred to as 'macros,' are the nutrients that our bodies need in large quantities to provide energy for our physiological systems and to provide the raw structural materials needed for body maintenance. Protein, fat, and carbohydrates are macronutrients" (FitAtMidLife 2018). And balance is key. Macros are essential for health maintenance, growth, reproduction, immunity, and healing. Too little or too many of any macronutrient may compromise these processes, resulting in a variety of poor health outcomes that vary, depending on the life stage and health condition of an individual. My immobility and rehabilitation situation required me to heal as best as possible through balanced nutrient absorption and daily exercise and without further weight gain.

My dietary focus was and still is to eat carbohydrates, protein, and fats in amounts and proportions close to the acceptable macronutrient distribution ranges (AMDR) as discussed in chapter 5. However, I often consume more proteins in relationship to carbohydrates. Nevertheless, I've never restricted simple and complex carbohydrates from my diet.

Many popular rapid weight-loss plans restrict calories or macronutrients or limit food choices. Then the purveyors of these plans advertise half-truths based on science that supports the product, plan, or service. But the other half of the truth—the health risk—is not emphasized.

For example, fad or restrictive diet plans designed without saturated or animal fats sell because they have twice as many calories as carbohydrate- and protein-dense meals. Or high-carbohydrates diets filled with fiber provide a feeling of satiety. Or high-protein diets with little to no carbohydrates cause satiety through the release of a gut hormone.

That's right. Research has discovered that a gut hormone plays a key role in regulating appetite by sending signals to the brain indicating fullness. The hormone, called peptide YY (PYY), is increased via the consumption of high-protein foods. Increasing levels of this hormone reduces hunger and food intake. Researchers in London found that, in both obese and normal weight subjects, a high-protein diet brought about the highest levels of PYY and the greatest reduction in hunger (Perry 2014). But outside of moderation, "In addition to heart disease, studies suggest that eating high amounts of protein can contribute to high cholesterol levels, gout and may put a strain on the kidneys, especially those who suffer from kidney disease" (MyHealthNews Daily 2012).

The truth that needs to be told about rapid weight-loss diets is they restrict balanced nutrients through limited food choices. Also, by design, they cause an unhealthy psychological relationship with food and contribute to sporadic weight changes known as the yo-yo affect. Those are the diets you love to hate because they appear to work at first and then eventually lead to broken metabolisms and obesity.

Gaining knowledge about both unhealthy weight loss and the importance of balance also enables you to learn and understand how fad diets are created and resold under different brands to get repeat sales. People desperate to lose weight don't know the products that failed them in the past are made new again under different brand names and marketing ploys. Then the cycle of unsustainable and unhealthy weight loss and weight gain repeats itself.

In order to make my point, I'm going to take you through the process of creating, marketing, and selling the next popular weight-loss product.

I'll call it the Ultimate Seafood Weight-Loss Diet Plan. I'm the diet product creator, in partnership with a market maker who promotes and sells this new, innovative weight-loss fad. To find likely customers, the market specialist uses consumer shopping habits and sales data, centralized obesity population case statistics, social media and online surveys, and so on to target its audience. Then the market specialist sells the revolutionary diet product to a captured population.

The advertisements used to sell the captured audience include testimonials and pictures of subjects claiming miraculous results—while using the product, some experienced a sixty-pound weight loss within a three- to six-month period. These are the results the target audience identifies with, and that identification motivates them to purchase the product whether the testimonials are true or not.

So I've targeted my audience, selected my results and subjects, and have a marketing plan that includes personal testimonials.

Here's the Ultimate Seafood Weight-Loss Diet Plan I've sold to the marketplace claiming a whopping sixty-pound loss in ninety days with a thirty-day satisfaction guarantee. And to accomplish this only required me to tell half-truths. Learn how a thirty-day guarantee sells products and makes market makers rich, even when the product doesn't work (chapter 4, "Fitness, Diet, and Antiaging Gimmicks Are Profitable.")

My Ultimate Seafood Weight-Loss Diet Plan allows you to choose any three seafood meals per day in various combinations. You simply choose the meals you want and they're dropped off at the doorstep weekly. Very convenient, wouldn't you say? These meals include various fish and shellfish portions and assorted fruits and vegetables, along with whole grain baked goods, noodles, cheese, beans, and rice plus dessert options. And you're allowed to drink as much water, coffee, and tea as you want, plus one four-ounce glass of wine per day. The prepackaged seafood meals are preseasoned in a proprietary blend of Mediterranean spices. Just heat the meals up, and they're ready to serve.

Some of you are thinking, this sounds like my kind of diet plan. I'm all in, especially if I can lose fifteen to twenty pounds per month eating my favorite seafood dishes and consuming wine.

But remember, you can't eat or drink anything else for three months. Or you'll go off the plan. How many of you could actually consume only these food choices for thirty days without cheating? After all, this plan is very limited in choice, is it not?

If you restrict yourself to balanced, healthy whole food choices of certain types during weight loss, isn't this just another restrictive weight-loss plan? Is it sustainable and healthy in the long run? And for those who manage to stay on a like diet for years, what toll could this have on health?

Before answering these questions, let's use another type of prepackaged meal well known to those who've served in the military. These packaged ready-to-eat meals are easily found in the marketplace and prized by food preppers, hunters, and logistic field planners.

They are what I consider limited in taste, smell, and aesthetic appeal and full of preservatives and taste-intensifier chemicals. Weight-loss diet plans like the Ultimate Seafood Weight-Loss Diet Plan have similarities to MREs (Meals, Ready-to-Eat), which are also restrictive food choices.

Want to know why restrictive food choices don't work in the long term? Repeating the regiment of eating the same types of foods daily numbs our senses and excitement about foods in general. The mind and body reject limited food choices, which ultimately causes us to eat less when there is no other choice available. In turn, this causes unhealthy weight loss and starves cellular tissue of needed nutrients.

For example, during military field training exercises, which I know former veterans can relate to, for weeks, soldiers are fed MREs. Each soldier is issued three per day at approximately 1,250 calories each. The meals appear to be fairly nutrient balanced and at first don't taste or smell bad—especially when you add Tabasco, which is in every meal. As I learned later, there's a reason that Tabasco comes with each meal (kind of like the proprietary "special" blend of Mediterranean spices).

Within three days, soldiers, including myself, were eating only one or two food packs out of the MRE daily ration. And by the fifth and sixth day, the main meal, which came in numerous varieties of casserole-like dishes in individual bags, became repulsive, especially if you didn't add the Tabasco. The rest of the side dishes, also wrapped in plastic, were mostly discarded or traded for other preferable foods in the MRE, like coffee, sugar, and powdered creamer—the hyperpalatable stuff. Regardless of the food variety in the MREs, all of them smelled and tasted similar and repulsive after the third to fifth day.

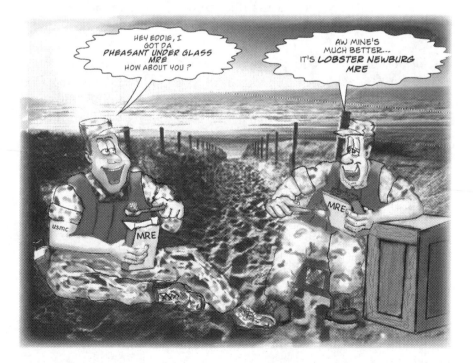

With the thousands of calories burned during field training, you'd think the body would want to consume the whole MRE. But I can tell you from personal experience this was not the case. Those meals that tasted reasonably good at first became repulsive in terms of sight, smell, and taste.

Now about that Tabasco. It was the pungent condiment sauce made from hot peppers that hid the unnatural smell and taste of the main meal. This condiment was actually addictive and made it possible to get calories into the body after the third day. I've often wondered which rocket scientist figured that one out.

Since my mind and body rejected consuming those meals, it was easy to ignore the hunger pains until they eventually went away. A similar situation occurs within any premade diet meal plan—like the blended Mediterranean spices used in my make-believe seafood diet plan. Around day four or five, the spices, like the Tabasco, ultimately become offensive to the senses. In either case, many would be repulsed, throw away food, and lose more weight than originally planned because they don't eat the whole meal. This speaks to that miraculous sixty pounds some lost in three months. This is not healthy weight-loss success.

From a limited food perspective, highly processed meals don't satisfy the mind and body for long. From a weight-loss plan perspective, MREs were considered a success for those in the field who wanted to lose weight. In fourteen days, like many other soldiers, I'd typically lose ten pounds when MREs were the only food source. If I was served the Ultimate Seafood food product in the field, I'm sure the result would not have been much different.

Although these chemically preserved meals caused soldiers to lose weight as a result of disinterest and disgust, there were other contributors to weight loss in the field. For instance, consider the physically intense training stress on the digestive, immune, neurological, and hormone systems, which affect the brain's hunger center and the body's metabolism. After all, military training is definitely not a walk in the park. It is mentally stressful and physically tough.

The point is, even if you choose to go on an MRE diet or choose a diet strategy like the Ultimate Seafood Weight-Loss Diet Plan, there is no guarantee you'll lose weight. For example, a few soldiers in the field were not repulsed by the MREs. They actually liked the meals and ate additional food other soldiers gave them. Similarly, a person on the Ultimate Seafood Plan may cheat by eating out a couple times a week. And since dieters can lose significant weight on restrictive diet plans, they sell. But what most consumers eventually figure out is that, after extreme weight loss follows weight gain. This is the yo-yo dieting habit that is so unhealthy for the body.

I know some of you have had miraculous weight-loss success by cutting protein or carbohydrates or fats from the diet or by severely limiting total daily calories or food choice. Maybe you have done so using a prepackaged weight-loss product and plan.

But keep this in mind: No quick weight-loss product or plan provides unbelievable results for nothing. These programs do not form healthy eating habits and behavior. How does Newton's third law of physics go? "For every action, there's an equal and opposite reaction." This law holds true relative to balance of calorie nutrients the body needs to naturally lose weight safely while supporting good health and long-term well-being.

For those who can tolerate a restrictive diet plan, you may lose weight quickly and sustain that loss for a long period of time. But eventually, this unnatural practice cannot be sustained. Let's put Newton's law into perspective. Using unnatural diet practices with limited food choice repeatedly for too long will affect metabolism and cellular health and increase risk of illness and disease.

Chapter 10

Choose Favorite Foods to Lose Weight

Successful weight loss does not require abstinence from the foods you love.

—MirrorAthlete Principled Fitness and
Healthy Lifestyle Philosophy

Tired of using weight-loss products that don't work and having weight gain increase? If this is the case and you're ready to make changes that can remove stubborn belly, hip, and thigh fat once and for all, it's time to learn about an innovative concept that allows you to eat your favorite foods to lose weight.

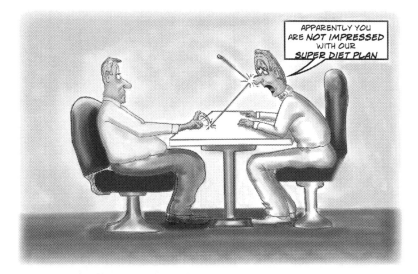

Sharing a favorite food plan to naturally and safely lose weight is revolutionary and powerful information indeed. In this chapter, you'll learn in detail how to create three favorite nutritional meals per day, have fun doing it, and ultimately achieve a sustainable ideal body weight. But the best takeaway is learning how to identify, relate, and create a favorite foods diet plan you'll love to eat while losing that stubborn body fat once and for all.

Throughout the chapter, there are challenging calorie counting and favorite food concepts and interesting ideals. If you need help relating to the following information, refer back to previous client cases and examples. Recall Marvin (chapter 5), Kate (chapter 8), and Tom (chapter 9).

Now you'll learn how MirrorAthlete: Pick a Favorite Healthy Meal Plan can become part of a successful weight-loss strategy that allows you to eat the foods you love and not gain weight. Once you commit to a favorite foods habit, you not only see the excess body fat and weight disappear; you also understand how to keep it off in the long term. And you'll do it without paying hundreds of dollars to achieve the goal. Could natural weight loss really be this simple? The answer is a resounding yes.

I've found anyone can apply MirrorAthlete: Pick a Favorite Healthy Meal Plan to lose weight naturally, improve overall health, and increase fitness levels and well-being. However, there are always a few caveats to any dietary program. For instance, due to food allergies or other medical conditions or ongoing drug treatment you may not consume certain foods. Regardless, this does not restrict one from choosing a plethora of other foods to satisfy the palate.

By applying principles we've learned in previous chapters, here's how I used the favorite food plan to lose weight. Using myself as the subject, I determined I could consume 3,300 calories per day of my favorite foods without gaining weight during my personal fitness challenge. I calculated at this time that I burned 900 of those 3,300 calories performing daily mobility and physical therapy exercise.

To lose weight, I needed to reduce my caloric intake or increase my daily exercise activity. I chose to reduce caloric intake by 300 calories a day. Since I was physically challenged during this time, I was at a mobility disadvantage when it came to losing weight. Since this was the case, I cut back on calories.

I counted food calories and plotted them on a favorite daily meal plan worksheet. After a month of applying a favorite food plan, I had a good feel for how much I could consume without gaining weight. The healthy whole foods I'd enjoyed during childhood were the foods I chose.

If you've experienced and enjoyed healthier eating habits at one time in life, it is easier to reflect back to that time period, relate it to your current situation, and create a favorite foods plan based on those memories. I grew up on a mix of traditional Western and European comfort foods during childhood.

I recall a lot of meat, chicken, fish, cheese, milk, potatoes, corn, squash, other vegetables and fruits, home-baked bread, and casserole and Crock-Pot dishes. The ingredients were purchased from local mom-and-pop stores and farms. We even received our milk and butter at the doorstep delivered by the milkman from the local dairy. We raised chickens and bartered and sold eggs, farmed many of our own fruits and vegetables, and canned and stored them for later use. We also farmed, canned, and sold pumpkins by the ton seasonally to local stores. It was a way families back then provided additional sustenance to the table.

Reflecting on the healthy meals I ate as a child, I was able to relate to those food memories. I knew that, back then, I'd loved fresh foods, and it wouldn't be difficult to find those same options in the local markets.

The goal was to lose thirty pounds in approximately one year. In order to do this, I calculated I could consume 3,300 calories per day without gaining weight. This meant, if I stayed within 3,000 calories each day, I'd be at a 300-calorie deficit daily. At this rate, I calculated my possible weight loss according to the equations we learned earlier:

300 cal loss/day × 7 days = 2,100 cal loss/week

2,100 cal loss/week × 4 weeks = 8,400 net cal loss/month)

8,400 cal loss = 2.4 lb. loss/month (3,500 cal = 1 lb.)

Remain mindful that, for many, including myself, losing weight more quickly than this may not be sufficiently comfortable, healthy, or habit forming to sustain desired weight loss and achieve and retain desired body weight over the long term.

I planned my three main meals at approximately 800 calories (2,400 calories/day). This left around 600 calories (2,400 + 600 = 3,000 cal/day) for other high-nutrient, low-calorie snacks if I got hungry.

I selected some fillers to alleviate hunger between meals when I needed them. These included protein bars and drinks with high fiber, yogurt, peanuts, fruits, and vegetables. I also did not consume any alcoholic beverages during this time.

Examples of my favorite foods were calculated from food labels and nutritional resource indexes and then plotted on the food calories worksheet. Refer to form 10.1 "MirrorAthlete: Pick a Favorite Healthy Meal Plan." The food calories per serving on the worksheet came from two food nutrient and caloric data sources. The first was *Understanding Nutrition*, Whitney and Hamilton, Appendix H, Table of Food Composition (Whitney, Hamilton, and Boyle 1987). Then I cross-referenced many of those numbers with a popular online internet nutrition site (FatSecret 2016). If you have older nutrition books and software, use them. The nutrient and caloric values haven't changed much since they've been available online.

Next I present my favorite food and meal examples broken down by fats, protein, and carbohydrate macronutrient and caloric data. To plot your favorite food macronutrients and calories, copy blank form 10.0 "MirrorAthlete, "Pick a Favorite Healthy Meal Plan" (see appendix).

Since I'm a carnivorous creature by habit, the best food choices for me to focus on were proteins. I selected lean animal products and removed nonessential fats, including visible cholesterol fat from meat dishes.

Although a vegetarian diet is not my cup of tea, I know it is for many. If you'd like to create a vegan favorite foods plan, simply substitute meat and dairy dishes for other high-protein food sources—beans tofu, whole wheat bread, broccoli, brown rice, peanut butter, almonds, cashews, assorted lentils, soy milk, soy yogurt, veggie burgers, or spinach, to name a few.

Measuring food calories also require awareness of by-the-gram weight-to-calorie conversion. Nutrient information is often listed on labels in grams and not always calories. I'll show how I averaged out the daily macronutrient percentages within the AMDR (acceptable macronutrient distribution range) previously covered in chapter 5. Refer often to form 10.1; the following data is plotted on that worksheet example (see appendix).

The favorite foods exercise begins by providing a grams-to-calorie converter at the top of each favorite food (dinner, other meal, or snack) choice listed below. The foods I love to eat are broken down by their macronutrient caloric composition. Later, I'll show you how to build a favorite meal plan using this knowledge to achieve a weight-loss goal naturally.

My Favorite Protein Foods

Macronutrients gram-to-calorie conversions:

> 1 g fat = 9 cal
> 1 g carbohydrate = 4 cal
> 1 g protein = 4 cal

- An 8-oz. 20% lean sirloin (14 g fat = 130 cal + 0 g carbohydrate + 66 g protein = 264 cal) = 394 total calories/serving
- An 8-oz. buffalo sirloin steak (3.5 g fat = 31.5 cal + 0 g carbohydrate + 35 g protein = 140 cal) = 171 total calories/serving
- An 8-oz. Atlantic salmon (24.60 g fat = 221.4 cal + 0g carbohydrate + 45.11 g protein = 180.4 cal) = 402 total calories/serving
- A 4-oz. (1/4-lb.) grounded beef patty 20% lean (20.2 g fat = 181.8 cal + 0g carbohydrate + 29.2 g protein = 116.8 cal) = 299 total calories/serving

Eggs – On average, I eat no more than six whole eggs per week. If high cholesterol is of concern, remove egg yolk and consume egg white. You can also purchase organic, cholesterol-free egg substitutes. One egg has approximately seventy-two calories. Realize that one egg yolk has 171 milligrams of cholesterol, almost your daily requirement of two hundred milligrams daily. If you separate the egg white and toss the yoke from a large egg, then you're down to about seventeen calories per egg without the cholesterol.

Tasty breakfast tip – Egg whites make great low-calorie, high-nutrient veggie omelets.

My Favorite Dinner Dishes

Crock-Pot cooking – I use a Crock-Pot to cook what, in my opinion, is one of the best tasting and most convenient meals to make. Simply combine any meat, poultry, or fish with any combination of rice, noodles, potato, beans, or vegetable in a Crock-Pot. Season to taste. Add one pint of water and let it stew for six to eight hours on low heat while at work. Then dinner's ready to serve when you get home. Let the meal cool to skim the fat off the top of the liquid surface, reheat, and serve. You can also snack on these leftovers to curb your appetite throughout the week. Once you get into the Crock-Pot habit, you'll never stop because the meals you can prepare taste so good and literally take minutes to prepare after cooked.

Pick up a Crock-Pot recipe book to see all the great meal possibilities. One of my favorite Crock-Pot dishes is a slow-cooked roast with cabbage, onion, mushrooms, carrots, and potatoes, along with two tablespoons of virgin olive oil and seasoned to taste.

Casseroles are another favorite. These dishes are similar to Crock-Pot food recipes but take a little longer to prepare. They have nearly the same calories per serving cup. Combine potatoes, rice, noodles, and assorted vegetable or cheese mixes with chicken, tuna, and eggplant. Casseroles range from 200 to 350 calories per cup serving.

Beef stew with potatoes, carrots, broccoli, and greens in a tomato-based sauce gives you approximately 200 calories per cup (FitDay 2015).

My Favorite Dairy Foods

Macronutrients gram-to-calorie conversions:

1 g fat = 9 cal
1 g carbohydrate = 4 cal
1 g protein = 4 cal

- A cup of 1% milk (2.37 g fat + 12.18 g carbohydrates + 8.22 g protein) = 103 total calories/serving
- A cup of plain yogurt (3.5 g fat + 16 g carbohydrates + 11.9 g protein) = 143 total calories/serving

- A slice of American cheese (7.39 g fat + 1.97 g carbohydrates + 5.37 g protein) = 96 calories/serving
- A cup of small curd cottage cheese (10.15 g fat + 6.03 g carbohydrate + 28.1 g protein) = 228 calories/serving

I consume low-fat yogurt, low-fat milk (1%), or low-fat buttermilk or condensed/dry nonfat milk for casserole recipes. I prefer low-fat cottage cheese or cheese labeled with no more than 5 to 7 grams of fat per ounce over high-fat cheeses, such as cream cheese or processed cheeses, as well as cheddar, brie, Swiss, blue, and American cheese. If casserole recipes call for soups, it is okay to *infrequently* cook with cream soups made with nonfat or 1% milk.

My Favorite Carbohydrate and Protein Mixed Foods

Macronutrients gram-to-calorie conversions:

1 g fat = 9 cal
1 g carbohydrate = 4 cal
1 g protein = 4 cal

- A slice of multigrain wheat bread (1 g fat + 12 g carbohydrates + 2.6 g protein) = 67 total calories/serving
- A cup of granola-type cereal (29.72 g fat + 65.6 g carbohydrates + 18.14 g protein) = 602 calories/serving
- A cup of raisin bran (1.56 g fat + 42.74 g carbohydrates + 4.87 g protein) = 204 calories/serving
- A cup of grounded beef chili (14.2 g fat + 19.68 g carbohydrates + 13.46 g protein) = 260 calories/serving

Although I consider chili more or less a balanced macronutrient meal, if beef is left out of the chili mix, the macronutrient values change caloric value. For instance, many popular chili bean brands (without beef for the vegetarian) have macronutrient values per cup in the rage of 10 grams fat, 13.9 grams carbohydrates, and 17.4 grams protein.

I also enjoy whole multigrain wheat bread, which is far healthier than white bread. I don't recommend white bread at all because of the added sugar and additional chemical process it goes through. Pumpernickel, rye, English muffins, and rice crackers are good healthy choices. Plain pastas and rice (white, brown, or wild) prepared with low-fat cream, butter, or cheese sauces re okay. Beans, split and black-eyed peas, kidney beans, navy beans, black garbanzos, lentils, soybeans, vegetarian refried beans, and tofu are all good choices. Choose granola and raisin-bran-type cereals. Hot cereals and most dried fibrous cold cereals are also healthy complex carbohydrate food choices.

Yes, pizza is one of my favorite foods. I enjoy it weekly. I love pepperoni with a good tomato sauce, topped with cheese, green peppers, onions, and mushrooms. Order or make a fourteen-inch regular crust. One slice (10 g fat + 36 g carbohydrates + 12 g protein) = 288 calories. That means three slices contain 864 calories.

My Favorite High-Fiber Carbohydrate Fillers

Macronutrients gram-to-calorie conversions:

1 g fat = 9 cal
1 g carbohydrate = 4 cal
1 g protein = 4 cal

- A cup of mixed vegetables (corn, lima beans, peas, green beans and carrots) (.27 g fat + 23.82 g carbohydrates + 5.2g protein) = 118 calories/serving *(8 g fiber*/serving) (Certain vegetables provide higher dietary fiber concentration. Find food fiber per serving values online and within book nutrition table listings.)
- A medium-size apple of any type (.24 g fat + 19.06 g carbohydrates + .36 g protein) = ~80 calories/serving (3.3 g fiber/serving)
- A cup of brown rice (1.74 g fat + 44.42 g carbohydrates + 4.99 g protein) = 213 calories/serving (3.5 g fiber/serving)
- A large potato with skin (.37 g fat + 57.97 g carbohydrates + 6.2 g protein) = 260 calories/serving (8.9 g fiber/serving) (Most of the nutrients and fiber are in the potato skin.)

My Favorite Snacks

Macronutrients gram-to-calorie conversions:

1 g fat = 9 cal
1 g carbohydrate = 4 cal
1 g protein = 4 cal

- Tasty popcorn, popped at highest range temps in 50 percent olive oil and 50 percent butter (the fats don't burn this way), lightly salted (5.27 g fat + 7.27 g carbohydrates + .96 g protein) = ~80 calories/cup serving
- Pretzels (1.18 g fat + 35.89 g carbohydrates + 4.65 g protein) = 173 calories/cup serving
- One tablespoon of butter (11.52 g fat + .01 g carbohydrates + .12 g protein) = 104 calories/tbsp serving; on toasted wheat bread (67 calories/wheat bread slice + 104 calories/tbsp butter) = 171 calories
- Sherbet (3.86 g fat + 58.67 g carbohydrate + 2.12 g protein) = 278 calories/cup serving

Other favorite sweets and snacks – Granola bars, frozen desserts, juice bars, Popsicles, fig bars, gingersnaps, Jell-O, fresh fruit, and honey are all good sweet treats. Angel food cake, homemade cookies, and pies are fine in moderation. Avoid cooking or purchasing baked goods that use vegetable oils labeled "partially hydrogenated" and/or that claim to have "0 trans fat."

Other healthy low-fat baked snack choices include saltine crackers, breadsticks, pretzels, graham crackers, RyKrisp, matzo, melba toast, and corn tortillas. Be sure to pay attention to nutrient listings on baked snacks. Some of these foods are healthier than others.

Fresh fruits and vegetables are all good sources of complex carbohydrates, fiber, and essential nutrients. Fresh fruits, vegetables, and juice concentrates (as long as you choose those with fewer sugar additives) are also options that are low in cholesterol and high in dietary fiber. Be careful to avoid overconsumption of olives and avocados. Both have a high vegetable fat content, so use them sparingly when balancing daily caloric intake.

My Favorite Fats

If you use cooking oil, you likely prefer one or more of the following most popular cooking oils found in households to sauté and fry foods—corn, sunflower, soybean, cottonseed, safflower, sesame, canola, olive, and peanut oil.

However, vegetable oils must be used sparingly. One tablespoon (1 oz.) averages out to 120 calories per serving. However, when I cook certain foods—eggs over easy, for example—that don't absorb the oil, I count half of the cooking oil calories. However, if I mix the oil into a recipe, I count all the calories. "Olive oil is widely known to be high in monounsaturated (good) fat. It contains zero trans (bad) fats and is lower in saturated (bad) fat than other commonly used ingredients such as shortening and butter" (SALOV 2016).

Use monounsaturated and polyunsaturated vegetable oils to cook with instead of butter, lard, or shortening if cholesterol is a health concern.

If you cook with oils, you also need to learn about *smoke point* and how cooking temperatures can denaturize (destroy) the healthy nutrients in them (see chapter 11, "The Impact of Cooking Oils on Health"). After reading chapter 11, you'll understand why I personally prefer animal fats and monounsaturated virgin olive oil as my cooking fats of choice.

My Favorite Daily Meals

Next I provide examples of my favorite meals from the favorite foods previously listed. Keep in mind, the following meal examples represent a small sampling of meal varieties I created and consumed during a period of time when my goal was to lose weight.

Although 800 calories per meal was the objective, think of your daily calorie intake as a target you strive to achieve rather than a rigid rule set in stone. Sometimes calorie intake will be over or under your calculated estimates. The goal is to average out close to your daily caloric needs.

Favorite Breakfasts

1. Two cups of raisin bran (408 cal) and two cups of 1% milk (206 cal) = 614 calories
2. Two eggs (soft boiled or over easy) (144 cal), two slices of multigrain bread (134 cal), and two slices of American cheese (192 cal), plus whole banana (105 cal) and fruit yogurt (180 cal) = 755 calories
3. One cup of granola (602 cal), one cup of 1% milk (103 cal), and one apple (80 cal) = 785 calories

(Note that, with these three breakfast options, macronutrient intake averages around 17 percent fats, 62 percent carbohydrates, and 21 percent proteins.)

Some mornings, I'd make two pieces of toast with butter or only peanut butter or have a bowl of oatmeal with raisins added and then add more calories later between meals if needed. The point is to put balanced nutrients into your body at least three times a day. Otherwise, it will be hard to resist overeating at the next meal, especially if you skip one.

Before and after breakfast, I love to drink coffee. Both coffee and tea alone have literally no calories (2 cal/cup), and water has no calories. I drink as much coffee and tea as I like without creamer or sugar added. Coffee and tea are also great antioxidants. But for those who are caffeine intolerant try drinking noncaffeinated low-calorie drinks and receive the flavor and antioxidant benefits.

Favorite Lunches

1. Quarter-pound hamburger, 20% lean hamburger on two slices of wheat bread with all the veggies and condiments (540 cal), one slice of American cheese (96 cal), one cup of low-calorie yogurt (150 cal) = 786 calories
2. Two cups of Crock-Pot or casserole comfort food (~600 cal), two medium-size apples (160 cal) = 760 calories

3. Two cups of small curd cottage cheese (456 cal), one cup of fruit cocktail (drain syrup) (150 cal), one cup of pretzels (173 cal) = 779 calories

Each of the three lunch option macronutrient averages are 16 percent fats, 46 percent carbohydrates, and 38 percent proteins.)

Favorite Dinners

1. A large potato (260 cal) with 1 tbsp of butter (104 cal) and two cups of chili (on top of potato) (520 cal) = 884 calories
2. A large potato (260 cal) with 1 tbsp of butter (104 cal) and two cups of mixed vegetables (on top of potato and seasoned to taste) (226 cal) = 590 calories
3. An 8-oz. 20% lean sirloin (394 cal), a large baked potato (260 cal) with 2 tbsp of sour cream (62 cal), and two cups of broccoli seasoned to taste (on top of potato) (60 cal) = 776 calories

(For each of the three dinner options, options averages are 15.5 percent fats, 57 percent carbohydrates, and 27 percent protein.)

The macronutrient averages when factoring in all nine meal choices listed above are 16 percent fats, 55 percent carbohydrates, and 28.6 percent protein. (See "Macronutrient Calorie Intake Balance per AMDR" in chapter 5: Adults [19 years and older] Fats 20–35%, Carbohydrates, 45–65%, Proteins 10–35%.)

I plotted a favorite meals plan for one day on form 10.1. Now you know how you can create more. I created twenty-one favorite meals from which I randomly selected three daily.

Once you make three meals a day for one week using form 10.1, you'll have created a system that makes meal selection interesting and fun. Fold the form in half, put it into a box, and pick one for the next day's meal plan. Then put it back in the box for the next day or for weekly meal plan drawing.

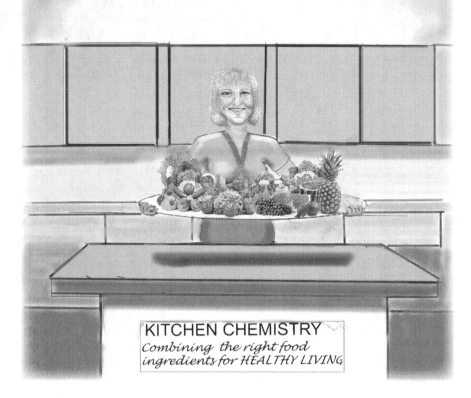

KITCHEN CHEMISTRY
*Combining the right food
ingredients for HEALTHY LIVING*

This process takes the decision-making out of what the next day's favorite meal will be and allows you to shop and prep for them in advance. It's a fun way to stay on a balanced favorite foods course while losing weight and developing healthier eating habits.

I had more than one box to pick from. I had three—a favorite breakfast, lunch, and dinner box to draw from. This was my daily way to pick a favorite healthy meal. I randomly selected three separate meals daily. Then I threw them back into the boxes and repeated the practice the next day.

As illustrated on form 10.1 under calorie analysis (see forms section at the back of the book), I calculated that I could consume 521 more calories on January 1 or accept the additional calorie deficit. When I had a calorie deficit, I often ate various fruits, vegetables, and other snacks throughout the day or evening before 8:00 p.m.

The secret to painless weight loss is to identify and plan to choose favorite natural whole foods that are high in nutrient and volume density and also provide satiety and energy needed during a weight-loss period. Healthy weight loss and sustaining it in the long term is not about restricting yourself from the foods you love. Instead, it's just the opposite. Feeding the brain and body what it needs and then sustaining those healthy habits will create change that lasts long term.

Personal Fitness Challenge: "Healthy Weight Loss Requires Habit Change"

Losing weight safely isn't just about understanding how to calculate daily calories. Nor is it an issue that can be resolved by some quick fix. It isn't that easy, or so many people wouldn't be struggling with obesity. Until unhealthy habits change, sustaining healthy weight loss will not occur—especially when you can't see beyond an attractive package or resist the temptation to eat hyperpalatable, addictive foods.

I'm not going to tell you balancing a healthy diet plan is simple. It does require a bit of willpower and discipline initially to change food choice habits and shopping behavior. But if you're able-bodied and have no medical or health issues, it is reasonable to predict a one- to two-pound weight loss per week applying a favorite whole foods plan while performing low-impact exercise for at least thirty to forty-five minutes daily.

During my personal weight-loss challenge, I knew if I stayed the course I could lose approximately 28.8 pounds in one year. Since I had long periods of pain management incidents after surgeries, followed up by physical therapy, I knew this goal would be challenging.

It actually took me longer to lose weight because of my inability to stay consistent with aerobic exercise due to pain. But at least I was losing and not gaining weight throughout the duration. The favorite foods plan provided a feeling of control and hope that I'd eventually lose the weight I wanted. Outside of favorite food selections, I found other ways to reduce calories, and it didn't take a lot of effort.

For instance, I found creative ways to remove unessential fatty cholesterol from meat dishes. I began the practice of removing extra cholesterol fat calories before and after cooking. You've noticed that, when meat cools, you see the wax-like hardened fat substance coagulated around it. Or if you cook a pot of meat, after the broth cools, the fat floats on top. This is easily seen and can be skimmed off (extracted from) any meat dish with a spoon. It is also easy to separate the skin from chicken and turkey or trim it off before you cook it. Separation of fat in this way will not remove all the cholesterol fat calories but will make the meat very "fat lean," with little cholesterol.

When I chose to make burgers or casserole dishes with ground beef, I'd select products with 15 to 20 percent fat content. However, if ground beef is above 20 percent fat, tilt the pan at an angle just after cooking, leaving the bottom of the pan clear to gather fat juices. Then spoon out the liquid fat before adding meat to the casserole or whatever dish you're creating. Or put the cooked ground beef or meat in a strainer to separate and drain the fat into a disposable container while it's hot. Or let the dish cool and separate the "waxy" fat later.

Other than hamburger dishes, I chose lean cuts of pork tenderloin, steak, poultry, and fish to diversify my protein dishes. Good sources of low cholesterol and saturated fats rich in omega-3s include tuna, cod, salmon, and scallops. Wild game such as elk and deer are very fat lean and sources of high protein. Also, buffalo and emu meat have come back to the marketplace in a big way and are fat lean, very tasty, and satisfying. Ask your local butcher about specialty meat orders.

Prepackaged and unhealthy fatty sauce mixes – Be mindful of butter, cheese, cream, whole milk, or rich sauces to bake and enhance food flavors. Use these sparingly. Many of them are processed with high saturated fat and/or partially hydrogenated trans fats that equate to unnecessary and unhealthy calories and cholesterol. Try balancing your diet by adding in more complex carbohydrates with 50 percent less of your favorite sauce mix. When you start discovering your own brand of favorite organic spice mixes, you'll crave them over hyperpalatable food chemicals.

Beverages – Stay away from carbonated drinks with artificial sweeteners. Avoid high-fat drinks such as milkshakes, 2% and above milk, heavy creamers, and eggnog. I still drink soda once in a while. But I drink only those I know are sweetened with cane sugar. Since sugar sodas are high in calories, I drink very few of them. I'll also drink a glass of red wine here and there. Not only is this healthy in moderation, but it also really brings out the taste in Mediterranean-style meals.

There is only one type of alcoholic beverage science has documented having a health benefit when moderately consumed. Red wine is the healthy alcohol beverage when you consume *no more than* one to two five- to eight-ounce glasses in a day. I know this is good news for wine lovers.

Here's what we do know about drinking red wine in moderation. The resveratrol found in the red grape skin, seed, and vine has been shown to increase HDL and lower cholesterol. Plus, it has antioxidant benefits, minimizes blood clot risks, lowers blood pressure, and reduces stress, while assisting digestion and preventing plaque from forming on the artery walls. Keep in mind, wine does have calories and preservatives in varying quantities and can have a negative impact on the way you feel and your overall health.

Caloric tip – A five-ounce glass of wine has around 85 to 125 calories in it.

Guidelines on Restaurant Foods

Fast food places should be avoided or infrequently visited. This is especially true for those whose body weight or high cholesterol and/ or triglycerides in blood tests reveal an increased health risk and those who have dietary restrictions.

However, if you choose to eat out, salads; broiled or grilled meat; fish, seafood, or chicken; vegetables and fruits; and sandwiches and hamburgers light on mayonnaise are okay in moderation. Avoid foods (including vegetables) that are fried and breaded and french fries. Also avoid fast food breakfast or grilled meat sandwiches and ordering "super" or "extra" anything, including fattening processed drinks to wash down the meal.

A rule of thumb I apply even to this day—never eat out more than once a week and never choose all-you-can-eat food bars and buffets. If you go out with family or friends, choose a restaurant you know prepares healthy, wholesome foods. Ask your waiter or waitress for the healthy choice menu.

Also retain this tidbit of information—when ordering, ask if the dish is prepared fresh by the chief. What you're asking is whether the whole foods were purchased fresh in the local marketplace and not processed and/or frozen and then microwaved or heated up on the stove. When foods are packaged and received from a storage warehouse, assume those foods and drinks are likely processed with hyperpalatable preservatives and additives. Many processed and preserved foods are high in sodium, fats, and sugars and chemically engineered.

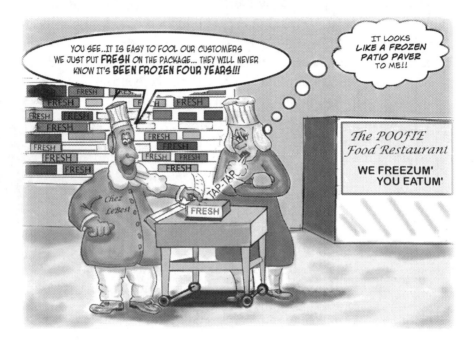

Today I'm no longer in a rehabilitative and severe pain management state. My physical activity levels allow me to add another 1,200 food calories per day without gaining weight. And believe me, that's a lot of good comfort food. I haven't had the need to calculate calories for years. Once you start eating healthy and exercising daily, there is really no need to worry about counting calories. The body will adjust and self-regulate at an efficient metabolic rate to sustain desired body weight and fitness levels.

Chapter 11

The Impact of Cooking Oils on Health

> Select cooking fats benefit weight loss, health, and fitness goals.
>
> —MirrorAthlete Principled Fitness and
> Healthy Lifestyle Philosophy

Vegetable oils are typically considered a healthy food source and are commonly used in baking, sautéing, or frying foods. By the end of this chapter, you'll understand how consuming a balance of various and select dietary fats can support weight-loss, fitness, and health goals.

One very popular and healthy cooking oil used today with a long nurturing lineage is olive oil. Olive oil's benefits have been inherently known by Mediterranean cultures long before science could study and prove that distinction. Our European ancestors understood olive oil as a healthy food source and, in addition, applied it to the body in ceremonial practices. The traditions around farming and production of this food for trade have bound people socially, economically, and culturally over thousands of years.

From the rustic villas of Roman times to present day, olive oil has been used and traded as a fuel source for light and heat; for medical and cosmetic purposes; and, of course, for its high nutritional value. It's long been used for seasoning and cooking traditional Mediterranean foods.

Today, modern science confirms what Mediterranean people knew long ago. "Medical studies have demonstrated that olive oil is very effective in preventing various diseases including diabetes, obesity, cancer, and aging. Furthermore, the collected data show that olive oil has excellent therapeutic qualities in the prevention of cardiovascular diseases, because it reduces cholesterol in the blood, decreases the risk of thrombosis and, consequently, the risk of a heart attack" (Macine Del Trasimeno 2017).

Five thousand years ago, the Greek island of Crete began production of olive oil. That heritage and ancient vineyard stock was passed on and took root in California's orchards. The state is a major producer of Tuscan oil products with centuries-old ratios of Frantoio, Leccino, Pendolino, and Maurino olives providing consumers high-quality virgin olive oil. Aside from cooking oil, olive oil is used in a number of other products, including soaps, cosmetics, and skin moisturizer and highly prized for its high omega-9 oleic acid content.

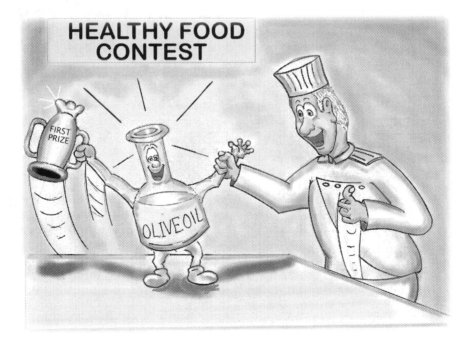

Throughout Europe's southern region, cooking traditional meals with olive oil is "the most emblematic food of the Mediterranean culture" (Botanical-Online 2016). If you were born in this region or into a Mediterranean heritage or similar culture, olive oil is likely a food staple.

The benefits of oleic acid were put on the map when it was famously used as the principle ingredient in *Lorenzo's Oil*. In 1992, this movie told a true story about the powerful health properties of oleic acid. It was developed for young boys who came down with adrenoleukodystrophy (ALD), a disease similar to MS (multiple sclerosis). ALD is a disease where the myelin sheath (electrical conductor insulators in the nerve cells of the brain) becomes compromised.

High concentrations of oleic acid, along with other omegas and vitamin E are found not only in olive oil but also in other types of oils, including grape seed, canola, sesame, poppy seed, and peanut oil. This fatty acid is said to boost memory and reduce blood pressure, to name a few healthy attributes. "For millions of people with diagnosed diabetes and pre-diabetes, consuming foods rich in oleic acid may be beneficial in controlling the disease" (Richardson 2015).

Monounsaturated fatty oils with oleic acid are found in animal products, fruits, and vegetables. Oleic acid (omega-9) is a pale yellow, oily liquid with a lard-like odor. Monounsaturated fats have great natural preservation and storage properties and are less susceptible to spoilage.

Hydrogenated vegetable oils (polyunsaturated fatty acids), on the other hand, "are considered damaged if at any stage in the manufacturing or transport and handling or use the oil has been exposed to excessive oxygen or heat. The same goes for nuts or seeds with a high PUFA content, although they are slightly more self-protected than naked oils" (Fairchild 2012).

Mindfulness of cooking oil type, quality, storage, and handling is important to understand for health-conscious consumers. Why? Understanding these things can reduce health risk.

For instance, quality PUFA oils appear to lower cholesterol but also appear to lower HDLs (the good fat), as seen in a recent study. "As expected, the results of subjects on the PUFA diet showed 9.4% lower concentrations of *total cholesterol*" (Kralova Lesna et al. 2008). This is an important study and consumer consideration when high cholesterol may be problematic. However, the study also shows that too many PUFAs in the diet lower both HDLs and LDLs simultaneously and, therefore, causes a counter health benefit effect.

Therefore, a balance of PUFAs in the diet would be prudent to sustain the healthy nutrient balance and benefits. Now to further identify, define, and relate to cooking oil, it's necessary to cover manufacturer process, oil type, and healthy nutrient differences and sensitivities during handling and storage.

It is beneficial to know that "the best oils are cold-pressed. The oil is obtained through pressing and grinding fruit or seeds with the use of heavy granite millstones or modern stainless steel presses, which are found in large commercial operations. Although pressing and grinding produces heat through friction, the temperature must not rise above 120°F (49°C) for any oil to be considered cold-pressed" (The George Mateljan Foundation 2016).

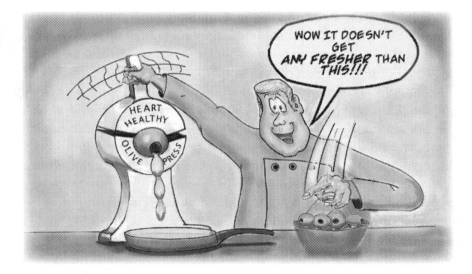

Pressed vegetable and fruit oil temperatures are an important part of the manufacturer process, why? Because when overheating any oil—most specifically polyunsaturated fats—the oil properties change in ways that are unhealthy.

"Nutrition scientists, biochemistry professors and oncologists agreed that excess heating of vegetable oils and multiple use release carcinogens and long exposure to these elements may cause cancer" (Deccan Chronicle 2017). It is especially bad when PUFA omega-3s are overheated. High concentrations of alpha-linolenic acid (essential omega-3 fatty acid), if overheated, can lead to the formation of carcinogens and mutagens. "Avoid food cooked in any oil over 15 percent PUFA content: soy, canola, perilla, safflower, sunflower, corn, walnut oil, rice bran oil, and peanut oil … Canola oil is about 21%

linoleic acid, and 7–10% alpha-linolenic acid; and alpha-linolenic acid is an omega-3 PUFA which should *never* be heated" (Fairchild 2012).

To help you understand healthy cooking oils, I've included "Cooking Fats and Smoke Point (SP) Data" (see appendix). This will help in comparing and choosing the healthiest fats for meals.

Looking at the data makes it clear why butter and virgin olive oil are some of the healthiest cooking fats. I feel comfortable in making this statement based on the high concentration of MUFAs and low to mid PUFAs, decent omega-6:omega-3 ratio balances, and of course taste and smell preferences. If you choose to use other cooking fats and want to minimize dietary fat health risk, refer to "Cooking Fats and Smoke Point (SP) Data" to help make a healthier fat food choice.

Analyzing the table data will enable you to more easily understand how Americans have an omega-6, fried fatty foods habit. "Most experts agree that the omega 6 and 3 ratios should range from 1:1 to 5:1. The sad reality is that it now ranges from 20 to 50:1 for most Americans. They are getting too many omega-6 fats" (Mercola 2012). I'd bet you can guess what foods those might be. Just consider the fried foods ordered in restaurants or fast food places and the processed foods available in local stores.

Why is a proper dietary balance of essential omega-3s and omega-6s so important? "The results of cell culture and animal studies indicate that omega-6 and omega-3 fatty acids can modulate the expression of a number of genes, including those involved with fatty acid metabolism and inflammation" (Linus Pauling Institute 2016). If our gene modulation can express itself in a healthy way through balanced diet, it can also express itself in an unhealthy way.

This does not mean you should stay away from omega-6 fatty acid oils. Omega-6 is essential to the diet and beneficial for overall health. However, since the fatty acid is abundant in the average diet, deficiency is rare. And consuming too much of this fatty acid is known to lead to health problems like arthritis, heart disease, and even cancer.

On the flip side, experts proclaim you can't overconsume omega-3s. Omega-3s have a powerful anti-inflammatory capability and appear to be the counterpunch to alleviate inflammatory discomfort caused by overconsumption of omega-6s. Omega-3s can alleviate other symptoms of illness and disease such as bowel disorders, heart disease, arthritis, asthma, high blood pressure, psoriasis and even lower triglycerides.

Deficiencies of omega-3s are also "linked to decreased memory and mental abilities, tingling sensation of the nerves, poor vision, increased tendency to form blood clots, diminished immune function, increased triglycerides and 'bad' cholesterol (LDL) levels, impaired membrane function, hypertension, irregular heartbeat, learning disorders, menopausal discomfort, itchiness on the front of the lower leg(s), and growth retardation in infants, children, and pregnant women" (Rotella 2006).

Aside from omega-3 deficiencies, lacking a balance of both essential fatty acids may lead to other medical problems, including impaired visual and neurological development (preterm infants), depression, diabetes, stroke, sudden cardiac death, bipolar disorder and schizophrenia, and Alzheimer's disease and dementia, to name a few.

To reduce risk of oxidative inflammatory stress on cellular integrity and to feel better while losing more weight, consider limiting the following cooking oils—palm, corn, cottonseed, soy bean, safflower, sunflower, and others with unhealthy nutrient ratios.

This recommendation is specific to select oil types that contain a high PUFA percentage with unstable omega-6:omega-3 ratios that easily spoil through lipid peroxidation. "Lipid peroxides are unstable markers of oxidative stress which decompose to form complex, reactive by-products" (Cell Biolabs 2016). Lipid peroxidation "most often affects polyunsaturated fatty acids, because they contain multiple double bonds in between which lie methylene bridges (-CH$_2$-) that possess especially reactive hydrogen atoms" (Wikipedia n.d.).

This peroxidation effect through oxidative stress is caused through improper handling and storage and exposure to high temperatures during the manufacturing process. Consuming spoiled or rancid oil products means they are metabolized, and cellular tissues absorb them, further increasing the rate of oxidative molecular harm within the body. This subject is fully covered in chapter 14, "Processed vs. Organic Food." Dr. Andrew Weil agrees that testing for rancidity or spoilage is an important quality assurance process that should be conducted prior to oil being sold to the public.

The oil industries know how to test for rancidity. "If we suspect that the oil could be close to this stage other complementary analysis such as UV absorption are recommended. Based on international rules IOC [International Olive Council] Codex, extra virgin olive oils must show a peroxides value under 20. Nonetheless, it is expected that fresh and well processed oils should show peroxides value less than 12" (Australian Olive Association 2016). In his book *8 Weeks to Optimum Health*, Dr. Andrew Weil says, "Rancid oil can also cause damage to DNA, accelerate aging, promote tissue degeneration and foster cancer development" (Weil 2007).

Oil blends used in restaurants and fast food places present other challenges for health-conscientious consumers. You now know it's not easy to compare healthy fry oils in general. Now imagine a health-conscious consumer trying to wrap his or her head around fry oil blends and proper cook temperatures. This is where fry oil type, temperatures, and nutrient quality knowledge is valuable for those who want to lose weight and stay healthy.

As illustrated, knowledge about omega-3 and omega-6 ratios is valuable to health-conscientious consumers, especially when choosing foods that have been fried.

Case in point, I've observed through time contradictions between popular hamburger chains where, in past promotional statements, the chain has first said they used corn oil and then said it's no longer in the blend. The fact that they switched to canola oil—rich in omega-3—is a good thing. The fact that they blend it with hydrogenated soybean oil is very bad. Similarly, another popular hamburger chain at one point was even sparser in its omega-6 disclosure. The point here is that you have to read labels and ask about oil blends. What is an establishment using to fry its foods?

Refer to "Cooking Fats and Smoke Point (SP) Data" (see appendix) and then compare the fatty acids in canola, palm, and soy oil to understand why the latter two are unhealthy in comparison. Hint—compare the MUFA and PUFA percentages.

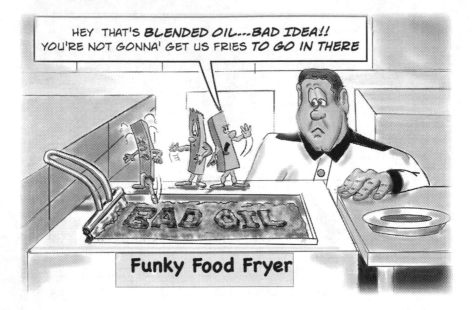

Dietary fats are always an interesting topic during consults because there are so many misunderstandings about them in general. However it becomes easier to choose a product once you understand the nutrient property and conditional differences.

To help better understand those differences, I'm offering the following tidbits of cooking fats insight from the experts and will summarize those recommendations to help you make wise cooking fat choices. "Ideally, choose oils that have a PUFA content of 10% or less for cooking. The higher the PUFA content of an oil, the more delicate it is, and the more carefully it should be handled. This means it needs to be kept airtight and refrigerated" (Fairchild and Noland 2012). If you haven't noticed within "Cooking Fats and Smoke Point (SP) Data," corn oil has a 46.1:1 omega-6:omega-3 ratio. In other words, its PUFA content far exceeds the suggested 10 percent value. This is a major reason I don't use corn and soybean oil if at all possible.

If you choose to forgo cooking oils or use them infrequently and prefer to eat foods high in essential omega-3, the following foods are high in alpha-linolenic acid—walnuts and Brazil nuts; sesame, flax, hemp, pumpkin, and mustard seeds; avocados; fish; leafy green vegetables (mustard greens, Spanish, kale, collards, and purslane); grains; and spirulina.

"Oily fish, such as salmon, mackerel and sardines, contain two types of omega-3 fats—DHA and EPA—that have been shown to reduce blood fats called triglycerides and possibly prevent dangerous heart-rhythm disturbances. Because of this, the American Heart Association recommends that adults eat fatty fish twice a week, and that people with heart disease consider taking fish oil pills to get extra DHA and EPA" (Ndri.com 2016). "There are different types of omega-3 however. Alpha-linolenic acid (ALA) is found in plant sources and eicosapentaenoic acid (EPA) and docosahexaenoic acid (DHA) are found in marine sources. EPA and DHA have shown the most cardio-protective effects" (Harris 2014).

Native Americans historically used seed oil high in gamma-linolenic acid (GLA) from the herbal plant *evening primrose* to treat internal body swelling. Today, evening primrose oil (EPO)—"which is obtained from the plant's seeds via cold expression or solvent extraction—is better known for its ability to reduce inflammation in a variety of systemic conditions" (Christensen 2010).

Omega-9 was lightly touched on because it is a nonessential fatty acid, meaning the body can synthesis it from other foods in the diet. But to shed a little more light, "Monounsaturated fatty acids (MUFA), also known as omega-9 fatty acids, offer a functionally stable alternative to these 'bad' fats and provide valuable health benefits protecting against metabolic syndrome and cardiovascular disease" (DOW AgroSciences n.d.).

Dietary fat manufacturers and food industries have acknowledged the connection between health risk and unhealthy dietary fats. Consumer awareness and demand of healthier food choice has also risen as a result of consumer safety advocates and dietary watchdogs holding the industry and manufacturers accountable for unhealthy food products that cause increased health risk. And for these reasons, those industries have been promoting and offering healthier cooking fat choices within the marketplace. For example, "Omega-9 canola oil, a high MUFA oil, has replaced more than 1.5 billion pounds of trans and saturated fat from the North American food supply since 2005" (DOW AgroSciences n.d.).

Although canola oil is a healthier choice than other cooking oils, remain mindful that consuming too many highly concentrated and overheated PUFAs can increase health risk (refer to "Cooking Fats and

Smoke Point (SP) Data" (see appendix). Note that approximately 33 percent of PUFAs are found in canola oil.

A diet high in MUFAs, as opposed to one with SFAs and unhealthy PUFA ratios, can reduce health risk as well as body fat weight. If you need to watch your cholesterol, cooking oils high in MUFAs and balanced omegas may be a healthier choice than saturated animal fats.

However, if your blood cholesterol and body weight are within normal ranges, you may consider other healthy dietary fats. Ghee, certified organic butter made from grass-fed and ethically raised cows, is one such option. My take on butter versus margarine—any organic butter is healthier than margarines and tastes better on toast, baked potatoes, and vegetables. Ghee, unlike other butters, also fries great at high temps without splatter. Or try using free-range lard as an option to unnatural and overly processed vegetable shortening and fry oils.

Personal Fitness Challenge: "Fried Foods Moderation"

Prior to injury, I mostly used margarine and vegetable oil for baking, corn or canola oil for frying, and olive oil for sautéing. Almost everyone we knew fried foods with corn, soy, and canola oil.

Before I was injured, I really never put too much thought into dietary fats, especially fry oils. I more or less consumed them in moderation, understanding that including too many fats in the diet was not healthy.

I also didn't put any thought into genetically modified and engineered food crops used to produce fry oils. Had I at the time, I would've been alarmed to learn how much of our food source—including fry oils came from genetically modified crop seeds. If you're not aware already, you need to know that a large percentage of cooking oils in the marketplace are produced from these genetically modified food crops.

It is known that approximately, "93 percent of soybeans and 90 percent of corn grown in the U.S. are genetically engineered, and sugar beets (95 percent of which are genetically engineered) account for 55 percent of U.S.-grown sugar. Soybean oil, canola oil, cottonseed oil and corn oil made in the U.S. come from crops that are almost entirely genetically engineered" (Deike 2014). Knowing this is another reason to choose cooking oils wisely and use them in moderation. More details on genetically engineered and modified food crops can be found in chapter 14, "Processed vs. Organic Food."

My past and present saving grace with regard to fatty foods is that I always ate them in moderation. But I'm also aware of the foods I love to eat and have a tough time stopping once I get started. Those foods are french fries and tater tots. I have to admit, like many of you, I have a weakness for any type of fried spud. They're so good. Unfortunately most places you purchase them from fry them in corn, soy, palm, or unhealthy oil blends.

Although I rarely eat out, I realize others may not have that choice for one reason or another. I recommend if this is the case, don't order the fried foods. Purchase a hamburger, sandwich, or salad. Don't order the meals. You won't be able to resist eating the fried spuds.

Further advice—if you can, try to limit the fast food habit to a one-time-per-week indulgence. Although I don't frequent fast food establishments, that does not mean I don't like the taste of those foods. But I learned long ago that sustaining good health requires not indulging in too many Genetically Modified (GE) fried foods.

If a convenience or fried food habit becomes the norm, it will be a tough one to break because of the lab-farmed, hyperpalatable fats in the foods you love to eat. And regardless of exercise activity, if an unhealthy fats habit is not brought into moderation, body weight will likely continue to increase to unhealthy levels.

Another healthy tip I can provide is to cook fried foods without using oil. I love fried foods just like you but need to moderate when it comes to consuming them. Try using an air fryer. My wife picked one up about two years ago. The foods are cooked using air convection at high heat, which creates the crispy food layer. The fries, or any other food, taste as good as or better than the same foods fried in oil. You can now enjoy *"Fry-Like" favorite foods* without oil, and the taste is marvelous. Pick up an air fryer and recipe book, and you'll not be disappointed. We now cook all our protein—steak, fish, pork, poultry, and so on—in this easy-to-use device and have cut our cooking oil consumption in half.

Chapter 12

Many Habits Were Formed Day One

Childhood experiences influence adult habits and behavior.

—MirrorAthlete Principled Fitness and
Healthy Lifestyle Philosophy

Many habits and behavior were learned and formed long ago. For better or worse, they influence lifestyle choices as adults. While changing a bad habit is certainly possible, it often seems impossible for many to do—especially until they recall the connection to the origin of a bad habit or behavior.

Behavioral therapists tell us bad habits are learned behavior. "The behaviorist does not look to the mind or the brain to understand causes of abnormal behavior. He assumes that the behavior represents certain learned habits, and he attempts to determine how they are learned" (Bustamante, Howe-Tennant, and Ramo 1996). By knowing when, where, and how a bad eating and sedentary habit began, *I believe* it is easier to change an unhealthy lifestyle course and move toward a more positive one.

For example, it is known certain toxins and chemicals have a negative effect on behavior. If your weight problem revolves around a frequent habit of binging on junk foods, you may not understand how hyperpalatable foods keep you addicted to them and how that affects brain chemical balance. "Dietary changes can bring about changes in our brain structure, which can lead to altered behavior" (Magee 2009). This, in turn, makes it hard to break an addictive food or drug habit.

Junk food bingeing, in my opinion, falls into a similar addictive category as alcohol, smoking, illicit drugs, pharmaceutical abuse, and the like. All of these things have an effect on brain-body chemistry and can lead to undesirable behavior and weight gain. Unhealthy signs of food habit dependency may include depression, sadness, overzealousness, high excitability, anxiousness, feeling out of sorts, lack of energy, low tolerance and patience, and low ambition and productivity levels. Chemical dependency amps up or slows down the brain-body metabolic communicative connections and affects the way people feel, behave, and appear.

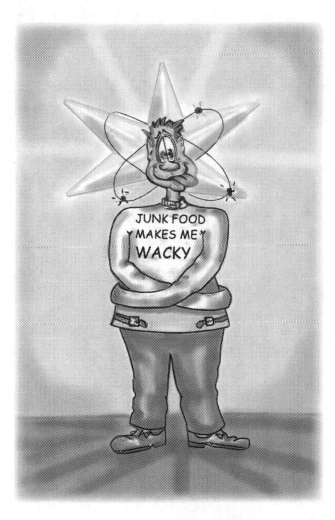

Experts in the medical and health professions have known for years that treatment for eating disorders may involve behavior therapy that seeks to modify existing food and exercise patterns (Katch and McArdle 1993). Through behavior modification, it is possible for long-lasting change to occur. But to fully succeed requires an understanding of how the habit or behavior began in the first place.

We are also genetically wired at birth and then further developmentally and behaviorally influenced by others and environment. For example, maybe you hated vegetables as a child for whatever reason, and to this day you still avoid them. Maybe a parent kept you at the table until the plate was clean, and that was a bad experience. So as an adult you avoid them. If you continue to repeat this avoidance behavior in front of your children, what do they learn? You got it; they repeat the behavior. However, if they learn whole foods are essential to good health and actually taste good, they learn to value, appreciate, and demand them as adults.

A cultural behavior or habit change occurred in the latter half of the twentieth century; it had a significant social impact, specifically on food choice at dinnertime. Do you recall the frozen TV dinners developed by C.A. Swanson and Sons in 1953 (the name in full was TV Brand Frozen Dinner)? Do you remember eating them while watching television instead of sitting at the dinner table? If you grew up during the '50s and decades to follow, you'll likely agree the meal innovation also influenced, *in part*, the unraveling of traditional family communication by changing social behavior. This behavioral change occurred through the habit of eating dinner and watching TV.

Although a lack of family communication at dinnertime can be problematic in building strong family bonds, I believe it's the convenient processed food habit that should be the focus here, especially if body weight is a problem and health is at risk. As if the convenience meals of the sixties and seventies weren't bad enough, now more premade, hyperpalatable food choices filled with unhealthy food chemicals flood the marketplace.

These chemicals include preservatives, taste and smell intensifiers, and dyes to retain fresh and attractive-looking food characteristics. The addictive draw to some of these chemicals makes it harder than ever to break unhealthy addictive food habits. Unbeknownst to many, they alter behavior, increase weight, and cause disease, including diabetes and cancer.

For instance, "high fructose corn syrup (HFCS) is a highly refined artificial sweetener which has become the number one source of calories in America ... HFCS packs on the pounds faster than any other ingredient ... and contributes to the development of diabetes and tissue damage" (Bosch n.d.).

Another additive, "sodium nitrite is widely regarded as a toxic ingredient, and the USDA actually tried to ban this additive in the 1970s but was vetoed by food manufacturers who complained they had no alternative for preserving packaged meat products ... It's actually a color fixer, and it makes old, dead meats appear fresh and vibrant" (Bosch n.d.).

I grew up more or less, like many of you, in a farming community. My food preferences are still farm-to-stove fresh foods, as opposed to highly processed ones found in fanciful and colorful packages with ingredient names you can't pronounce. Today's processed foods have exceedingly long shelf or freezer life, where organic foods don't. They also are surprisingly addictive to smell and taste.

You'll know which ones they are because you can't stop eating them, even when you're full! Organic whole foods, on the other hand, taste naturally good, satisfy hunger, and provide the brain and body what they need to function well. You feel good, lose weight, and stay healthy.

I understand some of you have a tough time identifying healthy foods that will help you lose weight. I assure you, once you target the addictive food habit nemesis, you'll begin to lose weight, increase activities, and achieve a set fitness goal.

Science shows us that, once you're lighter on your feet, you become more physically active, feel better about life, and portray a positive attitude reflected in behavioral change. An article by Kirsten Weir for the American Psychological Association quotes James Blumenthal, PhD, a clinical psychologist at Duke University: "'There's good epidemiological data to suggest that active people are less depressed than inactive people. And people who were active and stopped tend to be more depressed than those who maintain or initiate an exercise program.'" The article also quotes Michael Otto, PhD, a professor of psychology at Boston University, who noted, "'Usually within five minutes after moderate exercise you get a mood-enhancement effect'" (Weir 2011). The point here is that daily exercise activity is just as important as healthy eating habits. The two work hand in hand.

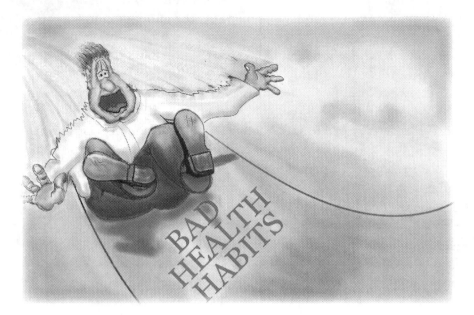

If you've become overweight or obese and nothing has worked in your attempts to lose excess weight, I have to say, "Don't be so hard on yourself." There are many reasons weight gain becomes problematic. Fortunately for many, successful weight loss is possible through mindful reflection of bad habit origin—why and how it began in the first place. Once a behavior's origin has been identified, reversal of the habit is more than possible. It is also life changing and, for many, lifesaving.

For instance, were you rewarded as a child with certain foods for a job well done? And does a daily pat on the back now cause a bad eating habit or behavior that is keeping both you and your children overweight?

"When we are children we are taught by our parents to associate rewards with food. For example when we do well in school, pay attention to our parents, or do our chores etc., we are given praise by our parents and then rewarded by candy, cookies or McDonalds. This reward system begins to change the child's outlook of food. Instead of seeing food as a simple way of giving our body the energy that it needs we begin to look towards food as a reward. As adults this behavior stays with us and we reward ourselves with food" (AOTA 2016).

Now you're able to relate to how food rewards learned during childhood influence habits and behavior as an adult. The willpower to break an addictive food-reward habit may require behavior modification therapy, especially if it has caused a severe eating disorder and increased risk to health. "Behavior modification is the systematic use of principles of learning to increase the frequency of desired behaviors and/or decrease the frequency of problem behaviors" (Gerrig and Zimbardo 2016). Modifying behavior may also require distancing oneself from a triggered food response or environment that causes it. And the place you shop is no exception.

Do marketers know a thing or two about impulsive behavior and shopping habits during seasonal events? Sure they do. During Christmastime, what do you see heavily promoted and stocked in grocery stores? You got it—turkey, champagne, favorite movies and songs, assorted seasonal candies and baked goods, decorative knickknacks, favorite boys and girls toys, and on and on. What about Black Friday? Same thing. Marketers understand people's shopping habits and behavior and how to trigger a purchase response whenever their marketing departments require one. I've had many discussions with clients on this topic.

Marketers are not mind readers. However, they are behavioral prediction gurus and know how to target consumers and lure them in to ensure repeat sales based on past shopping habits. Recall the Personal Fitness Challenge found in chapter 9, "Health Risk Prediction and Prevention."

Below I've listed and targeted common traditional, emotional, and environmental triggers that keep many people overweight and unfit throughout the year. If any of these *origin-triggers* have contributed to an unhealthy habit or behavior and your health is now at risk, changing course may now require specialized medical treatment:

1. *Last year's resolution to lose weight failed* – You know why your weight-loss goal from previous years was unsuccessful. You did not resolve to change your eating, drinking, drug, social, or activity habits and behaviors. Nor did you seek help for your addiction-related problem that now affect relationships, career,

and health. For whatever reason, the idea of seeking professional help is still too painful to confront. I will not pretend to know what you are going through. However, until you come to terms with those emotional triggers, you'll not likely achieve your fitness goal and will instead increase your health risk.

2. *Obesity and pain relationship* – Bodily pain often has a direct connection to unhealthy body weight, habits, and behavior. If you're grossly obese and do not seek medical treatment, excess body weight will cause more pain and damage to the nervous system; internal organs; weight-bearing joints; immune, digestive, and circulatory systems; cardiopulmonary function, and on and on. It is for these reasons you *must* become proactive and seek medical treatment and consultation.

3. *Stress complicates weight loss* – People get stressed out living in a fast-paced environment, and that takes a toll on the encompassing being. We not only lose sleep; we forego daily exercise activity and eat unhealthy foods. You must make time for sufficient rest, participate in daily exercise, and eat healthier to support stress reduction, improve mood, and reenergize the body. Without proper rest, the body's metabolism, along with energy levels, slow down. Change sleeping habits to get seven to eight hours of sleep per night. If insomnia or suspected sleep apnea (excessive snoring is a symptomatic indicator) is preventing a good night's sleep, see your doctor for sleep apnea study and treatment for insomnia.

4. *Every day and weekend is a food fest.* This habit can last throughout the entire year. Social sporting events such as football, hockey, basketball, soccer, and baseball seasons are loaded with reasons for weekly food and drink celebration. First and foremost, you must understand that frequent parties will likely influence your daily behavior and food habits. If you're not willing to give up weekend party events but still want to lose weight, at a minimum, learn how to manage calorie consumption habits and modify behavior. Recall chapters 7, "Substitute Addictive Habits," and 10, "Choose Favorite Foods to Lose Weight." If you can't change unhealthy food habits on your own, you may have a serious eating disorder and need professional help. Remain mindful of some telltale symptoms if body weight

continues to increase. "Symptoms of compulsive overeating: hiding food, binge eating, eating when full, eating in private, fixation with body weight, shape or size, eating more rapidly than normal, habitual dieting, rapid fluctuations in weight" (Rader Programs 2014). These sorts of habits are complicated and difficult to change without medical treatment. "As with most other mental disorders, there is no one specific cause for binge eating disorder. Rather, it is the result of a complex group of genetic, psychological, and environmental factors" (Dryden-Edwards 2016).

5. *Holiday food habits* – Too many Americans consume fast food, especially during the holidays. Here lies the crux for much of overeating and obesity problems in America. During the holidays, everyone is in preparation for the main event—an all-day feast. During this time of year, there is a spike in food and alcohol sales. Yes, business booms almost in every sector of the economy, and fast food places are no exception. Unhealthy food habits often begin during holidays and then continue throughout the year. Learn more about changing unhealthy food habits in chapters 7, "Substitute Addictive Habits" and 10, "Choose Favorite Foods to Lose Weight."

6. *Love of baking* – I know many have a love of baking—and there is nothing wrong with healthy baking habits. The pitfall is when you like everything you make just a little too much. We also know kids love your baked cookies, cakes, and pies as well. Too much sugar, fats, and salts are not good for anyone, even kids with fast metabolisms. If you're having a tough time with whatever is tugging at your apron, try changing up the dessert menu by serving more fruits, Jell-O, pudding, yogurt, granola, and other healthier options. Also purchase a low-fat, low-sugar desserts cookbook.

7. *Empty nesters cook for an army* – Regardless of seasonal sentiment, there are many empty nesters who continue baking for an entire family after the children are gone. There are many emotions tied into traditional meal memories, which trigger emotions tied into volume cooking, and this is a tough habit to break. If your goal is to lose weight, learn to cook for one or two and freeze leftovers for another meal.

Personal Fitness Challenge: "Dark Horse"

To be frank, I developed some bad habits that influenced a change in behavior at various stages, including disease discovery, preparation for surgeries, and during a long rehabilitation and partial mobility period.

At certain points, I allowed medical opinion, advisement, and recommendations to convince me I could not physically do what I had once taken for granted. Of course, this news was depressing, and my state of mind was affected. I reacted accordingly. I was difficult to be around and began isolating myself from the outside world and didn't like anything about my situation. I also became horribly depressed. At the time, I self-identified as a "dark horse"—one who couldn't win a pain-free mobility and recovery race.

Once you experience physical or mental trauma, bad habits are likely to form and behaviors are likely to change. But these habits and behaviors can be positively reversed *once you recall how they were triggered*. My mental trap and reactive, unhealthy behavioral trigger initially began with my belief that I couldn't get better and improve my mobility situation.

The evidence—substantiated disease and injury diagnosis—showed I'd likely need permanent mobility assistance. I was told to prepare to unload weight-bearing joints to alleviate radiating body pain in both the hips and back. And I was told I could expect to use mobility aids for the long term. Although the word *indefinitely* was never used, I couldn't see any way to improve the situation anytime soon. Nor could I envision being able to gain the same mobility function. This was very dark news for me, and those who've suffered similar losses can relate.

Believing permanent disability was my lot in life, I mentally categorized myself as a "cash cow disability person." I coined this term in 2004 after I had the left hip bone graft surgery. I further defined it as "one who is financially dependent on the government and others because of limited mobility and unable to hold full time employment for some period of time." And with no hope of reversing the bone disease (AVN, avascular necrosis of both hips) and certain to go through two total hip replacements at some point in time …

At this time, I didn't give a 100 percent effort to improving my predicament. I also took too many painkillers, didn't care about my diet, and quit exercising for months. To make matters worse, I really didn't care if I lived or died at one point. I suppose, if I hadn't previously broken my lower back prior to the hip surgeries, the pain complication wouldn't have been as bad.

Chronic pain is a terrible thing that jolts the brain into depression and alters behavior and habits. This particular type of situation requires specialized pain management treatment, physical therapy, and counseling, especially if destructive behaviors manifest and drug abuse ensues. *Yep*, I was there at one point—and I understand the need for this type of treatment. I would do it all over again if need be. Why? Because I understand what a dark horse needs to cross that finish line.

I didn't want to see or talk to anyone because I felt trapped within a broken body full of pain at the ripe old-young age of forty-four. These events changed me and my outlook on life for years in ways that were uncharacteristic of who I was, what I was about, and what I believed in. I lived in a depressed abyss and felt like a dark horse put to pasture. And to make matters worse, I felt I had no one to talk to who could understand or relate to my predicament. But after I sought specialized pain management and psychosomatic therapy, things began to change.

Through this process, I realized that uncontrolled pain was only part of the problem. I also felt sorry for myself and needed to do something about it. I had to stop the flood of negative emotions and become focused on how to positively move forward. I had the skill sets necessary to improve my physical body. But the question was how would I mentally increase my willpower and motivate myself enough to heal my encompassing being?

First of all, I needed to accept a tolerable amount of pain in order to increase exercise activity. To do this required (1) a decrease in painkillers that enabled me to think clearly and (2) a halt in overconsumption of unhealthy foods, especially if I was to begin reducing my body weight.

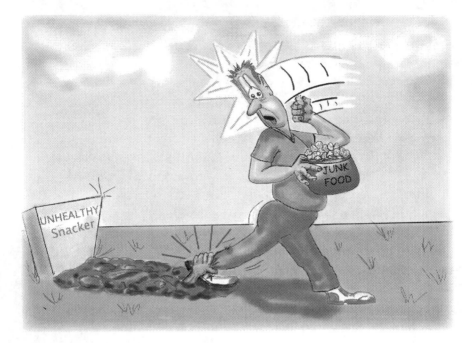

The hardest thing for me to do was manage pain, an area in which I'd never been scholastically trained. And believe me, pain management is easier said than done. It was mostly about applying a different state of mind that involved accepting a certain amount of pain during daily therapy and exercise activity. In other words, what pain tolerance level was I willing to accept? What were the lifestyle changes I was willing to make? And if I did reinjure myself trying, could I get back into the race and cross that line?

During my military career, I was motivated to *move with purpose*. I came to believe this past mind-set could be used once again to motivate purposeful, healing change. Those memories were the driving triggers that allowed me to accept the situation and gave me the willpower needed to motivate a change in behavior and focus more positively on the task at hand.

Long ago, I learned how to endure laborious, uncomfortable, and often grueling mental and physical team challenges. Those challenging military exercises often resulted in lessons learned and field entrenched survival memories I could reflect upon and use when needed. I only needed to recall a few situations and experiences and then make those memories relevant to my immobility challenge. I began to focus and meditate on the mantra I coined and described in Chapter 5, Personal Fitness Challenge: *Black Cloud* – while serving in the Army Guard: *Don't stop until your mind tells you to stop.*

This singular oxymoronic memory helped provide the willpower needed to change my life—it enabled me to believe that I could slowly free myself of mobility aids one step at a time, literally! Imagine the stupidity of this mantra. Where nothing else had seemed to mentally fire me up, it pushed me ultimately to move forward and free myself of walking aids. Why? Because it was connected to an inspirational *recalled emotional trigger*—one that proved that what seemed physically and mentally uncomfortable and impossible at the time was possible. I had done the impossible many times in another lifetime, as have many of you. Why wouldn't you apply those motivational and emotional triggers to healing yourself and enjoying life to the fullest?

I specifically recalled that, while serving, there was nowhere else to go but forward and that I had to endure the suck like others. Quitting was never an option. Those who've experienced a challenging field training exercise or active duty deployment understand what I'm talking about.

To me, this mantra basically meant *never stop trying to change a bad situation into a better one.* I had believed at one time that, through exceptional effort, a successful outcome was more than possible if there's "no quit." So why wouldn't I believe it possible to use that mentality to improve a current fitness challenge or life adversity or immobility situation?

During the worst state of pain and depression, I meditated on that mantra, in short, to also mean, there's a time to rest, recuperate, heal, and get over it. I eventually realized a worse outcome was inevitable if I didn't change my behavioral habits. I called this behavioral change process a "light bulb *on* recall experience." This recall process allowed my mind to free itself of *can't* and say *can.*

I believe everyone has a light bulb *on* memory processor that can be tapped into when needed to make a life-changing decision that will propel him or her to heal sooner, rather than later. Even when you feel all alone and hope seems lost, you are not and it isn't!

If you're open to mental exploration of the past, it does reveal life lessons taught to us at an early age or at some junction in life. Simply recall what mental or physical trigger motivated you to excel during better times. Then make it relative to a current day adversity situation to provide the willpower *and* power forward. I reached the healthy lifestyle finish line as a white horse and you can too by recalling a light bulb *on* moment.

Don't stop till your mind tells you to stop—which is never!

Chapter 13

Leveraging Healthy Habit Change

Commit to healthy habit change and achieve weight-loss goals.

—MirrorAthlete Principled Fitness and
Healthy Lifestyle Philosophy

After working with clients over the years, I came to a conclusion—it was undeniable that many needed help changing unhealthy habits in order to achieve a weight-loss goal. This required a unique fitness programming approach and toolbox choice for some clients.

I understood that, for some, achieving a fitness goal required programming compromise—which I coined *leveraging healthy habit change.* And isn't a concept fitness consultants and trainers typically cover as far as I'm aware. Leveraging healthy habit change through programming compromise is an important concept to master in application, especially when weight-loss failure has become an all-too-common theme.

Leveraging a healthy lifestyle habit is a slower process than removing a bad habit cold turkey. It is a habit change technique that takes longer to achieve the goal but allows a programming compromise, or *infrequently occurring indulgence,* whereas the objective is achieved at some point in time. The application of compromise—or permission to cheat on your weight-loss progress once in a while—provides just enough flexibility in what's often perceived and feels like a *regimental fitness program approach and process.* That perception, for many, is a major cause of weight-loss failure.

Throughout the years I've learned what healthy habits work best to sustain long-term well-being and fitness results. In my opinion, a leveraged healthy habit process can work to achieve a fitness goal. This approach, when relatable and applied in moderation, can provide sustainable life-changing results when nothing else seemed to work.

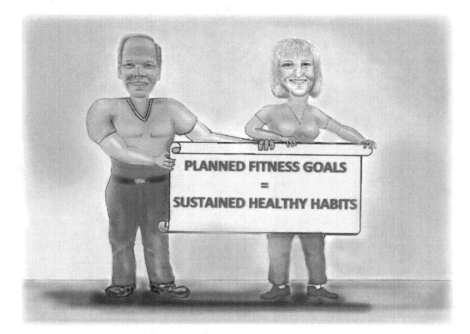

However, if leveraging healthy habit change doesn't work for you, it's likely for one of the following reasons—addiction to something consumed, an unhealthy environment, an underlying medical condition, use of the wrong fitness program, or you're not ready to quit a bad habit or behavior.

The truth is you don't have to suffer to achieve safe and natural weight loss. When you achieve balance through healthy habit, no suffering is required to stay the course. For some, I suppose any change in lifestyle *at first* presents a form of suffering. This is especially true if sedentary habits have kicked in and you're addicted to something and unable to quit on your own. If this is the case, seek medical help.

Although you don't need to calculate or track calories or fitness results through a healthy habit change program, at some point, you may want to. If you do, I highly recommend using the worksheets found in the back of the book after reading chapters 5, 10, 13, and 18. If it's relevant and applicable to your fitness goals, use the leveraging concept within a customized healthy habit program to achieve weight loss and other fitness goals.

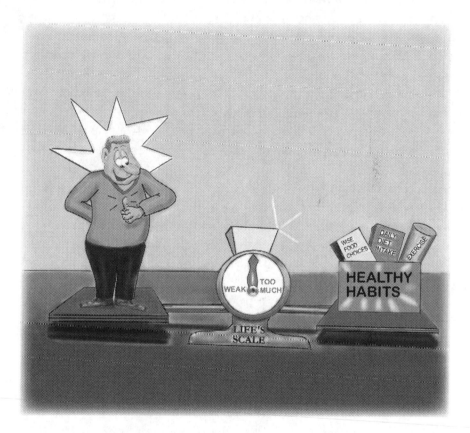

As a healthy lifestyle consultant, I felt it important to cast a large healthy lifestyle program net that would allow anyone to achieve a desired fitness result.

From a *leveraging* perspective, to ultimately achieve the objective, I knew I was on track. For instance, when your lifestyle is rife with bad habits, what are the odds of achieving and sustaining a desired result without healthy habit change awareness or mindfulness? When one understands and is aware of how to target, leverage, or remove a bad habit, one is more apt to achieve the goal and sustain it for the long term.

Yep, I gave my clients permission to let go of the guilt for a day or modify an unhealthy habit to a better one—one step and one day at a time.

As I've explained to clients, I'm happy to maintain a neutral weight-loss result over a holiday or an occasional night out on the town. If I happen to add a pound because I've modified my diet or exercise activity for one day, these pounds are easily shed in a short period of time—provided the commitment toward living a healthier lifestyle is leveraged no more than two days a week.

Now this line of reasoning works for me and for many others. You may not want to add a pound or have weight that temporarily increases during a programmed weight-loss period. That's entirely up to you. I'm simply saying that, if you choose this strategy, you won't beat yourself up mentally when a neutral period happens or slight weight gain occurs unexpectedly. The key is not to repeat the leveraging tactic daily or on weekends. In other words, leveraging unhealthy indulgences two days in a row or on weekends is a no-go! One day on a Friday or Saturday is fine. Why not both days? Typically on weekends, people overindulge. Need I say more? And leveraging on average must be moderated, "not in excess," on any given day.

You'll have to balance this type of logic relative to your lifestyle and set goals. But I think it is important to remember, when you restrict yourself too long from the things that make life enjoyable, even the best diet and exercise plan will fail without self-permission to splurge once in a while. Learn how to forgive through habit modification. Take a break from the grind, and if an infrequent indulgence causes a negative body weight result, don't beat yourself up.

Some may reason that the diet modification or leveraging tactic is similar to an indulgent food-reward practice. The difference between this leveraging tactic and a food-reward system is it's not attached to a good behavior. In other words, you simply give yourself a little breathing room to adjust to habit change and make a smoother transition toward healthier habit choices.

I see how cutting loose once in a while motivates people to stay a healthier lifestyle course—by not excluding everything that makes life enjoyable. Some consultants may see this as heading down the wrong road. I consider it a reasonable risk to allow the practice if it will help someone make a healthier lifestyle commitment.

But if leveraging causes food bingeing or reinforces other unhealthy food behavior, habits, or disorders, the practice should be avoided completely. Within a period of one to three months it becomes obvious whether leveraging a weight-loss program is right for you. The weight results will speak for themselves.

The importance of committing to weight loss and getting more fit is often recognized when a New Year's resolution is made. It's typically at this point in time people need and want physical change and will commit to trying just about anything to make it happen.

For those of you who achieved the weight-loss resolution goal and sustained it throughout the following year and beyond, congratulations! However, if the loss was achieved using fad diets, diet pills, restrictive diets, and/or unhealthy drug-like supplements, consider these tactics unnatural, unhealthy, and unsustainable in the long term. And know that they increase health risk. If you don't know by now, I'll say it again, *rapid weight-loss products, in the long run, will cause more pain and suffering that need not be.*

Tina was a former New Year's resolution client of mine. Prior to committing to a healthy habit change program, Tina had repeatedly failed her weight-loss goal. Per choice, she committed to specific habit change choices to lose weight naturally over the following year. Tina's desired result was to lose fourteen pounds of body fat safely over a three-month period.

I emphasized at first that she should commit to half the healthy habit list I had to offer. She initially chose a few changes and ultimately signed a contract *with herself* to commit to most of these healthy habits over a three-month period. During this time, Tina leveraged specific habit changes based on her lifestyle. In other words, some of the habit choices she chose were not followed exactly as written—she modified some of them to accommodate her social habits. But the fact is, she leveraged most of the healthy habit choices in a three-month window to achieve her weight-loss goal.

After three months, Tina lost the fourteen pounds and, thereafter, discontinued my consulting services because she felt she could sustain the effort without any further fitness consultation. I wished her all the best. I know some fitness professionals would say I lost a repeat paying customer by not selling an advanced fitness program. I like to think of it as a success story that provided more client referrals seeking similar services.

Our session covered the healthy habit choices listed in the following section [Healthy Habit (HH) 1-14]. Tina's selections were recorded on the Healthy Habit Commitment Form (13.1) to refer to; and I've also included blank form (13.0) if you'd like to make use of it (see appendix).

Healthy Habit 1 – *Don't Go to Any Meal Hungry!*

Never—I repeat *never*—go to any meal in starvation mode! The habit of not eating a little bit before a holiday feast or special event seems to be engrained within the American culture. A small meal or snack prior to the main meal can be of great value. I know too many people repeat the ritual of starving themselves in anticipation of overeating. You'll continue this gluttony habit unless you change your behavior.

When we starve ourselves, we eat too quickly and get overfull. Then we end up lying around like beached whales on a lido deck. It makes good sense to eat a snack prior to the meal. The point is, when you get to the table, you won't be starving and won't eat as much.

Another technique includes food grazing—visually looking over the table and then choosing a few small portions of certain foods to consume slowly to reach satiety. Grazing as a weight-loss practice has similarities to snacking. I prefer and recommend applying plate portion control and eating favorite foods to cut calories. That works for me and for others and is worth trying if grazing is not your cup of tea ((refer to Healthy Habit 6 plotted on form 13.1 (see appendix)).

In my opinion, a weight-loss strategy that includes grazing or a daily snack without a satisfying meal in between is not a good plan because, for most, it's not sustainable.

Case in point, how many of you could go to the king and queen's ball filled with many scrumptious food delights and not overconsume—especially if the only food plan is to graze and select a few appetizers or snack a little here and there throughout the event? I know. Some of you put this to practice often, and it works. For others, they end up snacking more than grazing and consume more than they would have if they had eaten a satisfying meal.

I'm not saying we're all undisciplined. I am saying there aren't many who can restrict food choice and quantity this way. For those of you who can turn off the feeding frenzy by using a low-calorie, high-nutrient grazing or snacking technique, my hats off to you. You have willpower most of us can only dream about.

Those I spoke to who graze foods admitted they were miserable doing it long-term. Every one of them also said, "I ended up going back to my old eating habits and gained more weight."

Is there a place for grazing in a weight-loss program? I'd say yes, but leverage this caloric consumption technique in moderation.

Food grazing and snacking behavior has similarities to weight-loss practices that include minimeals but differ in quality, quantity, and frequency of consumption. Minimeals typically consist of 200 to 400 calorie per servings, five to eight times per day. The problem with minimeals, like grazing at dinnertime, is that they're not typically satisfying.

Writer Simone Cave made some very good points on how grazing and snacking habits cause people to change behavior and ultimately gain weight because these things are not as satisfying as three meals per day, among them:

> The problem with grazing is that many people ignore the bit about eating only a little, hearing only the message to "eat often"—the result is we've become a nation of snackers ...
>
> They [nutritionists] say snacking makes us even hungrier; it also interferes with the body's ability to burn fat, leads to obesity and type 2 diabetes, as well as tooth decay.
>
> What we should really be doing, it seems, is going back to three proper meals a day, with no snacks in between.
>
> For many, snacking is a major cause of weight gain, says Professor Stephen Atkin, head of diabetes and metabolism at Hull York Medical School. (Cave 2010)

The words *grazing, snacking,* and *minimeals* alone do not inspire or get anyone excited about changing dietary habits. I do agree that eating three proper meals a day is important for healthy weight loss. But I disagree in part with Cave's statement this should include "no snacks in between." For some, I believe leveraging a midmorning, afternoon, and light evening snack between meals *can lead* toward a healthier three-meal-a-day habit if applied correctly. But note the key words in my statement—*can lead*.

For particular clients, I found it necessary to provide a compromise or leveraging of consumption techniques. Otherwise, not all clients would agree or commit to significant habit change for the necessary duration, and some would ultimately fail at their weight-loss goal.

Healthy Habit 2 – *Eat Three to Four Fruit and Vegetable Servings Per Day*

Plain and simple, we need vitamins and minerals to sustain healthy brain-body function and metabolism. For example, "Vitamin D helps your body absorb the amount of calcium (a mineral) it needs to form strong bones. A deficiency in vitamin D can result in a disease called rickets (softening of the bones caused by the body's inability to absorb the mineral calcium). The body cannot produce calcium; therefore, it must be absorbed through our food … The best way to get enough vitamins (A, B, C, D, E, and K), calcium, iron, magnesium and other trace minerals [for example, chromium, copper, iodine, iron, selenium, and zinc] is to eat a balanced diet with a variety of foods" (CDC 2005).

Vitamins and minerals have a unique role to play in our well-being, metabolism, weight loss, and overall health. For instance, if you can't get three to four fruit and vegetable servings per day for whatever reason, consider supplementing the daily diet. Learn more about superfoods and supplements and their antioxidant roles in cellular protection and healthy longevity (chapter 14, "Processed vs. Organic Foods").

Healthy Habit 3 – *Don't Drink Alcohol Prior to a Meal*

You don't drive and drink do you? Well, what makes you think you could overeat and drink without injury? Although I'm being a bit facetious, I'm also serious in the way I want to make my point. Alcohol is a depressant, painkiller, relaxant, taste intensifier, and willpower inhibitor all rolled into one. Also alcohol adds additional calories to the daily caloric intake (alcohol has seven calories/gram) plus calories from mixers used in those drinks.

Like smoking and drug addiction, alcohol is addictive and affects behavior and health negatively. If you don't want to stop consuming alcohol and are concerned about calorie intake, consider changing a liquor or beer habit to drinking a couple of glasses of red wine instead. No, I'm not advocating for anyone to become a wino. I'm simply saying that one may be able to modify or leverage a bad habit through a lessor of two evils. However, you're better off drinking more water than alcohol if you're *serious* about healthier lifestyle and weight loss. Get behavioral modification and alcohol addiction help if drinking is the cause of poor health or unhealthy behavior.

Healthy Habit 4 – *Drink Plenty of Water before, during, and after Any Meal*

Water is a natural solvent and absorbs well in the stomach and intestinal lining, which assists the body's digestion to process food more efficiently. Plus, water makes you feel fuller faster during meals. There are many metabolic benefits, which include flushing toxins out of the body. We hold approximately 66 percent water weight. So it stands to reason that water is very important to our health, fitness levels, and weight-loss goals.

If serious about weight loss, focus on drinking about two liters of water throughout the day and more during mealtime. To learn how important water is to the fat burning engine read the Personal Fitness Challenge: "Water the Elixir of Life."

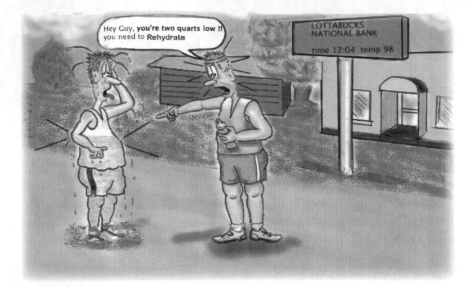

Healthy Habit 5 – *Leave the Dinner Table after Eating the Main Course*

Do not stay at the table after eating dinner or a holiday meal. This is where most of us fall prey to adding on the pounds. It was very difficult to resist picking at the holiday turkey, cranberry, mashed potatoes, sweet potatoes, pies, and olives. Oh, the dressing and gravy. Give me a break! I'm dying here. I think I just made myself hungry. See how hard this is, and I'm supposed to be giving you advice. Look, I never said I wasn't human or that this would be a cakewalk—no pun intended—which is all the more reason to have a premeal battle plan! Move your conversations away from the table after eating what's served on the plate.

Healthy Habit 6 – *Plate Portion Control Is Key*

I've previously talked a little bit about portion control. Moderation and balance of food portions on your plate is important. When I say portion control, I'm not talking about counting calories, grazing, eating minimeals, or snacking. I'm talking about surface area on your plate as a food portion control gauge. For example, you might reduce food portions served on a plate by a quarter of the normal serving. You don't need to track these calories if you don't want to. You've already reduced a typical serving size of your favorite foods by 25 percent.

Or if you currently serve meals on a plate of a certain size, you can serve yourself less than a full serving or try using a plate that is 25 to 50 percent reduced in diameter (Katch and McArdle 1993, 306). Now load it up with your favorite foods the same way you would with a plate of "regular" size. Try selecting foods that provide a macronutrient balance whenever possible. Limit yourself to one plate during main meals. Also, don't increase the food height on the plate.

Right off the bat you've cut your calories by a quarter to a half. True, this is not rocket science, but it will reduce food calories and body weight.

Healthy Habit 7 – *Take Twenty Minutes to Eat Your Meal*

Make sure you take at least twenty minutes to eat a meal. It will take the brain this much time to realize the stomach is satisfied. To help slow down your eating pace, have a sixteen-ounce glass of water on the table and practice more social engagement. Do not skimp on adding more water during the first twenty minutes. It will help you achieve a feeling of satiety while enjoying good company.

Healthy Habit 8 – *Eat Sensible Meals by Reducing Unhealthy Food Choices*

I like the taste of certain hyperpalatable unhealthy foods too. But you *must* try to avoid eating too many of them.

Remember, you're not saying *no forever* to unhealthy food favorites. Your long-term goal is to commit to healthier food choices that can include occasional indulgences. For example, Tina leveraged a healthier food habit by committing not to eat french fries more than twice per month. She wasn't told they were off limits; she simply learned how to leverage the indulgence by eating them less frequently.

Healthy Habit 9 – *When Ordering Fast Food, Limit Selection*

I know some are hooked on ordering a full meal deal. Changing this unhealthy behavior requires a change in your food ordering habit. For example, order a burger; give up the fries; and substitute the soda for a coffee, water, milk, or natural juice. Sodas and juices high in sugar, sodium, and unnatural chemicals and fried foods cooked in unhealthy fry oils will only make it more difficult to lose weight.

I didn't restrict my clients from eating favorite foods or drinks when going out on the town. I simply recommend they reduce frequencies, quantity, and/or substitute healthier choices.

Healthy Habit 10 – *Never Eat Dessert Right after a Meal*

Never—I repeat *never*—eat dessert after you've eaten a meal. This may add insult to injury. As previously stated, your stomach needs at least twenty minutes to register satisfaction. If you eat dessert before the brain registers satisfaction, you may overeat.

Wait an additional ten minutes after the meal before getting dessert. If you're still hungry at this time, have dessert. Consider a half portion of what you'd typically serve yourself.

Healthy Habit 11 –*Don't Eat after 8:00 p.m.*

Your metabolism slows down significantly at night. If you feel hungry after 8:00 p.m., eat an orange, grapes, apple, banana, yogurt, or fiber bar, or have a fiber drink. If you're diabetic, talk to your doctor about other low-calorie, high-nutrient alternatives. Even too many natural sugars can cause blood sugar to spike. This is not to suggest you can't have a favorite evening dessert. You just don't want to eat them often or after 8:00 p.m. Also, be sure to shut the lights off in the kitchen and store the food away after meals. This provides a psychological barrier by enforcing the rule that the kitchen is closed.

I've even had clients move refrigerators to the back porch or the garage to make it more inconvenient to snack. Although this approach seems to work for some, it is really inconvenient when you want to make a meal. I don't recommend moving the fridge out of the kitchen. I believe this can lead to other bad habits and behaviors, due to foods being inconveniently located.

Healthy Habit 12 – *Don't Take Leftovers Home*

If you can't turn down leftovers after leaving a family function or restaurant, have the discipline to freeze them immediately upon returning home. Do not leave these foods readily available in your refrigerator. If you do, it could lead to overeating. I know there is no way I could resist the temptation of ready-made holiday or restaurant foods in my refrigerator, and I'm sure you are no different. So remove the temptation to the freezer and plan to eat the leftovers at another time.

Healthy Habit 13 – *Don't Quit Exercise Activity, Especially during Holidays*

Find a daily activity that increases your metabolism fifteen to sixty minutes a day and three to five times per week. Start at fifteen minutes of duration per day and set frequency of activity at least three times a week. For example, choose walking, biking, hiking, gardening, house chores, walking the dog, dance, yoga, aerobics class, swim, fitness activity classes or home video aerobics, or any type of *low-intensity* activity that increases heart rate for a period of time. Doing so will contribute to your ability to achieve your weight-loss goal (chapter 5, "Caloric Exchange: A Balancing Act"). Record exercise activities on a calendar and plan to commit to them daily.

Healthy Habit 14 – *Get a Medical Checkup Annually*

If you're beginning a new diet or fitness program after years of inactivity, it is advisable to get a medical checkup. It is a good practice to see a doctor at least once a year. Medical consultation annually and prior to significant dietary and exercise change is a prudent thing to do (chapter 9, "Health Risk Prediction and Prevention").

Personal Fitness Challenge: "Water the Elixir of Life"

Currently on average, I practice at least six to eight of the healthy habits mentioned above, which supports healthy body weight, good fitness levels, and overall well-being. I highly recommend, if you change no other habit and you want to look and feel better, drink more of the elixir of life—water.

I've recommended to clients to prioritize drinking more water when it comes to developing healthy habits. And they look at me like, *I already drink a lot of water*. But in reality, none of us do, and most take it for granted. It takes time to develop a daily habit of drinking enough water to satisfy the body's thirst requirement. And for those like me managing neuro-musculoskeletal pain and *my* ideal body weight, drinking enough water throughout the day is a must.

Very soon you'll understand the importance of adequate hydration and why drinking more water, like daily exercise, should be a *lifestyle* priority. Without adequate hydration, it's more painful to exercise, you'll feel hungry more often, you'll lack energy, and you'll struggle to lose weight regardless of any other habit change you make.

There are varying opinions by experts on how much water one should drink daily. Environmental conditions can vary the body's hydration needs. So can diet, physical work, medical conditions, geographical location, drugs, and air pollutants. The question becomes, How does one know if he or she is properly hydrated? And why is water so important to how we look and feel? It is surprising how little people know about the body's water needs—and especially how clueless they are when the body is screaming for it.

Severe lack of water in the body (due to not drinking enough of it) is known to cause heat exhaustion, heat stroke, kidney stones, and other ill-health complications. Water is essential for many physiological, metabolic, hormonal, and cellular functions. It sustains healthy joints and creates a moist environment for our eyes, ears, nose, throat, and lungs. It retains healthy skin, hair, and teeth. Water also rehydrates us after we urinate and have bowel movements and replaces moisture lost through breathing and perspiring. Water is also needed to regulate body temperature, absorb food calories, burn stored body fat, and so much more.

There is really no rule on how much water one should drink in a day. But there are recommended hydration guidelines to follow based on scientific fact. Our bodies are made up of around two-thirds (66 percent) water, and maintaining that requirement is physiologically crucial for life-sustaining electrolyte balance and blood volume, toxin removal, and healing what ails us.

The daily average hydration consensus from experts appears to be 1.9 liters (eight 8-ounce glasses) per day. This recommendation by the Institute of Medicine, for example, is not supported by hard scientific data. Instead, this example refers to the baseline of an individual who exercises at least twenty minutes per day, weighs about 150 pounds, and lives in fairly mild to cool temperatures throughout the year.

Now looking outside this hypothetical baseline average, the kidney functions are capable of handling up to six gallons of water a day. Imagine consuming that much water a day. But an athlete, roofer, construction worker, and others who work very hard can exceed this volume easily, especially during hot summer months. I make mention of this because environment and workload change hydration needs above any hypothetical baseline or norm.

There is an easy way to know if you are not getting enough water. Be mindful of urine color. If urine appears dark yellow, drink more water. When urine is clear, you're getting enough of it. Another tidbit of information you'll want to be aware of is that nothing—not beer, coffee, tea, or any other beverage—is a substitute for water, but drinking one of those could make your urine appear clear. Your body still needs adequate water replenishment—period!

Now let's, for a moment, consider *overhydration*. Why? Because it is something most of us simply don't think about, let alone practice. In general, if we drink more water in a day than average, is it good for us? In almost all cases, drinking too much water is not going to be a problem. However, there are activities one could participate in where drinking too much water could have a fatal outcome.

Let's take a closer look at the overhydration scenario and what conditions or events could cause a fatal consequence. If you happen to drink too much water and then retain it, the electrolyte sodium concentrate will become too dilute in the body. When this occurs, a significant drop in sodium causes internal cells to swell. This dilute sodium electrolyte effect is known as *hyponatremia*.

If the body becomes *severely* oversaturated with water and electrolytes become out of balance, then the body is at risk of seizures, coma, or even death.

The cause and effect lie within the internal cellular electrolytes, sodium, potassium, chloride, calcium, and phosphate concentrations becoming overwhelmed with water. In other words, the inner cells retain more water, and lower concentration of these electrolytes can become life-threatening. Under this scenario, water retention can cause swelling within the brain cavity. The blood that travels through the brain can then be restricted or interrupted.

Fortunately for most of us, drinking too much water in a day is not going to be a problem. However, past news headlines featuring water drinking contests that resulted in "water-related" deaths put this topic on the map.

So the question is, How much water do we really need?

The answer appears to be rather simple. Drink as much as your body requires and no less than the average requirement of eight 8-ounce glasses of water per day for optimum physiological and metabolic function and good health. When you drink enough water, your body's thirst is quenched, and that supports hunger suppression and weight-loss goals.

The water hydration recommendation represents the ideal—If you don't drink enough water in a day, the body will find another way to hydrate itself through unhealthy food and drink consumption. When the body lacks proper hydration, the brain believes it's still hungry and will compel you to eat more. It is in this way the body extracts enough water out of other foods consumed through the digestive process. Once the body's quench is satisfied, then it tells the brain's hunger center it's also satisfied.

Until you are consistently drinking enough water, it will be much harder to lose weight. So how much food and drink do you need to consume to extract two to three liters of water in a day? I'd say a lot. Try drinking two to three liters of water in a day and see how much food you avoid eating. That may provide the answer you're looking for.

Tina chose two habit changes at first to achieve her weight-loss goals. They were similar choices I made when I began my personal rehabilitative fitness challenge—to expedite healing and increase mobility. She started out by drinking more water and began walking two to four miles per day, which were easy choices to commit to. Within two weeks, she committed to nearly all the healthy habit changes, as seen on form 13.1.

Like Tina, I continue to apply six to seven of the same healthy habit changes and leverage modification of habits as needed.

The top four healthy habit priorities for me still today are daily walks, caloric nutrient balance (consuming three meals per day), drinking two liters of water daily, and a daily vitamin and mineral supplement.

Chapter 14

Processed vs. Organic Food

> Chemically and genetically engineered foods increase
> health risk.
>
> —MirrorAthlete Principled Fitness and
> Healthy Lifestyle Philosophy

I shared how you could lose weight while eating your favorite foods in chapter 10. However, it is important to remain mindful that favorite foods often contain a mix of unhealthy chemical additives and genetically modified organisms (GMOs). These foods may also be promoted and marketed as healthy, wholesome foods that are good for weight loss. The marketplace doesn't make it easy for health-conscious consumers to identify truly organic food choices.

But you can take this to heart: When you come across foods sold in attractive packages and/or containing ingredients lists with items you can't pronounce, suspect they're loaded with unnatural and unhealthy toxins. Many of those food chemicals strangely addict you to them and make you want more even after they make you feel badly.

These foods have also been chemically altered to preserve, nutritionally fortify, and enhance flavor, taste, smell, and color—often leaving very few healthy nutrients within the finished product. The point is, the more food is processed and handled, the greater the likelihood the nutrients are rendered useless and eating them will put your health at risk.

In order to relate to healthy versus unhealthy food choices, it is necessary to identify unhealthy ingredients on labels and remain mindful of deceitful marketing practices. Just because a food is labeled and promoted as a *superfood* or as *organic* does not guarantee that this is always the case. Also, if you're concerned about eating organic, rather than genetically modified food crops, an organic certification will put your mind at ease. Organic certification *should* also guarantee no unnatural insecticides, pesticides, and fertilizers were used to farm the food.

Superfoods are typically referred to as organic, but may or may not have been farmed using GE (genetically engineered) seeds and may or may not meet other organic certification standards. Learn how to tell the purity and quality differences between organic superfoods and organic certification markers or stamps through familiarization with the following terminology: "Organic is a labeling term that indicates that the food or other agricultural product has been produced through approved methods ... Overall, organic operations must demonstrate that they are protecting natural resources, conserving biodiversity, and using only approved substances" (USDA 2016).

"Superfood is a popular term in the health food industry. It refers to foods that are low in calories and high in nutrients ... Superfoods include most fruits and vegetables as well as other foods like yogurt, salmon, and barley. Broccoli is one of the top vegetables because it contains calcium, folate, fiber, and vitamins A, C, K, E and the B vitamins, according to the World's Healthiest Foods" (Price 2015).

Superfoods are often and unfortunately used to promote and sell consumers on unsubstantiated health benefits. "The term 'superfoods' is at best meaningless and at worst harmful," said Catherine Collins, chief dietitian at St. George's Hospital in London (Pomeroy 2017). Superfood claims often lead some to put off lifesaving treatment or surgery, turning instead to natural cure solutions.

For those who are considering alternative treatment outside of Western medicine, in my opinion, if you now suffer with a chronic disease like cancer, time is not on your side to try a natural cure in the hope of putting it into remission. After cell damage occurs, treatment strategies to reverse or remit it must be carefully weighed through the advisement of an oncologist.

The second point I'd like to interject before continuing sharing information about terminology like *organic* and *superfood* is that healthy food choices should also include a proactive antioxidant prevention strategy. Incorporation of this healthy food habit knowledge can reduce free radical cell damage and cancer risk throughout the body.

"According to the free radical theory of aging, cells continuously produce free radicals, and constant radical damage eventually kills the cell. When radicals kill or damage enough cells in an organism, the organism ages." Antioxidants are important to the metabolism and overall cellular integrity because accelerated oxidization due to *free radical damage* in the body can increase or decrease depending on genetic means and dietary restriction (Nelson 2016).

Within my personal fitness challenge at the end of this chapter I'll define, relate, and apply the *free radical theory of aging* and antioxidant benefits of high-nutrient foods on a personal level. I'll also detail the free radical theory on aging, cell mutation, and cancer prevention. I digress. I'll now continue to expand upon the differences between *superfood*, *certified organic*, and *organic* foods.

Superfoods are often promoted as being high in antioxidants, which they typically are. That's not the same thing as *certified organic*, in which certified standards validate the food's place of origin; the farming practices used to grow it; the methods of processing, storage, and distribution; and so on. Those who want quality and purity of food nutrients at the table can take comfort in knowing that, when you choose foods labeled "certified organic," you're getting the real deal. This guarantee assures the consumer the product is as 100 percent true to nature as it gets in a developed country.

Certified means that "blue ribbon" panels, as in the National Organic Standards Board (NOSB), comprised of six subcommittees, guarantees quality standards have been applied by organic food farmers and processors. These subcommittees oversee crops, livestock, handling, materials, compliance, accreditation, and certification. Together, they create policy when they meet in public to develop recommendations and proposals for the full NOSB's consideration and develop regulations and guidance on certification, production, handling, and labeling of USDA organic products. Recommendations made by the NOSB are not official policy until they are approved and adopted by the USDA (NOSB 2013).

Organic certification assures organic foods meet the highest quality and purity standards. This includes things most consumers don't think about, such as clearing unhealthy bacteria found in water and soil during the grow phase and processing of fresh foods to market. It also seeks to eliminate contamination due to poor handling and sanitary practices after harvest and unacceptable storage and food process practices. "Some U.S. producers are turning to certified organic farming systems as a potential way to lower input costs, decrease reliance on nonrenewable resources, capture high-value markets and premium prices, and boost farm income" (USDA 2016).

In general, noncertified farmed organic fruits, vegetables, and animal products may be from a country farm and generally of good quality. But one or more standards for certification are not applied. For example, the farmed product may have been grown using chemical fertilizers instead of organic biofertilizers.

What are organic fertilizers? They are actually living microorganisms that increase the fertility of the soil. They are by-products from animal waste and organic materials, which replenish and correct soil nitrogen levels. When biofertilizers are used correctly, they protect plants from harmful disease and are safe for the environment. If you're interested in growing quality organic products in your garden, it is important to learn how to use organic fertilizers and insecticides properly.

Organic garden insecticides are made of *Bacillus thuringiensis* (Bt) and pyrethrins. They are derived from plants and found in most garden stores and used to kill insects on contact. One drawback is that overapplication of organic sprays can create a more toxic environment. Be sure to read labels regarding application and frequency of use of a product if you want to grow quality garden foods at home.

So how do consumers make healthier choices without organic certification? We all have to eat, right? My answer—almost any whole food purchased in a store is better than any heavily processed food as far as I'm concerned. But if that whole food was farmed using genetically altered seeds, this should be of concern. A lab-farmed seed alteration can't be detected in foods by appearance, smell, or taste.

A 2014 article, "Shopping Guide Helps Consumers Dodge Genetically-Engineered Foods," points out the difficulty of avoiding these products and attempts to make that easier:

> "Avoiding GE foods isn't easy because consumers are denied the right to know if foods in the grocery aisles have been genetically engineered or contain GE ingredients," said

Renee Sharp, Environmental Working Group's director of research. "It is our hope that EWG's new guide will provide shoppers with the information they need to make more informed decisions when shopping for themselves or their families."

Also, to help promote the anti-GE initiative, Environmental Working Group representative Scott Faber appeared on *The Dr. Oz Show* to discuss the alarming prevalence of such foods.

About 70 percent of food in supermarkets is genetically engineered or contains GE ingredients, according to some estimates. (Deike 2014)

I believe the EWG, like other consumer safety advocates, are concerned humankind will continue to genetically manipulate the next generation's seed and food banks and not adequately educate and publically disclose that information. This focus if not changed will result in increased consumer health problems and food insecurity concerns, including limited access to affordable quantities of certified organic and nutritious foods.

A Large Percent of Our Processed Foods Are Now Genetically Engineered

During the mid-twentieth and early twenty-first centuries, commercial farming and food industries have changed to meet the global food demand. That change now impacts how we farm and process huge volumes of products and how we bring those products to market. There is nothing more concerning to consumer watchdogs then genetically engineered and chemically washed and infused foods, as medical and health experts fear this will cause the next health epidemic.

What unknown health risk and disease could possibly occur? That's really hard to pinpoint. As you'll soon learn, our cells' DNA sequential code could be altered in ways that are yet undetermined with continued manipulation of crop seed DNA and unnatural farming practices and processes.

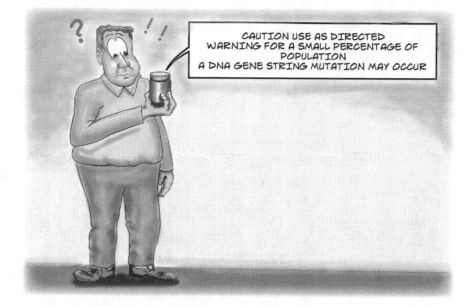

Humankind's manipulation of our seed bank and processed food supply, no doubt, will challenge medical professionals in the future to find cures for what ails us. And if pandemic disease is proven to result from unnatural growing and process practices, what impact might this have on a global scale?

In the words of scientist and broadcaster David Suzuki:

> Since GE foods are now in our diet, we have become experimental subjects without any choice. (Europeans say if they want to know whether GMOs are hazardous, they should just study North Americans). I would have preferred far more experimentation with GMOs under controlled lab conditions before their release into the open, but it's too late.
>
> We have learned from painful experience that anyone entering an experiment should give informed consent. That means at the very least food should be labeled if it contains GMOs so we each can make that choice. (Suzuki 2000)

To understand how the manipulation of farming and food industries got to this point, it is important to identify the origins of marketplace interests that got us here. And one of those interests is connected through constitutional law in recognition of large corporations required by shareholders to turn a profit.

"U.S. corporations have gained inordinate power over all our politicians by manipulating the 14th Amendment to the Constitution. The amendment was adopted in 1868 to protect the rights of newly freed Blacks, yet by 1886 the Supreme Court had begun recognizing it as a protection of the rights of the 'persons' called corporations—persons which do not breath, do not have consciences, and are mandated to make a profit for their shareholders" (Anderman 2011).

The Fourteenth Amendment illustrates how consumer health interests became compromised by shareholder profit mandates. As long as this mandate stands, corporations are required to make a profit, and consumers must trust corporations will do the right thing. If they don't, voters must apply political pressure to hold corporations accountable when they cause harm to consumer health.

In the end, you must know American corporations and science are destined to continue to find ways to increase harvest yields and shareholder profit in a global economy. And these political and economic interests will continue their course and take a toll on global health.

How does this mandate cause a compromise of national seed banks and a further decline of quality farmed products on a global scale? The continuous alteration of DNA seeds and the chemical sprays required to produce greater quantities of unblemished crop yield are also decreasing nutrient purity and increasing health risk.

Health risk appears more likely as DNA manipulation of crop seeds is necessary to produce superior pesticide and herbicide-tolerant (HT) crops. When a crop inevitably loses its tolerance to chemical sprays over a period of time, further genetic modification is required to enhance DNA-resistive properties for those same sprays. It is highly suspected that both GM crop seeds and highly concentrated chemical sprays are now harmful to human health.

Is it possible or likely that these super resistive, lab-farmed seeds are toxic to humans and could damage our DNA, thereby causing chronic illness or disease? I don't specialize in genome or genotype science or disease-causing pathological agents and the like. However, there are many scientific studies and experts around the world that have done the hard work for us. And the data appears to show that these foods could be problematic for healthy longevity. The data also shows powerful lobbyists and political interests have a lot to lose should they change crop seed, farming, and food processing practices.

It seems our food and drug agencies are less concerned about our health and more focused on something else. How come consumer protection laws don't cover GE food labeling, limitations or bans on certain crop seeds and dangerous food chemicals, and the like outright?

Could it have anything to do with our Constitution's Fourteenth Amendment as relative to corporations? Maybe. But there are other motivations in the marketplace that incentivize politicians and farming and food industries to behave the way they do. Could these behaviors have anything to do with the First Amendment?

"The United States Supreme Court held that the First Amendment prohibited the government from restricting independent political expenditures by a nonprofit corporation. The principles articulated by the Supreme Court in the case have also been extended to for-profit corporations, labor unions and other associations" (Wikipedia 2016).

This rule, applied to nonprofit and for-profit organizations alike, provides political speech protected expenditures—backed by deep-pocketed corporate and union power players. This includes the interests of political activity committees (PACs) supporting elected officials' positions on various topics. Let's look at example that shows how corporate interest, nonprofit, and for-profit consumer messaging is protected by the First Amendment.

"Monsanto and other biotech companies maintain that GMOs have cut the use of pesticides. The claim is highlighted by a Big Agriculture–funded campaign opposing California's Proposition 37, which would require the labeling of genetically modified foods" (Peeples 2012). This begs the question, why wouldn't Monsanto want to list on food labels the fact that GMO seeds were farmed using reduced pesticides and good for us?

The answer is easily found through the corporate's actions to defeat California's proposition 37. Monsanto Company was the top opposing contributor of the proposition's labeling campaign, spending $8,112,867. The proposition fell short in requiring mandatory labeling of GMO foods, with 47 percent of the voting electoral. Although the measure failed at the time, it had a huge impact on consumer awareness about GE foods and an effect on health. "Proposition 37 has exposed the dark side of Big Ag and Big Food, and their desperation to keep

U.S. consumers in the dark about whether or not our food has been genetically engineered, a fundamental right enjoyed by citizens in over 60 other countries" (Cummins and Paul 2012).

As you now know, many countries outside of the United States aren't drinking the Kool-Aid. Nor are they *willing* to be a part of our GE experiment. There are thirty countries around the world, including Japan, Canada, Australia, and *all* countries within the European Union that have significant restrictions or outright bans on the production or use of GMOs. And yet, here in the United States, approximately 86 percent of corn and 93 percent of soybeans grown are genetically modified, and a good percentage of these foods end up in our diet. "According to California's Department of Food and Agriculture, 70% of processed foods in American supermarkets now contain genetically engineered (GE) ingredients" (Organic Trade Association, n.d.).

It should be more apparent than ever to consumers why big agriculture, food manufacturers, politicians, and others turn a blind eye to GE food labeling laws. It's good for their interests and their bottom line.

GE Foods and Health Connection

Some research shows GE foods effect on human DNA may be manifesting itself after years of consumption. So how could consuming GE foods morph our genes into unhealthy ones? And what type(s) of known and current diseases, if any, and human DNA health risks has science connected with GMO consumption?

According to researchers in New York:

> Morgellons is the strange manifestation of unusual fibers seen in skin lesions that itch, and appear to "move." People with the affliction describe a crawling stinging sensation, just under the skin ...
>
> They suggest that the fibers are biological with floral root-like structures, and could be from cross contamination of DNA from plants and humans through GMOs.
>
> Some physicians are suggesting that Morgellons is an unusual morphing of Lyme disease ...

> There are well over 15,000 self-identified sufferers from 15 countries including the US ... The numbers are rising, not declining. (Gordon 2013).

In addition, it must be highlighted that there are experiments being performed in countries that study Monsanto's Roundup Ready corn with scientific research linking it to disease:

> While GMOs don't have what scientists call "acute" effects, what about "chronic" affects—those that come on gradually and can't easily be tied to one cause? The French study—the most comprehensive GMO safety assessment ever conducted—highlights that concern ...
>
> The researchers say their results show "severe adverse health effects, including mammary tumors and kidney and liver damage, leading to premature death" from Roundup-Ready corn and Roundup herbicide, whether they were consumed separately or together. (Philpott 2013)

Without relevant studies on GE foods proven safe for human consumption, more market places outside of the United States will likely limit or ban them. The "data presented here strongly recommend that additional long-term (up to 2 years) animal feeding studies be performed in at least three species, preferably also multi-generational, to provide true scientifically valid data on the acute and chronic toxic effects of GM crops, feed and foods. Our analysis highlights that the kidneys and liver as particularly important on which to focus such research as there was a clear negative impact on the function of these organs in rats consuming GM maize varieties for just 90 days" (De Vendômois et al. 2009).

Because of GE seeds, national crop seed banks have the potential to become intolerant to superbugs and superweeds. Thereafter, a country may become dependent on foreign growers, leading to unaffordable food prices and famine. So under this hypothetical situation, how could it manifest to national famine?

Since a large percentage of crop seeds are genetically engineered to resist harmful weeds, pests, and chemical sprays, scientists are concerned superweeds and superpests will evolve per Darwin's natural selection theory. The theory shows us, time and again, life has a way of surviving harsh environments—meaning GE seeds are likely to yield less food because of surviving superweeds and superpests that evolve.

If this scenario played out, future crop yields would not sustain a population without outside help.

Is this hypothetical situation factually occurring?

Data appears to show the effects of GE seeds on human population are more than merely hypothetical. Especially if our seeds lose resistance to agricultural spray applications, national crop production could fail in a catastrophic way. Thereafter, we'd not be able to feed ourselves if a *limited GE seed bank supply* became nonresistive to superbugs, superweeds, and chemical sprays.

The question everyone wants to know is does this reality already exist?

It appears our GE crops are becoming resistive to commercial crop sprays, as verified by data showing increased demand in herbicide use in the United States over a thirteen-year period (1996 to 2008) by 383 million pounds. Although much of these crops are used to feed livestock in wealthier countries, as opposed to people in poorer countries, the metabolized product in livestock is still being consumed within the world's markets one way or the other. "In 2008, GE crop acres required over 26 percent more pounds of pesticides per acre than acres planted to conventional varieties. And the equivalent of 318 million more pounds of pesticides over the last 13 years as a result of planting GE seeds" (Benbrook 2009).

The manipulation of crop seeds and foods is also having an impact on the *antibiotic-resistive* gene characteristic relative to health data. In other words, GE crop seeds have increasing potential to cause a rise of drug-resistant supergerms in human DNA.

According to an article by Sean Poulter:

> Scientists now fear that GM foods, which are often modified to be resistant to antibiotics, will leave Britons vulnerable to untreatable illnesses ...
>
> Geneticist Dr. Antoniou of Guy's Hospital, London said ... "Bacteria in the gut are going to take up genes that will make them resistant to potentially therapeutic antibiotics.

"The possibility is that someone who picked up the antibiotic resistance through food and then fell ill, that a medical antibiotic might not be effective." (Poulter 2016)

The focus here was not to prove GE seeds, processed foods, and crop spays are going to make everyone sick and lead to world famine. Instead, it was to realize these things are connected, and food choice may make a difference in how you look, feel, and behave.

Man-Made Foods and Ingredients to Avoid

A good rule of thumb is that, if you can't pronounce a label ingredient and/or don't recognize the word, it's likely a chemical preservative, additive, dye, bleach, or the like or a sight, taste, and smell enhancer. Or if you don't want to read labels or are short on shopping time, avoid purchasing highly decorative and attractive packaging or premade meals. Any whole foods without organic certification are much better than highly processed convenience foods or fast food. The more processed a food, the greater the odds it's loaded with unhealthy stuff.

What do I personally consider to be the "worst" of food ingredients likely to contain both GMOs and food chemicals—which significantly increase health risk and cause weight gain? I personally make an effort to stay away from certain foods or ingredients whenever possible.

The worst GE crop foods likely come from corn and soy and other crops grown in the United States and their oils. And the worst chemical additives often used to make hyperpalatable and addictive foods are HFCS (high fructose corn syrup), which is also likely processed from GE corn crops. Other bad food ingredients, as you're now aware, include any artificial sweetener and trans fats and should be avoided whenever possible.

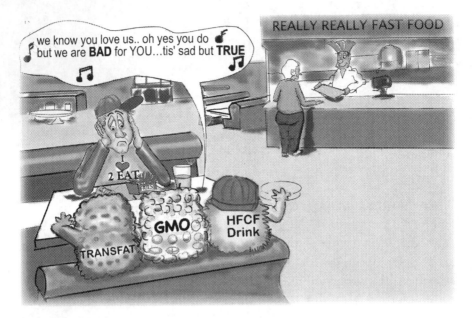

Other food chemicals are known to be unhealthy for us. Sodium nitrate, for example, is used as a preservative and is highly carcinogenic once in the digestive system. MSG (monosodium glutamate) is a highly addictive taste intensifier and causes us to eat more by disengaging the "I'm full" function of the neurological brain pathway. BHA (butylated hydroxyanisole) and BHT (butylated hyrdoxytoluene) are other preservatives that have potential to cause cancer and affect our neurological systems. Sulfur dioxide is an additive that is considered toxic by the FDA, and its use on raw fruits and vegetables is prohibited. Potassium bromate is used to increase volume in some white flour and breads and known to cause cancer in animals.

Food dyes vary in potential harm to health, which includes behavioral problems for children. The worse dyes appear to be Blue No. 1 and No. 2 (E133), Red No. 3 (and also Red No. 40) (E124), Yellow No. 6 (E110), and Yellow No 5 (Tartrazine) (E102). Laboratory studies with animals show these dyes cause forms of chromosomal damage and/or tumors and/or neurological disorder and are a potential cause of cancer (Bosch 2010).

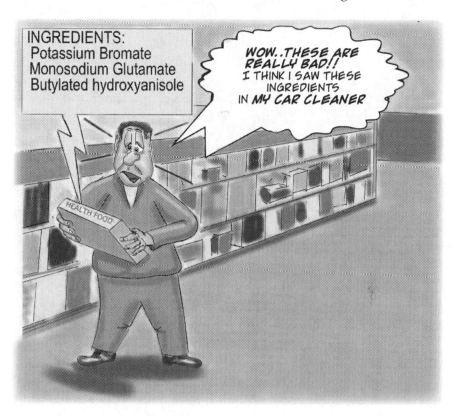

How GM Foods and Steroids End Up in Dairy Products

It's one thing to feed GM crops to livestock and another to inject hormones into dairy cows. Yes, humankind has even engineered drugs to stimulate dairy cows to produce more milk.

In 1990, Monsanto revealed a study that showed significant evidence of the growth-promoting effects of rBGH (recombinant bovine growth hormone—steroids). It revealed that systemic effects at low doses of rBGH in mature rats increased body weight, liver weight, and bone length. Regardless of the data, the product was approved for dairy milk production. And the FDA was reluctant to mandate labeling practices that showed consumers whether or not dairy milk products were produced using cows injected with rBGH. There were also many lawsuit attempts by Monsanto to stop producers and retailers from listing this information on product labels—similar to GM food label law measures.

The FDA continues to stand by Monsanto's synthetically engineered product(s) as safe for human consumption. It appears this company has a monopoly interest in our dairy milk production, as in its GE seeds and aspartame business as previously covered in chapter 7. Now you understand the Goliath consumers are up against and how deep those pockets are.

But this does not mean other countries have to purchase American dairy products like GE foods. Twenty-seven nations in the European Union, as well as Australia, Japan, New Zealand, and Canada, do not purchase American milk, yogurt, ice cream, cheese, and other dairy products that have been produced using rBGH synthetic steroids. "Hormone-treated milk is different from non-treated milk because it contains increased levels of the hormone IGF-1, which promotes cancer tumors" (Mercola 2010). The article goes on to say that, according to Dr. Samuel Epstein, "Excess levels of IGF-1 have been incriminated as major causes of breast, colon, and prostate cancers" (Mercola 2010).

"The European Commission commissioned two independent committees of internationally recognized experts to undertake a comprehensive review of the scientific literature on both the veterinary and public health effects of rBGH. The veterinary committee fully confirmed and extended the Canadian warnings and conclusions. The public health committee confirmed earlier reports of excess levels of the naturally occurring Insulin-like-Growth Factor One (IGF-1), including its highly potent variants, in rBGH milk and concluded that these posed major risks of cancer, particularly of the breast and prostate" (Epstein 1999).

The good news is there are now states within the United States that label dairy products with a "no rBGH" identifier.

Consumers Are Connecting the Food and Health Risk Dots

Today's public is very educated and concerned about the quality of foods their children are consuming. As a result, *organic* yesteryear farming practices are seeing a renaissance. School and community garden education, organic city growing gardens, and local farmers' markets are reaching an all-time high in popularity. This brings with it a renewed hope the US Department of Agriculture and US Department of Health and Human Services will continue to make positive policy changes for the sake of healthy food education and choice. This effort is partly the result of a changing federal government farm bill. The bill provides the resources necessary to communities that benefit organic farmers, farmers' markets, and healthier food choices in school cafeterias. This includes outdoor garden growing education and practices offered within K–12 schools.

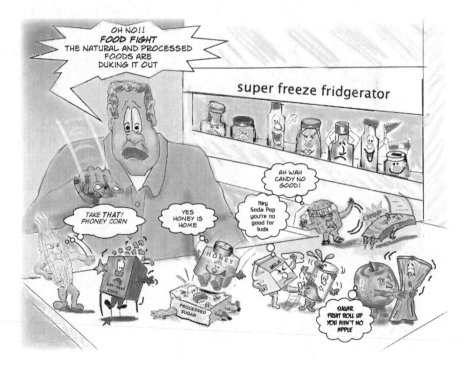

The bill also provides resources to local farming communities and an assortment of qualified organizational and regional food distribution centers that can apply for federal farm-to-market program grants.

As of 2012–2013, under the Obama administration, the farm bill in its development looking forward had a wish list of thirty-five provisions supported by 260 organic farming and educational organizations who endorsed a revised farm bill for the following five to seven years. "The Agriculture Act of 2014 passed the Senate with an overwhelming bipartisan majority of 68–32 on February 4th, 2014. The Farm Bill was signed into law on February 7th, 2014 and sets national agriculture, nutrition, conservation, and forestry policy" (US Senate Committee 2014).

Complementing a great farm bill, schools began a unique fitness campaign on February 9, 2010, led by Michelle Obama. The campaign focused on resolving childhood obesity. Her campaign mission was to encourage healthier food choices in schools, better food labeling practices, and more physical activity for kids.

This campaign initiative is a clear indicator that Washington recognized our country had a childhood obesity problem and that communities required healthy lifestyle education and program resources to reverse what some health experts now fear is an era of childhood obesity epidemic.

I attended Michelle Obama's Let's Move Phase II program— as presented during the National League of Cities Conference, in Washington, DC, March 9–13, 2013. During the conference the First Lady spoke of an expanded initiative to reverse childhood obesity, with the goal of encouraging students to engage in at least sixty minutes of exercise activity daily. The second phase also included a public-private partnership that sought to involve fifty thousand school nutritional food programs nationwide over the next five years.

Regardless of political views, it's hard to disagree these policies wouldn't have a net positive impact over time on the health and productivity of future generations.

Personal Fitness Challenge: "Remit Disease Naturally"

Although I couldn't save one hip from replacement, the thought of losing the other motivated me to find a way to preserve its functional integrity as long as possible. I believed it was possible to slow down avascular necrosis (AVN) progression and put it into remission, provided I made some lifestyle changes.

What exactly is AVN and what is the mechanism that destroys the hip and other long bones in the body? "Avascular necrosis is the death of bone tissue due to a lack of blood supply. Also called osteonecrosis, avascular necrosis can lead to tiny breaks in the bone and the bone's eventual collapse. The blood flow to a section of bone can be interrupted if the bone is fractured or the joint becomes dislocated. Avascular necrosis of bone is also associated with long-term use of high-dose steroid medications and excessive alcohol intake" (Mayo Clinic 2015).

When I was diagnosed with avascular necrosis, I immediately wanted to know what had caused it. The cause of my AVN disease was determined by substantiated medical evidence and findings confirmed by military medical review board. The cause was the use of steroids (prednisone and cortisone) prescribed by medical doctors over a period of time—around eight years. The steroids were used to treat severe reactions to contact dermatitis during field training exercises (service connected). In other words, I'd frequently had an allergic reaction to poison oak, ivy, and sumac during field training exercises prominent in the Northwest.

There were behaviors and habits I changed to give the body a fighting chance to preserve the salvageable hip—especially after bone graft surgery. However, I wasn't 100 percent sure at first what type of fitness activities, diet, and other lifestyle changes I'd make to prolong the health and durability of that hip.

After many medical consultations, I learned it was possible to have a successful bone graft that could last long-term. Although I understood the graft would be painful (and would include a long recovery window and no guarantee of success), I went for it. Later on, I also believed that, if I didn't make certain lifestyle changes, I'd lose the grafted hip to another total hip replacement, which could possibly lead to a worse mobility situation.

Eventually I concluded that, if I practiced what I preached, I might be able to further preserve bone health and integrity and possibly remit disease for a longer period of time. It was clear that sitting on the sideline and continuing a sedentary lifestyle was not a choice.

The way I went about making healthier lifestyle changes was based on medical, health, nutrition, and other scientific data. And I checked myself on my current behavioral habits.

I first began the process of researching and targeting obvious GE foods and food chemicals that could be removed from the diet. Then I focused on healthy bone nutrients, which led me to study free radical activators and antioxidant supplementation.

I also researched articles that studied the relationship between oxygen and cancer. "Nobel Prize winner Dr. Otto Warburg famously hypothesized '… the prime cause of cancer is the replacement of the respiration of oxygen in normal body cells by a fermentation of sugar,' meaning, cancer is caused by a lack of oxygen. Today's modern cancer cell biology has shown he was on the right track as mitochondrial health and shifting to a more oxygen-rich environment may protect healthy cells and further neuter cancer cells" (Envita Medical Center n.d.). If cancer can't survive in an oxygenated environment, I reasoned, then maybe AVN could be put into remission through more aerobic walking activity, which would circulate more oxygen-enriched blood into the hip area. There are no scientific studies that correlate directly to my line of reasoning. I was grasping at straws.

Regardless, I immediately gravitated toward low-impact aerobic walking exercise to increase oxygenated blood flow to the hip area and to also reduce excess body fat.

I did find a lot of circumstantial evidence that connected antioxidants, aerobic exercise, balanced diet, and habit changes—a combination *I believed* would keep this disease from progressing to other long bones of the body. Maybe the cure for me was 50 percent belief. Who knows for sure? I did believe, and I still do today, that antioxidants have powerful healing agents found in certain foods and supplements. And those antioxidants have earned the coveted *super* in my vocabulary for their healing benefits.

Why do we need antioxidants in our diet? According to Harvard School of Public health:

> We … extract free-radical fighters from food. These defenders are often lumped together as "antioxidants." They work by generously giving electrons to free radicals without turning into electron-scavenging substances themselves.
>
> There are hundreds, probably thousands, of different substances that can act as antioxidants. The most familiar ones are vitamin C, vitamin E, beta-carotene, and other related carotenoids, along with the minerals selenium and manganese. (HSPS 2016)

To be sure I gave my grafted hip a fair shot at survival, I abstained from alcoholic beverages for five years and avoided prescription steroids like the plague. Why? These are two ways long bones in the body can be compromised by the disease. If there was any possibility alcohol or steroids would act as a chemical oxidant accelerator in my grafted hip, I wanted no part of it. That's how important it was for me to save it over the next five years following surgery. Why did I pick five years? I just picked a number.

There was no medical doctor who could guarantee my lifestyle changes would save the grafted hip and prevent it from collapsing like the other one. But not one of the doctors I consulted said it could hurt. I was convinced I'd likely extend the life of the grafted hip if I changed my lifestyle. I believed I could improve the situation. That belief gave me the courage, strength, and willpower to accept a long-term recovery and pain challenge to get healthy and get mobility back sooner, rather than later.

Only time would tell if I'd made the right decisions. I was strong in spiritual faith and believed it possible to achieve the impossible. And should I fail, I could accept a higher power had other plans and purpose for me. However, *I didn't focus on failure.* Throughout those five years, I challenged myself to increase my walking distances. Some warned me not to get my hopes up or advised me to slow down, lest I worsen my condition, or issued other words of caution.

I know those who emphasized caution wanted to protect me and didn't want to see me in pain or cause further health risks and complications. But I felt I had good factual information and resolve most couldn't relate to. For instance, I knew our bodies naturally produce free radicals on a daily basis from stress, bad health, contaminated air, viruses, bacteria, and chemicals from foods and drugs that greatly increase the oxidative burden on healthy cells and cells under repair.

By deductive reasoning, it was not so hard to relate to how our biochemical transmitter exchanges and cells could be influenced, irritated, and inflamed through environmental pollutants. Nor was it hard to see how these environmental oxidative burdens increase the risk of acquiring any number of diseases—including AVN. (For related topics, see chapter 15, "Antiaging and Physical Performance-Enhancement Truths".)

After all, "oxidative damage and free radicals are associated with a number of diseases including atherosclerosis, Alzheimer's disease, cancer, ocular disease, diabetes, rheumatoid arthritis and motor neuron disease. Many studies have shown the benefit of antioxidants in the prevention or delaying the course of these diseases" (Hajhashemi et al. 2010).

It just made sense—if antioxidants could prevent or delay rheumatoid arthritis and other immune diseases, why not AVN? So I ate fruits and vegetables every day and took a multivitamin and other antioxidant supplements—which I still do to this day.

Antioxidant protection and aerobic exercise as preventative medicine in a clean-air and low-stress environment are now a large part of my lifestyle. What I've learned is that environment has far more free radical generators than most are aware.

Environmentally, things have changed for the worse over the last two hundred years. We have more external toxins, called "free radical generators" by researcher Jeffrey Blumberg, PhD, professor of nutrition at Tufts University in Boston. "When you follow the USDA's advice to eat multiple servings of fruits and vegetables, you're compensating for the effects of environmental toxins. Your body simply doesn't produce enough antioxidants to do all that, says Blumberg" (Davis 2006).

And the effects of these oxidative burdens on bodies are greater in big cities, partly related to air quality. If you live in a big city, you are more likely to develop cancer, lung or heart disease, and Alzheimer's and Parkinson's disease because of the environmental oxidative burden.

"Multivitamins and vitamin supplements can provide the body with an antioxidant boost. Fruits, vegetables, whole grains, legumes, and nuts contain complex mixes of antioxidants, and therein lays the benefit of eating a variety of healthy foods, says Blumberg" (Davis 2006).

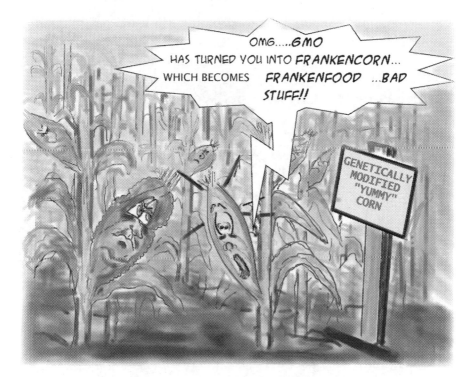

Data on antioxidants show they have potential to significantly slow down oxidative damage at a cellular level. Therefore, antioxidant supplementation may serve as a good prevention practice to keep the body's immune system in tip-top shape and decrease the risk of disease.

But in the same breath, I also understand that, because of genetic predisposition, disease is not always preventable, regardless of preventative practices. For example the oxygen from the air we breathe "can produce highly reactive compounds called reactive oxygen species (ROS). Many such reactive species are free radicals containing an unpaired electron. They have a tendency to either accept or donate an electron and are, therefore, unstable and highly reactive" (Hajhashemi et al. 2010). Through the mere act of breathing, we may inadvertently take in various free radical air species of various compositions that may affect DNA cell health and cause disease when we are predisposed genetically.

There is no test to determine who's genetically sensitive to ROS. However, with genome technology advancements, one day it may be possible to prescribe an antioxidant treatment cocktail that targets and repairs cells at the atomic level to slow down disease and aging and extend life.

Exactly How Do Antioxidants Work?

Thinking of the human cell as an apple in analogy makes it easier to understand how antioxidant food varieties sustain better health and improve longevity and mobility.

For example, when the skin of the apple is removed, the apple begins to oxidize and turn brown quickly after exposed to air. At this point, the fruit cells begin to spoil and die. The protective skin of an apple slows down the cellular oxidization process. Let's break down this concept to an atomic level:

> The nucleus of an atom is surrounded by a cloud of electrons. These electrons surround the nucleus in pairs, but, occasionally, an atom loses an electron, leaving it with an unpaired electron. The atom is then called a "free radical," or sometimes just a "radical," and is very reactive. When cells in the body encounter a radical, the reactive radical may cause destruction in the cell. According to the free radical theory of aging, cells continuously produce free radicals, and constant radical damage eventually kills the cell. When radicals kill or damage enough cells in an organism, the organism ages. (Nelson n.d.)

When cells age prematurely or die within a grouping of healthy ones, it is then possible for disease to proliferate to malignancy and then metastasis to another area of the body. As our apple analogy can predict, one bad apple can spoil the bunch. However, when enough antioxidant shielding, or replacement electrons are provided, like replacing bad apples with good ones, the risk of disease or progression of spoilage may be significantly slowed down or put into remission.

Oxidation is a natural process of metabolism. And through this process, 1 to 2 percent of our cells get damaged daily and need repair to acquire a missing molecule to keep free radicals, more or less, from causing severe damage to other cells around them. When an oxygen molecule (O2) becomes electrically charged or radicalized, it tries to steal electrons from other molecules. "The damage to cells caused by free radicals, especially the damage to DNA, may play a role in the development of cancer and other health conditions" (NIH 2014). And I believe this includes AVN disease.

You now know that the oxygen you breathe, the company you keep, place you work and exercise, and the foods and drugs you consume *all* affect cells electrically and chemically and may alter DNA. If antioxidant insurance is not part of the healthy lifestyle equation, one way or the other, cellular health is at increased risk of compromise.

What you need to know is that antioxidants can be found in a large variety of organic plant and animal foods that can be consumed to protect cells from the worst oxidative damage.

It is also noteworthy that antioxidants are not interchangeable and don't shield all oxidative damage occurring throughout the body. An abundant variety of natural whole foods can balance out the body's antioxidant needs. "When the amount of antioxidant substances equals or exceeds the amount of pro-oxidants, the body can prevent cellular damage and maintain stability. If pro-oxidant chemicals increase well beyond the level of antioxidants, the body is unable to keep up and oxidative stress results" (Lee 2016).

Another way to look at this is that it takes a village of antioxidants from organic whole foods to fortify immune system and cellular DNA health. Although it's inevitable that our environment will cause us to become sick at some point in time, it is also true that a variety of dietary antioxidants is more likely to delay the scourges of aging, as opposed to accelerating it.

In 2008, I sold my Sacramento home and moved back to northern Oregon, partly because of the bad air and water quality I felt was detrimental to my long-term recovery and mobility challenges.

I further reasoned that by keeping pro-oxidants at bay with more antioxidants, it was possible to keep the grafted hip for a longer period of time. Since I understood the bad apple in a barrel analogy, I knew if I didn't shield the bone graft at the cellular level, it might not take or last for the long term.

I believe the lifestyle changes I made remitted and slowed the progression of AVN, since it was diagnosed in 2003 in both hips. To this day, the salvaged hip is still holding its functional integrity, despite the fact that the disease had destroyed the other hip before diagnosis. I feel the healthy lifestyle changes paid off. Doctors originally told me the 2004 bone graft might last at best five to seven years. Thereafter, I'd likely need a second total hip replacement.

Although I'm challenged with progressive arthritis in the grafted hip, the AVN is still in a state of remission and has affected no other long bones in my body. As far as I'm concerned, I found a silver bullet lifestyle solution that continues to keep the disease at bay.

In closing this section, I'd like to share a small sampling of foods with high antioxidant properties I enjoy—foods that also support weight-loss goals.

It is encouraging to note there are multiple findings mentioned in medical journals and institutional research papers that show us foods high in antioxidants can provide protection against disease and slow down aging. Recall, "abundant evidence suggests that eating whole fruits, vegetables, and whole grains—all rich in networks of antioxidants and their helper molecules—provides protection against many of these scourges of aging" (HSPS 2014).

However keep the following information in perspective. Just because I list a food as high in antioxidants, as well as popular with some dieters, does not mean I'm recommending these foods for losing weight quickly (see chapter 5, "Caloric Exchange: A Balancing Act). Hopefully, the following food tips will encourage you to seek a plethora of other healthy food choices high in antioxidant nutrients.

Below I've listed two high antioxidant foods that also provide quality protein—two out of hundreds I could have listed—and one good antioxidant drink. The choices below were part of my weight loss and antioxidant favorites food plan but not specifically listed in chapter 10, "Choose Favorite Foods to Lose Weight":

Pumpkin – There are many weight-loss recipes based on pumpkin because it provides a high source of fiber and low fat, with high concentrates of vitamin A, beta-carotene, antioxidants, and iron. Health benefits include reduced risk of heart disease, lowering of cholesterol, improved vision, improved digestion, and a feeling of fullness. It also supports healthy immune system, lungs, and kidneys (Corleone 2014). Enhance flavor with cinnamon (a blood sugar reducer) for a filling and delicious treat.

Range-fed beef – Range-fed beef is a great organic food choice that doesn't contain antibiotics and is not raised on genetically engineered crops or injected with steroids. It is a high source of protein, lean in fat, and has more conjugated linoleic acid (which means reduced risk of heart disease and cancer). Range-fed beef is high in omega-3 and has more vitamins, such as vitamin E, than does its non-range-fed counterpart. "Grass-fed beef may have some heart-health benefits that other types of beef don't have" (Mankad 2014).

Green tea – Green tea is rich in antioxidants; promotes healthy heart, digestion, blood sugar regulation, and body temperature; raises metabolic rate; and accelerates the fat-burning process. Five cups a day is said by some to be the ultimate fat and weight-loss solution by boosting metabolism. Green tea is also a natural relaxer and relieves stress. Research shows preventative health properties in atherosclerosis; high cholesterol; cancer (bladder, breast, ovarian, colorectal, esophageal, lung, pancreatic, prostate, skin, and stomach); inflammatory bowel disease; diabetes; liver disease; and more.

"Researchers think the health-giving properties of green tea are mostly due to polyphenol chemicals with potent antioxidant properties… that give it its somewhat bitter taste. In fact, the antioxidant effects of polyphenols seem to be greater than vitamin C" (UMMC 2016).

I understand that my disease is permanent; it's simply not progressing. And those bone cells, like apples in a barrel, can become tainted very easily and reactivated at any time to destroy the grafted hip or spread elsewhere in my body.

I know that, if I can manage and remove unnecessary free radical generators through daily aerobic exercise and sustain a balanced antioxidant diet in a clean-air environment, I feel I have control over this particular disease. And that peace of mind alleviates stress on other parts of my encompassing being and sustains my state of well-being.

Chapter 15

Antiaging and Physical Performance-Enhancement Truths

> Physical activity releases natural body chemicals that support fitness goals.
>
> —MirrorAthlete Principled Fitness and
> Healthy Lifestyle Philosophy

A major fat burning and antiaging truth resides within our body's ability to release natural stress-reducing, pain-relieving, fat-burning, and mood-enhancing chemicals during and after exercise activity. And when exercise is performed with frequency, activation of natural body chemicals also provides the motivation and willpower to repeat the habit daily.

Regardless of your fitness level or physical capability, it is important to keep in mind that any "exercise reduces levels of the body's stress hormones, such as adrenaline and cortisol. It also stimulates the production of endorphins, the body's natural painkillers and mood elevators. Aerobic exercise is the key for your head, just as it is for your heart. It has a unique capacity to exhilarate and relax, to provide stimulation and calm, to counter depression and dissipate stress" (Harvard University 2011). And when body chemicals are in balance, they are the catalysts that sustain the willpower needed to achieve and sustain good health, well-being, and a good fitness level.

To achieve any fitness goal, willpower researcher Roy Baumeister, PhD, a psychologist at Florida State University, describes three necessary components: First, he says, you need to establish the motivation for change and set a clear goal. Second, you need to monitor your behavior toward that goal. The third component is willpower. "Willpower is the ability to resist short-term temptations in order to meet long-term goals" (APA 2016).

By learning more about chemicals that are naturally produced by the body, you not only learn their effect on well-being, behavior, and willpower; you also understand how important they are to the regulation of body metabolism and brain function. And when those chemicals are out of balance, unhealthy habits, negative mood, and health risks often ensue.

So how many body chemical substances and reactions occur within the approximately 37 trillion cells of an adult body? Well, there are too many to list to tell the truth. But one need only require knowledge of a few key neurotransmitter substances and their effect on metabolic function to relate to how important total body chemical balance is to the way you look, feel, and behave.

"There are many types of chemicals that act as neurotransmitter substances" to excite or inhibit movement of internal signals at neuron gaps. "Communication of information between neurons is accomplished by movement of chemicals across a small gap called the synapse" (Chudler 2014).

To further explain the importance of these internal neuron signals and body chemical balance, I'm integrating a personal story. The relative points made will further divulge how the antiaging and physical performance-enhancement industries target products to young and old alike. And it will demonstrate how people's health and well-being continue to be compromised as a result of man-made chemical products.

Competitive Sports and Bodybuilding and Remembering Sam

My brother Mike and I and a few close friends worked out with a chap named Sam in the late seventies. This was an era when bodybuilding was in its growth stage, and the internet was still decades away. The mentality of the day, as it still does, held that the more ripped and bulked in appearance, the bigger the boost to egos and admiration of others.

During the day, I recalled looking into gym mirrors to monitor my lifting technique and note improved muscular tone and development. Hence the term mirror athlete was born. That is, we weren't all athletes, but we looked the part.

Many believed that if they could achieve ripped muscular symmetry and a powerful-appearing stature, they were equivalent to athletes. But nothing could be further from the truth. For instance, posing in a bodybuilding competition didn't mean the bodybuilder had the skill sets or motor control to be a sports competitor. Nor was the person necessarily healthy.

It was Darrel "Mouse" Davis, a retired American football coach and former player, who laid out the value and worth of athletic appearance versus competitive skill sets. After an impressive yard-gaining scrimmage for the fullback position with Portland State Viking football in 1979, I asked him, "Why did you place me second string?"

Without blinking an eye, he made the snarky remark. "Did you see the size of Goodman's arms? I have to play him."

This response entertained a few student athletes who were on a work-study program at the college and overheard the conversation. This egged him on to continue the same lame logic, which he did. "Look. He's on scholarship, and you're not. Plus, those guns—I have to play him."

I struggled to understand the meaning of the conversation in the moment. Eventually it would make sense. I shared those snarky remarks with other players who didn't place on the first-string roster—where some of them, like myself, should have been. In essence, I learned they'd received a similar message from Davis. Although he never mentioned steroids, athletes understood the meaning of his message. I believed Davis's statements were code for "Get on the juice, or you can't compete at this level of play." Now maybe he was oblivious to steroids during the day and had strange logic in placing players on first string, but that was not the word on the street.

In my opinion, Goodman moved like a slug and looked like a bodybuilder on steroids. He could carry three players one to two yards past the scrimmage line before he dropped. I guess that was worth something.

After preseason training and tryouts, my assumptions would prove to be true. Although I outscrimmaged Goodman for yardage during spring tryouts, that didn't matter. I was placed on the second-string roster because I didn't have a scholarship and didn't have the physical bulk of Goodman. Davis's statement and actions spoke loud and clear to me in 1979.

I eventually decided I wouldn't stick around to sit on the sidelines or risk my health to make first string on the football team the following year. At this time I made the decision to stop playing football and pursue other interests. For me, this was a hard decision. After all, I was considered an exceptional player—with the state high school stats to prove it. I had received five scholarships from college football scouts—handed to me by Tigard High head football coach Deno Edwards. I could play at a college of my choice.

Later, I'd regret not taking one of those opportunities to play football at a smaller college. In short, I wanted to stay home close to family and friends and didn't see any reason I couldn't compete as a walk-on at a larger college. But unbeknownst to me, the odds were stacked against me by athletes who cheated to gain a physical and performance advantage.

I also tried out for the Portland State baseball team as a walk-on and was in contention for first-string catcher. My father didn't know this because I never told him. Weeks before the first game, I informed the baseball coach I was quitting the training camp. The head baseball coach was very upset with my decision. He informed me I was walking away from a starting lineup. It wasn't that I didn't want to play either sport. I just felt so betrayed by Davis's words and actions and the gravity of the situation. In the moment, I just wanted out of sports.

Alas, the dream of getting drafted onto a professional football or baseball team slipped through my fingers, as it had for so many other athletes and for different reasons.

Although many bodybuilders would claim their profession is a sport, I'm not here to argue that point. I understand the way bodybuilding, fitness enthusiasts, and athletic and sports-minded people think and act and what motivates them. Whether bodybuilding is a sport or not, it was something I enjoyed doing and could continue outside of organized sports. And it wouldn't take long to connect the steroid dots used in high school and then college all the way up to the professionals—once I began dabbling with the idea of becoming a competitive bodybuilder.

Again disappointment struck. Natural bodybuilding competitions weren't sacred; they had cheaters as well.

I followed the most famous bodybuilders—Arnold Schwarzenegger, Rachel McLish, Lou Ferrigno, Lee Haney, Dorian Yates, and Ronnie Coleman—and copied their exercise routines. Arnold was the most famous, starring in movies such as *Conan the Barbarian, Terminator,* and *True Lies* and becoming California governor, not to mention that he was a seven-time Mr. Olympia champion (1970–1075, 1980). Rachel McLish took the Ms. Olympia title twice (1980, 1982). Lou Ferrigno starred in *The Incredible Hulk* series from 1978 to 1982. Competitive bodybuilder Lee Haney was an eight-time Mr. Olympia titleholder (1984–1991). Dorian Yates took the Mr. Olympia title six times (1992–1997). And Ronnie Coleman held the Mr. Olympia title eight times (1998–2005).

Almost everyone I spoke to knew of these famous people and worked hard to achieve physiques like theirs. And quite frankly, some, including myself, believed we could achieve those results once we acquired and applied similar diet and exercise knowledge.

The bodybuilding industry continues to churn out a few Mr. and Ms. Olympia winners each year. And of the many who try, only a handful succeeds. Those who don't make the big league have less stellar careers as sports coaches, bodybuilding trainers, fitness trainers, healthy lifestyle or wellness coaches, or similar positions with other creative titles.

Don't get me wrong, many of these professions provide excellent fitness, health, nutrition, posing, and competitive sports training services and products, and many of its practitioners make a good living at it. But it's those who care more about profit than client that one needs to be leery or suspicious of.

Those famous bodybuilders, as well as current ones, promote training secrets within one of many Joe Weider magazines, for example, *Muscle & Fitness, Flex, Men's Fitness,* and *Shape.* Today there are a plethora of other magazines and internet site knockoffs with similar information selling the same pitches and products.

The most popular bodybuilding go-to source I recall at the time was Weider's *Muscle & Fitness.* The magazines, featuring those training routines, were shared in strength-training facilities like the ones I used for thirty plus years. Today, those gyms have been mostly replaced by fitness franchises and HIIT (high-intensity interval training) programs, including "ninja warrior" obstacle courses and the like.

Back then, if you wanted to compete in bodybuilding you'd seek one-on-one training services from a semiprofessional bodybuilder, sports athlete, or gym owner. As I later learned, these people had direct pipelines to steroids from shady pharmaceutical dealers in Mexico. The last place bodybuilding hopefuls would go to get a steroid fix was a doctor, because it was difficult to get a prescription. To be blunt, doctors weren't likely to prescribe a hundred to five hundred times an average steroid dose, even if there was medical reason. I did hear that some doctors would agree to prescribe those dosages, but patients had to allow the doctor to monitor their health weekly—and with a hefty price tag attached.

Looking back, I see that the odds of my making it as a natural athlete in professional football or the professional bodybuilding circuit were against me. I was very lean and muscular at a range of 188 to 192 pounds, standing five foot eleven. At the time, I needed to gain at least ten pounds of muscle and improve my forty-yard sprint speed, moving it from 4.8 seconds to 4.6 or 4.7 second in order to have a shot at professional football playing the position of running back or defensive safety. And that wasn't going to happen naturally within a three-year period no matter how hard I trained or what I ate. Because of my body type and metabolism, I may have been able to get there using steroids. But at what cost?

I know some were willing to risk their health and possibly life for the opportunity to achieve the riches and glory they craved. And Sam was one of those people who bought into this ideal—hook, line, and sinker. He wasn't even what anyone would've considered a competitive athlete of any type. He became the poster boy of all that could go wrong trying to achieve the big-man-on-campus dream.

Sam was five foot five and weighed approximately 190 pounds. He was short in stature and somewhat chubby, with no striking facial features. My friends and I also noticed he'd often make negative statements about his physical attributes. He seemed desperate to change his appearance and followed Arnold Schwarzenegger's diet and exercise programs found in the monthly Weider magazine.

Here's what I saw—a nice guy with a great sense of humor. Sam was a person you'd what to hang around with because of his good nature and charismatic personality. Even though he was slightly chubby, he was also fairly strong for his frame, with better-than-average looks.

Sam had what you'd call a short man's complex. He'd always say things like, "If only I could grow another five inches and have 22.5-inch python biceps like Arnold."

He often talked about the look-alike Arnolds in the gym in an unflattering tone. It was obvious he envied their physiques. He was fixated on what muscle-bulking and strength secrets they were hiding from everyone else, only known to a small inner circle.

After a period of time, Sam stopped working out with our group of regulars, which included Ron, Kevin, and Mike.

He pursued an aggressive strength- and power-training routine after he entered the lair of bodybuilding enlightenment. Training with a popular instructor in the gym, he now had connections to other bodybuilding information and products we didn't have. Sam had taken his bodybuilding program to a whole new level, and we weren't invited. Basically, you had to pay to play as I eventually discovered. And this membership wasn't cheap. It cost about $400 a week in 1979!

In a short period of time, Sam's muscle and strength gains were impressive, unlike his changing personality. He appeared to put on fifteen pounds of muscle mass and lost a lot of body fat. His bench and squat presses increased at least a hundred pounds within a six-week period. He also became very aggressive, angry, and difficult to be around. My friends and I suspected he was taking some kind of steroid, which altered his physique and personality, but we couldn't prove it. He wasn't spilling the beans.

Since Sam was not very pleasant to be around at this time, we mostly stayed away and jokingly named him the angry Atlas. To tell you the truth, we began to get a little jealous of his gains. We wanted to know what he was doing. He wasn't sharing, and quite frankly, it pissed us off. In retrospect, I realize it was good he didn't share. We learned a valuable lesson through his recklessness, which kept all of us from thinking twice about sampling the Kool-Aid.

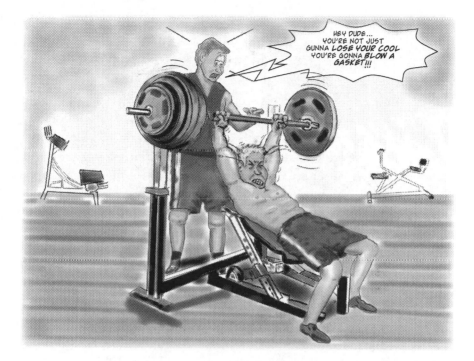

What was frustrating and hard to accept was that Mike and I were naturally more muscular and stronger than Sam. At the age of nineteen, I could free-weight bench 325 pounds, one to three reps unassisted, at 190-pound body weight. Ron and Kevin also stood taller and were more muscular than Sam. Their body weights and frames were similar to those of my brother and I, and they could both bench respectable weight and reps as well. Mike, at eighteen, was also a natural bodybuilder. He could bench-press an amazing 435 pounds, easily at two reps unassisted, and he weighed around 210 pounds. If I hadn't seen it, I wouldn't have believed it.

Before the juice, Sam could barely squeeze out a single rep of a 250-pound lift unassisted. He now could bench an assisted 350 pounds one time. It appeared he was gaining on Mike, who had the advantage in both muscular weight and height (at six foot one). Mike truly could have given Arnold a run for his money had he decided to train and compete in a pro bodybuilding circuit. Of course, he would have had to droid up to do it. "A common term used meaning – take a steroid product if you want to compete."

Sam made us all question what were we doing wrong and why we couldn't achieve similar results. For a while we even copied his exercise routine. But it made no difference in gains. If anything we were exhausting ourselves and losing muscle mass. We were perplexed by Sam's quick results. Soon his secrets would be known by all.

At the time, steroid and high-concentrate growth hormone use was a professional bodybuilder's closet secret. As we later discovered, there was a lot of money to be made as a steroid distributor and trainer. And those using them never voluntarily admitted it or divulged the supply channel. Distributors typically found those who fit the prospect profile.

Often the sales hook went something like this: "The only way you will compete against professional athletes and bodybuilders is to juice up." Sound familiar? Simply recall Mouse Davis's snarky undertones—size trumps natural athletic ability and performance.

If you were a desperate prospect and had means, someone in the gym with connections would find you. The guy would approach you in the following manner. "Need a spot for your next set?" Of course this flatters the prospect—a popular persona has shown an interest in you.

As the conversation continues it always leads to, "I'll let you in on a secret. Take my product and follow my training instruction without question and don't share this information with anyone ..."

Once a trainer had you, you'd not risk losing the product fix and opportunity to remain with the enlightened one.

How did the product supply chain work? Through time, I learned gym owners moonlighted as steroid distributors. They'd make monthly runs to Mexico and then resupply their employees (paid trainers). If the owner discovered a trainer going rogue, those steroid connections were cut off, and employment was terminated.

Now all eyes were on Sam—just what his ego needed. He was in the inner circle. His muscle head dreams were now being realized as the mini-Schwarzenegger look-alike. But there was one thing he couldn't change, and that was his height. We believe this physical shortcoming ultimately caused an obsessive behavior brought about by a chemical imbalance in the brain through heavy steroid use. Although his muscle mass and strength gains were impressive, his bizarre behavior was undesirable and concerning to say the least.

When asking him what dietary supplements he was taking, he rudely said, "Well, du, I'm drinking Arnold's protein drink with raw egg mix and using his exercise routine. Check out the latest *Muscle & Fitness* mag he's in." This was easy to verify because the routine and drink was promoted in the latest Weider magazine. And for the most part, we could see he was using the same program.

So what did everybody start doing in the gym after Sam revealed some of these tips? We went out and bought the latest Joe Weider's *Muscle & Fitness* magazine. We copied the routines, bought the protein mix from the gym guy's display case, added raw eggs and bananas to the drink at home, and drank it before each workout. And we did whatever else the Olympia winner of the year would pedal. All that was missing were the secret ingredients—*injectable and oral steroids and growth hormones*!

We were motivated to keep up with Sam but, as stated earlier, couldn't make the gains. He still wouldn't reveal the secret he was hiding. After a while, we were done with Sam's antics and wanted nothing more to do with him. It became apparent his tips were as bogus as Weider's Olympic bodybuilding product testimonials (as we later discovered and still hold true today).

If you don't believe steroids aren't used for a competitive advantage— even at the high school level—please get educated on the facts for the sake of your son or daughter's long-term health.

There is no doubt natural bodybuilders and sports athletes train hard to achieve their fitness and performance results. But there is a competitive and health risk difference between athletes who chemically cheat to achieve a performance advantage over others and those who don't.

Lance Armstrong, one of the greatest cyclists of all time, is a perfect example of someone who used illegal drugs to achieve riches and fame. He was caught cheating and stripped of his seven Tour de France championships and his Olympic bronze medal (2000 Sydney Games) for using steroids and a blood booster called EPO, also known as erythropoietin. EPO is a glycoprotein hormone that controls red blood cell production. He also administered blood transfusions, better known as blood doping, as reported by the US Anti-Doping Agency. Thereafter, Mr. Armstrong was banned for life from professional cyclist circuits for using performance-enhancement drugs.

Sam was cheating in ways that were similar to the methods of other famous steroid users.

It wasn't long before we discovered Sam's steroid secret—after he no longer showed up at the gym. This was also about the time I had my conversation with Mouse Davis after tryouts for the football team. All this information came together within the same period of time, including my decision to quit college sports.

The jig was up, and Sam didn't want to talk to anyone about it. He just disappeared from the weight lifting scene. We finally confirmed his secret as revealed by a gym member who wised up to the dangers of steroid use. He wanted nothing more to do with it and came clean. This was an eye-opener for all who knew very little of such things.

Two months more had past, and no Sam. He wouldn't even answer phone calls from Mike or Kevin, who were considered his closest buddies. It was as if he had disappeared from planet earth.

Late one evening and months later, a broadcast from the county sheriff's department came on between television programs. I had recognized the individual with the mug shot in the Washington County prison uniform. My eyes instantly gravitated to the short, pudgy man with glasses. It was Sam, who ironically worked within the same county sheriff's corrections facility he was jailed in!

I found out that Sam had been arrested that evening on attempted murder charges and was being held without bail. This was simply unbelievable. What were the details? One could only speculate at the time. I was glued to the set until the news broadcast finished.

The next day, a dead calm hung over the gym. There was no audible chatter, only light whispering and the clinking of weights. The word was out that someone in the gym had been supplying Sam with high concentrates of illegal steroids and growth hormone transported in from Mexico. This was a shocking revelation at the time.

To this day, I don't know if Sam's supplier/distributer ever faced criminal charges. However, gym gossip highly suspected that the gym owner and/or a well-known trainer were involved. Not long after the local police investigation began, a popular trainer no longer worked at our gym. Like Sam, he just disappeared.

At some point after Sam's departure and prior to his arrest, he'd done the unthinkable. While stopped at a street intersection, he had pulled his service revolver from the glove compartment. He'd attempted to force a woman at gunpoint into the vehicle. Those who followed the trial heard from the prosecuting attorney that his intentions were to rape the woman. To the best of my understanding and recollection of the time, the victim defied his order to get into the car and ran away. As she did, Sam panicked and unloaded the revolver into her back. Luckily, she did not die.

Unfortunately for Sam, he got a steep prison sentence, lost his freedom, and his wife left him.

Why do I tell you this story? Everyone is motivated by something that steers his or her life in one direction or the other. This story serves as an example of how engineered chemicals addict and alter the body and brain.

Does this mean all performance-enhancement products will cause a psychotic episode or are some safer than others? I don't know how to respond to a question like that. I do know that genetically, metabolically, and hormonally the encompassing being is influenced and reactive to an imbalance of unnatural neurochemical substance changes. I also know that antiaging and enhancement products come in many chemical flavors, with an unknown degree of physical and mental health risk.

It's what people don't understand about human biology, unhealthy lifestyle, and consumer products that put some into a permanent hurt locker.

How Neurotransmitters and Hormone Chemicals Affect Brain and Body

Think of your nervous system as an integral communicator that makes use of electrochemical impulses through neural conduits or expressways from the central nervous system that influence physiological function within the brain and body. Fully comprehending this concept requires a basic understanding of how chemical balance or imbalance can increase or decrease healthy brain and body function and well-being.

For example, *dopamine* is produced by the brain and has an important neurotransmitter bodily function. It increases its synthesis production through exercise activity. It boosts positive behavior, cognition, motor activity, motivation, healthy sleeping patterns, good mood, learning capacity, and attention to detail.

Also during exercise, *serotonin* is synthesized within the CNS (central nervous system). "Research suggests that serotonin plays an important role in liver regeneration and acts as a mitogen (induces cell division) throughout the body." Serotonin's role as a neurotransmitter of the brain is to modulate anger, mood, aggression, sleep, sexuality, and appetite and optimize metabolism. This chemical is also found in mushrooms, plants, fruits, and vegetables (Depression Wiki, n.d.).

Then there's *adrenaline*. It is a production of two like chemicals—*norepinephrine* (regulates physical activity) and *epinephrine* (released through stress). Together, these two neurotransmitter chemicals activate and stimulate our fight-or-flight response by increasing pain tolerance and boosting oxygen levels through increased heart rate and blood pressure, designed so we can get out of a stressful situation or survive a shock injury.

Adrenaline is a neurotransmitter and hormone that acts on nearly all bodily tissues. It is produced by the adrenalin gland located above the kidneys and originates from neurons within the CNS (Boundless 2016).

Growth hormone (GH) function is to balance and sustain human growth and metabolism after puberty. Its role on body weight targets adipose (fat cells) receptor sites to stimulate the breakdown of the fatty triglyceride acids while suppressing body fat cells from absorbing more fat after you eat. "Fat cells (adipocytes), for example, have growth hormone receptors where GH stimulates them to break down triglyceride and suppresses their ability to take up and accumulate circulating lipids" (Bowen 2006).

"Growth hormone secretion is mainly regulated by the interplay of … neurohormones. In addition … many neurotransmitters and neuropeptides influence GH secretion mainly by acting at the hypothalamic level" (Ghigo et al. 1993). Men and women's development of healthy muscle and bone, body fat regulation, capacity for weight loss, sexual desire, and sense of well-being is largely dependent on the balanced release of several hormones by the pituitary gland via the hypothalamus.

"The hypothalamus receives information from many sources about the basic functions of your body … Among the information monitored by the hypothalamus is the level of various hormones in the blood … When these hormones drop below a particular level this stimulates the hypothalamus to release hormones. These hormones travel to the pituitary gland, acting as the signal to the pituitary gland to produce one or more of its hormones" (Harding 2015).

If the brain's hypothalamic sensory function does not release hormones to signal the pituitary gland to release needed body hormone(s), then that's going to have an impact on the body. The pituitary gland's primary signaling function is to regulate the thyroid gland.

The thyroid is a small gland in the neck no bigger than a medium-size butterfly. This gland's hormone influences other hormone-producing glands, which have an effect on weight and other important metabolic interactions and bodily functions. Without proper levels of *thyroxin* (the hormone produced from the thyroid glands), the BMR (basal metabolic rate) responsible for healthy body weight and overall well-being underperforms.

It is seen through patient and animal research that hypothyroidism (underactive thyroid gland) causes weight gain, depression, sluggishness, bad mood, unhealthy appearance, impotence, and water retention adding to excess weight and cellulite, pear-shaped figure, infertility, PMS, hardening of the arteries, cystic breasts and ovaries (including cancer), irritability, bad complexion, puffiness under the chin, forgetfulness, irritability, apathy, dry skin, intolerance to cold, and unhealthy hair, nails, and teeth. If only one-quarter of the thyroid hormone is produced, you may also suffer from chronic fatigue.

On the opposite end of the spectrum, hyperthyroidism causes an overactive thyroid gland condition that has the opposite effect on the body's metabolism. The "hyper" condition speeds up the metabolic process, causing underweight and hyperactive conditions for many who have this disorder.

Some may attempt to self-treat weight loss unsuccessfully, using diet pills or severely restricting caloric intake while performing high-impact exercise to drop weight quickly. Meanwhile, they may be unaware there are numerous overweight conditions caused by glandular and hormone malfunctions only treatable by an endocrinologist.

If the thyroid is normal and production of thyroxin is low, the cause of underperforming hypothalamus, pituitary, or thyroid glands may be other influences, such as diet, environment, bad habit, or genetic predisposition to specific illness and disease, to name a few.

Supply and Demand of Anabolic Steroids and Growth Hormone

Now you understand there are "many neurotransmitters and neuropeptides that influence GH secretion mainly by acting at the hypothalamic level" (Ghigo et al. 1993). And regulating multiple hormone production as naturally as possible is needed to keep the brain and body healthy.

Today, hormone treatment is considered by some the antiaging or fountain-of-youth science of the century. But these engineered steroidal or hormonal products and performance-enhancement products may not work. Or they might stop producing results once no longer taken. And artificially overstimulating natural hormone production may cause unwanted side effects and increase health risk.

Most of us don't need to supplement our bodies with a steroid or a like product, especially when we're not deficient of naturally produced hormones. However, this does not stop young and impressionable bodybuilders and athletes and anti-agers from pursuing and using GH and anabolic steroids without prescription, medical need, or supervision. Performance- and physical-enhancement products and those designed to give users a competitive edge are very tempting, especially for aspiring athletes and those in the antiaging community.

"Some athletes choose to inject HGH (human growth hormone) for its performance enhancing potential, though it is a banned substance in nearly every professional sport. I do not recommend injecting HGH however, due to the potential side effects, the cost and, more importantly, it's potential to cause more long-term harm than good. Besides, as we now know, taking such risks is unnecessary because if you eat and exercise correctly, you will *naturally* optimize your HGH" (Mercola 2013).

As medical doctors and scientists focus on the effects of HGH on humans and within animal studies, it is understood that this hormone, as well as the body's naturally produced androgen (testosterone) are very essential for good health. Not only do these hormones optimize metabolism; they activate the desired male and female characteristics— muscle mass, strong bones, sexual desire, reproduction, hair, skin, energy, obesity and diabetes prevention, and sense of well-being.

For instance, if a woman has lost the pituitary GH function because of a medical condition or surgery, this can be a major problem. The adrenal gland's signaling mechanisms to the ovaries is no longer telling them to stimulate the production of female hormones (GH, testosterone, progesterone, and estrogen). That's right. Small amounts of testosterone are produced in the ovaries and adrenal glands at one-tenth the amount produced in men's testes—which is essential for a woman's overall sense of well-being and good health (Rosick 2004).

The GH balance, like other interacting hormones within the brains and bodies of both men and women, is important. It too affects the way we feel and behave but can increase health risk, especially when self-administering without medical supervision.

Are Antiaging Products Bilking the Consumer and Increasing Health Risk?

Marketers and sales specialists often sell antiaging products that are not recognized by the American Board of Medical Specialties (ABMS) and the American Medical Association (AMA) as legitimate or that lacks approved studies to back claims about product benefits. This American Medical Board represents 150 certified medical specialties and has varying opinions on antiaging products, testimonials, and claims. The FDA, on the other hand, an agency of the US Department of Health and Human Services, regulates consumer products in the marketplace, such as food, prescription, over-the-counter pharmaceuticals, dietary products, tobacco, vaccines, veterinary products, and so on.

In chapter 2, antiaging was defined as science finding ways to slow down, prevent, or reverse aging through a more youthful, functioning metabolism. However:

> Anti-aging can be a difficult topic to address: a war is currently fought over the meaning of the term in research and medicine, and as a brand for products in an energetic and often fraudulent marketplace. Even mentioning anti-aging medicine is likely to prejudice many readers ...
>
> ... The issue is that these real anti-aging therapies don't exist yet: an entire industry of business and manufacture has

come into existence in advance of the products it should be selling, and somehow is still thriving. (Reason 2013)

What I want to make clear is that antiaging products and those who market and sell them are one thing. Medically approved treatment by medical doctors is something else entirely.

Consumers beware. Just because the FDA approves a product to market does not mean it's without health risk. The FDA also approves relabeling of products for treatment use other than originally intended. This is why due diligence in understanding what we put into our bodies is so important.

Seeing an American Medical Board stamp of approval on any antiaging or performance-enhancement product would be a powerful endorsement. But don't look for this stamp of approval on those products anytime soon. "Anti-aging medicine is not recognized as a specialty by the American Board of Medical Specialties. 'Using hormones to replace a deficiency is generally accepted by most physicians,' said Dr. Lawrence Phillips, an endocrinologist at Emory University Hospital. But using hormones to battle old age or improve health in non-deficient individuals is unproven'" (Rhone 2012).

Again, be leery of those who lay claim to the latest and greatest antiaging, weight-loss, and performance-enhancement drugs. If you feel a need to experiment with your body's metabolism, only do so under a doctor's watchful eye.

Although Sam's focus was not quick weight loss, his fitness goal was just as lofty. He wanted to develop bulk and strength rapidly. And for the most part, he did. Prior to recognizing Sam as a steroid user, we all talked about steroid users as engaging in a type of cheating; it was a conversation piece. Sam mentioned that he was appalled by them. That's why we didn't peg him initially as an abuser.

Most of us didn't know there was a pipeline of illegal steroids in our backyard. During that time, there was no internet, and we believed almost everything we read in the muscle magazines and what the gym owners and fitness trainers told us. Thinking back, I see that we were really naive about such things.

I saw Sam in a jail interview years after his incarceration. He was talking about his steroid use and how it had caused his behavior to change and why kids should steer clear of steroids.

The saddest part of all was that his crazy psychosis was only temporary, much like his strength and muscle size.

His demeanor during the interview was that of the same soft-spoken Sam everyone had known and loved prior to his detestable out-of-character act. Unfortunately, Sam's story is not unique.

It is factual to state that deaths, bizarre behaviors, and ruined lives have been the result of unfettered steroid and steroid-like product use. To learn more about steroid abuse and the associated health risks, simply type into any internet search engine a phrase such as "sports and steroid abuse," "athlete deaths and steroids," "steroids and health risk," or "youth on steroids." Tens of millions of articles will pop up.

Are There Legitimate and Safe Antiaging and Performance-Enhancement Products?

There is a small demographic that *may* need and benefit from hormone therapy administered by a medical specialist. However a risk-to-benefit medical analysis and quality-of-life discussion should occur between the patient and doctor to ensure safe treatment and use is applied to regulate hormone deficiency.

However, this type of use is not often the case. An article by Daniel DeNoon quotes the assessment Michael Pollak, MD, gave to WebMD: "Almost half of growth hormone sold today is not for hormone deficiency—it is for people who want to feel young again. They say, 'This may help me and it has no risks.' This study says, 'Nope, growth hormone at age-inappropriate levels may be dangerous'" (DeNoon 2002).

Unwanted health risk may present itself should anyone decide to treat with a relabeled brand performance and enhancement drug with or without medical supervision. One such enhancement supplement professional athletes sought out in the past is ASD (androstenedione). It was banned by the FDA. It was the consensus of medical doctors that supplements like DHEA (dehydroepiandrosterone) whose main ingredient is synthesized ASD require medical analysis and monitoring prior, during, and after use.

However regardless of the product used, none of them guarantee health risk won't occur. Being monitored and treated by a medical doctor doesn't remove risk. Instead, a patient should think of medically administered hormone treatment as having quality-of-life benefits with acceptable risk.

ASD was available over the counter up through March 2004, at which point it was banned for sale to the general public and then listed as a controlled substance by the FDA.

It was sold to the general public and heavily used during the nineties by the likes of record-breaking baseball slugger Mark McGwire. His steroid use eventually gave him unwanted notoriety after it was discovered he'd used illegal performance-enhancement drugs.

"You can't even buy testosterone with a regular prescription," said Dr. Gary I. Wadler, an expert in supplement use and assistant professor of medicine at Cornell University Medical College. "You have to get a triplicate prescription. It's a controlled substance by an act of Congress. The schizophrenia of all this is, product A, which is over the counter, becomes product B, which is a controlled substance" (Sports Illustrated 1998).

Adrostenedione is also a natural steroid hormone that is produced by the adrenal glands and gonads. This hormone stimulates production of testosterone and estrogens—estrone and estradiol.

Although ASD was banned by the FDA and listed as a controlled substance, it is still available through illegal means. You can also purchase an over-the-counter DHEA-like rebrand (relabeled) and/ or chemically altered product "B" that has not been identified as an androgenic-anabolic steroid.

Parents of young, impressionable athletes should be aware of these performance-enhancement "relabeled product Bs," which are sold using different and seemingly harmless relabels that target young athletes.

Unless you are in need of medically supervised hormone treatment, you should avoid steroid-like supplements like the plague because of the increased cancer risk alone.

"[Michael] Pollak, director of the cancer prevention unit at Canada's McGill University in Montreal, is coauthor of an editorial published alongside the Swerdlow study ... The study in the July 27 issue of *The Lancet* looks at nearly 2000 British patients who, as children, were treated with human pituitary growth hormone ... between 1959 and 1985 ... They took a hard look at the lifetime medical records of the children – now adults … The editorial supports Swerdlow's worry that HGH has a role in cancer—especially colon cancer" (DeNoon 2002).

When Is Hormone Therapy Right for a Man or Woman?

Blood tests can determine whether either men or women are low in testosterone and whether androgen therapy is right for either sex. When a male's testosterone drops below safe levels, the common medical treatments are performed and monitored by a hormone replacement therapy (HRT) specialist. Why should hormone treatment be monitored? Too much testosterone for men and women can have unwanted side effects. Most notable unwanted characteristics or side effects in women include facial hair, bad acme, lowering of voice, shutdown of menstrual cycle, infertility, and ovary and breast cancer, to name a few.

Testosterone studies are not well understood in the treatment for women, as opposed to that for men, since testosterone is a man's "primary" naturally occurring hormone, whereas a woman's is estrogen.

Normal levels of testosterone relative to age are important because a man's overall health is dependent on an average production. According to Dr. Matthew Hoffman, "Men lose about 1 percent per year of their testosterone levels after age 40. In middle age and later, levels can dip below the threshold of what's considered normal." Hoffman notes, "Low testosterone becomes more common with age, affecting millions of men in the U.S. Although it may cause no symptoms, low testosterone can also result in poor libido, erectile dysfunction, depression, and loss of energy." He adds, "It's a treatable condition." (2014).

If you're diagnosed with low testosterone levels and there is no other apparent cause of contributing symptoms, then these things can likely be treated through medically supervised steroid treatment. HRT for men with low testosterone production can improve male characteristics in those who are deficient of the naturally occurring hormone.

It is recommended by endocrinologists that men with borderline testosterone levels work toward raising hormone levels naturally through exercise before going on testosterone therapy, especially for those who border around 350 nanograms per deciliter (ng/dl).

If testosterone levels fall below 300 ng/dl, then the general recommendation is to regulate toward mid to normal range. If all other secondary causes of reduced testosterone levels are ruled out, then therapy can be beneficial to the quality of life for those with below-average testosterone production. "'The take-home [message] is treatment is safe as long as you get careful monitoring,' Hedges says. 'If there are known issues, patients should be treated by a specialist'" (McMillen 2016).

The healthy levels of testosterone typically found in the bloodstream for men ranges from 350 to 1,000 nanograms per deciliter (ng/dl). Levels lower than 300 to 350 can become a contributing cause to obesity, bone density loss (brittle bones), and muscle loss and may increase chance of a heart attack.

Science clearly demonstrates that testosterone has an important connection to body weight and possibly cardiovascular health. Increasing testosterone levels may be beneficial to the health and well-being of those who suffer with a number of medical conditions, including osteoporosis (thinning of the bones), diabetes, obesity, depression, heart and circulatory abnormalities, and others.

"We recommend making a diagnosis of androgen deficiency only in men with consistent symptoms and signs and unequivocally low serum testosterone levels ... We recommend testosterone therapy for men with symptomatic androgen deficiency to induce and maintain secondary sex characteristics and to improve their sexual function, sense of well-being, muscle mass and strength, and bone mineral density" (Bhasin et al. 95 (6): 2536).

The question you should ask yourself is this: Is HRT and/or GH supplementation something I need? If an endocrinology test reveals you have "unhealthy" levels of hormone(s) and increased risk to health without treatment, then there is a need.

"Every woman makes a small amount of Testosterone, just as every man makes a small amount of estrogen. For some women it is Testosterone that gives them their energy and libido. If HRT does not relieve all your symptoms a trial of Testosterone is worthwhile to see if you are one of the Testosterone tribe" (Admin 2014). So when a woman is treated for low levels of hormones, endocrinologists focus more closely on levels of GH, estrogen, and progesterone, which are the hormones responsible for reproductive and menopause health. Like in men, GH in women is produced through the pituitary. Adrenal glands for women are very important in that they stimulate other hormones necessary for overall good health, weight management, and sense of well-being.

Why Antiaging and Performance-Enhancement Products Sell

Antiaging and performance-enhancement products sell because *at first* for many, they often produce a feeling of well-being, increased energy levels, and/or improved physical appearance and physical performance. And they're easy to find and purchase without a doctor's prescription.

The current antiaging and performance-enhancement mind-set is no different than that of yesteryear's competitive bodybuilders, athletes, and antiagers. And the millennial generation is no different, but with one exception—they have global access to any product or service, along with a "now" consumer expectation.

Consumers want what they want, when they want it. If a local business doesn't provide them what they want now, they'll easily get it another way. Today with the swipe of a keystroke, they'll find what they want in the interconnected world (Bernard 2012).

The world is a consumer oyster in a connected marketplace. A plethora of antiaging and relabeled enhancement products and services is available to the "now" generation, allowing young people to experiment on themselves without medical supervision. So even with the best consumer safety protections and precautions, there is no assurance kids won't shop globally to acquire the goods.

As parents, teachers, and coaches, our first line of defense is to educate our kids on products that cause chemical imbalance and increase health risk.

Personal Fitness Challenge: "Steroids and Avascular Necrosis"

Although I was tempted many times as an athlete, bodybuilder, and fitness trainer to use steroids, I'm happy to say I never jumped on that bandwagon. I learned early on about the health risks associated with steroid use and made a conscious decision to never use them to enhance my fitness level or sports performance. To tell you the truth, those risks scared the hell out of me—especially after watching what happened to Sam.

If you have kids in sports, be sure to share this information or have them read this chapter. Educating youth on such things is a powerful deterrent against the temptation to chemically enhance oneself—getting a short-term benefit at the cost of long-term illness and disease. If a medical condition does not justify antiaging or physical performance-enhancement drug use, the gamble is akin to playing Russian roulette with your health.

Imagine if I had used steroids in the eighties to play football or during the peak of my amateur bodybuilding career. Would that have progressed the AVN disease, causing it to affect me twenty years earlier than its actual occurrence? I'll never know the answer for sure. But if I was genetically predisposed to get the disease, it seems likely that would have been the case.

Steroid use and acceptable risk is something to be discussed between doctor and patient. From what I know about illegal steroid use, including doctor-administered cortisone shots and prednisone prescriptions, there is no assurance that monitored medical treatment would prevent these treatments from causing AVN disease—as prescribed steroids did in my case. The approved medical treatment administered to me had health risks I was not aware of.

"Whatever may be the pathologic etiology for the avascular necrosis, so far an exact relationship between the dose and the mode of administration of steroid and the risk of developing avascular necrosis has not been determined." However, "the duration of steroid treatment, the total cumulative dose and the highest daily dose of steroids have been implicated as important factors in the development of avascular necrosis" (Mendiratta, Khan, and Solanki 2008).

I was aware early on during doctor consultations that steroid use to treat contact dermatitis brought on by poisonous plants had a risk to the pancreas. However, there was never any mention of AVN by any treating physicians who administered those steroids for nearly a decade before it caused the disease. I had no symptoms of any hip problems until the head of the femur bone collapsed during a military training exercise. I was shocked and in disbelief to learn how treating poison oak with cortisone and prednisone to heal the skin had caused the destruction of one hip and likely loss of the other at some point in time.

If you aren't an endocrinologist, immunologist, or orthopedic surgeon, you most likely can't grasp the proper information about *all* the health risks involved with any type of steroid use. Had I had access to the internet back in the early nineties, I may have made different choices in treating the acute contact dermatitis in order to avoid bone disease. Don't let the "now" expectation and market charlatans duke you into risking your health.

For anyone who has no justifiable medical reason to use steroid treatment and anyone who is considering steroid or growth hormone use without medical supervision, I leave the following thoughts:

Strive to find a balance when it comes to natural antiaging principles and practices that complement a healthy mind, body, and spirit. You may then be fortunate enough to avoid insidious disease during the aging process.

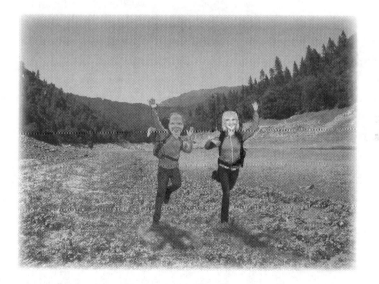

Be mindful—without good health you can't hope to experience life to the fullest or to age gracefully with your life partner or to avoid unnecessary pain and suffering.

—MirrorAthlete Principled Fitness and
Healthy Lifestyle Philosophy

Chapter 16

Don't Take Breathing for Granted

Oxygenate the body, burn more fat, and reduce illness and disease risk.

—MirrorAthlete Principled Fitness and
Healthy Lifestyle Philosophy

It is a fact that fresh-air environments during exercise activity motivate and stimulate the brain, body, and spirit in healthy ways. It is inherently known that taking in abundant outdoor air is refreshing, healthy, and good for us in many ways. Have you ever thought about why you feel more energized and active once you're outdoors and breathing nature's fresh air?

Many would say those who crave the outdoors are drawn to it because of a universal connection with nature, childhood memories, romance, beauty, reflection, meditation, relaxation, and any other number of reasons. Although these things are true, it is also true that moving about outdoors feeds us abundant oxygenated air our bodies need and crave.

However, all air quality is not of the same. And the pollutant levels in cities and large suburban areas are typically higher than those in rural and coastal environs and places with high elevation.

Does this mean city air has less oxygen in it than air in rural or remotely wooded hiking trails at sea level? No, it does not. The air we breathe is a mixture that contains primarily oxygen and nitrogen. The nitrogen generally makes up approximately 78 percent, while oxygen makes up 21 percent at sea level and decreases in value the higher one is in altitude. It is the air pollutants that are concerning to environmentalists, public health authorities, and respiratory health specialists. And if a medical doctor or personal trainer prescribes more exercise to help reduce body weight and improve cardio circulatory function, oxygen uptake and physical performance will be affected in environments where air quality is poor. This factor alone keeps many from participating in outdoor and indoor exercise activities.

When the body's lungs don't have to compete with air contaminants, it is more likely exercise will be sustained daily and fitness goals achieved. Believe me, the body knows when it's sucking in bad air. If outdoor air is heavily polluted with ozone, a colorless gas is produced by the action of sunlight on nitrogen oxides and hydrocarbons from automobile emissions. The symptoms of ozone decline in lung function "include chest tightness, eye irritation, sore throat, wheezing, coughing, shortness of breath and headache" (Sports Doctor 2000).

If you feel bad in the environment where you live, work, and play, then that place will not motivate you to exercise or move more. More than once, I've traveled five to twenty miles to walk or hike at higher altitudes during hot summer months to get out of the smog. Or I've sought shelter indoors to exercise as opposed to going outdoors. But being sure you exercise only in places where air quality is good does take some environmental awareness and planning, especially when you live in a high smog area.

While living in Sacramento, California, I worked out in a fitness center during the frequent hot summer days and walked two days a week when the air quality was better. On Saturdays or Sundays, I'd often head east toward Placerville or Reno to walk in elevated areas above the smog layer.

Exercising indoors may be no better than walking a busy street—especially if poor indoor air quality makes you feel bad. Buildings that have bad air quality are also defined as sick building syndrome (SBS) environments. Those who work within an office or home environment with unhealthy air conditions can develop respiratory illness after a short period of exposure and not know the cause of the affliction. Poor indoor air quality can be worse than a bad outdoor air day.

"People spend as much as 90 percent of their lives inside … The quality of our indoor air is not as high as the quality of outdoor air, which can lead to many health related risks and issues for everyone …

There have been studies that have shown that the levels of indoor pollutants can be 25%–62% higher than the levels of outdoor toxins" (Oliver 2008).

If your home air is full of cleaning product vapors and lacks good ventilation, how can you expect to feel well daily, especially if you're oversensitive to those toxins? If indoor or outdoor air quality makes you feel ill, then for the sake of your health, you must find a way to change the environmental condition.

It is seen in studies that, "when performing tasks in clean air, the ratio of body movement versus actual energy expenditure is larger than in polluted, or toxic air environments. We demonstrated a positive correlation between quality of indoor air and physical performance parameters, which may have implications for the individual's level of physical independence" (Snijders et al. 2001). This means there is less energy throughout the day to accomplish other tasks or daily exercise.

I can tell you that if I smell a high concentrate of toxin off-gassing indoors, I'm going to identify the source and correct the problem. That includes making sure my ventilation system is working as efficiently as possible to bring in more outside air. And to meet my daily outdoor exercise commitment, I'm going to walk, jog, or ride a bike when the air index quality is favorable to my activities (which means not during peak auto traffic time).

Finding a way to exercise lung capacity in clean-air environments is essential in order to sustain healthy lung function, overall health, and good fitness levels. Science proves daily aerobic exercise can remove many impurities from the body once unconditioned lungs become conditioned. For example, "when we don't inhale deeply enough, we decrease the amount of oxygen our breath delivers to our cells, reducing their ability to produce energy. In addition, deeper breathing removes more carbon dioxide, along with other potential toxins. Respiration also balances your body's pH, reducing the acidity that can impair immunity and other functions" (Rodale 2013).

If we take in ample clean air, whether exercising indoors or outdoors, our minds and bodies are motivated to repeat the habit daily. Recall what was learned from the previous chapter; more addictive and natural feel-good brain chemicals are released during exercise. Complementing the natural release of feel-good brain-body chemicals with fresh air-intake allows us to exercise longer, remain healthy, and remain more productive throughout the year.

Let's consider an office environment and its impact on employees' health and production. Do office workers typically get sick more often than non–office workers? This really depends on lifestyle, environment, and current health condition, among other factors. However, we do know that bodies in motion expand the lungs at greater capacity and transfer more oxygen to working muscles, while simultaneously removing foreign materials and toxins through the lymphatic system.

If you spend a lot of time indoors at home or in the office, air quality may have a negative impact on your health. If you notice coworkers or family members getting sick often, suspect building materials, cleaning or chemical agents, perfumes, hair spray products, and the like, along with poorly maintained air handling and ventilation systems or high levels of outdoor air pollutants or pollens breaching an indoor air space as a result of inadequate filtration and/or stagnant air circulation characteristics.

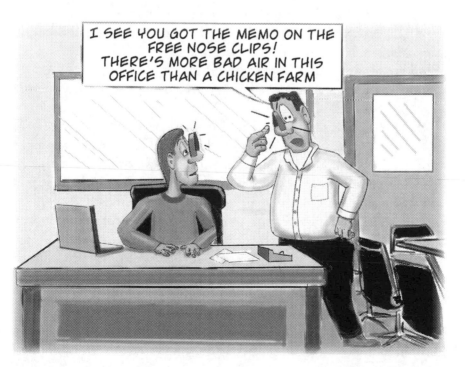

Most commercial and public building air standards require a 10 to 15 percent fresh-air makeup pulled from outside. Good HVAC (heating ventilation and air-conditioning) building maintenance practices should include adequate outdoor fresh-air intake, filtration, and sanitary preventative maintenance practices of all air-handling systems in accordance with OSHA and EPA safe workplace indoor air guidelines and standards. Your living space at home should be under similar scrutiny. Filters and condensate pans and coils need to be cleaned not less than quarterly or semiannually. And duct systems may require cleaning once annually to minimize poor air quality.

Aside from air quality concerns, office workers and sedentary homebodies should be aware of ergonomic posture and immobility habits. Without ergonomic postural awareness, office and telecommuter home workers and online gamers risk unhealthy lung function when poor sedentary habits become the daily norm.

Poor ergonomic posture also has a direct correlation to increased risk of carpal tunnel syndrome; back, neck, shoulder, and eye strain; and lung conditions related to shallow breathing. Ergonomic specialists in the workplace don't typically focus on breathing function. However, they do assess employee posture to reduce repetitive musculoskeletal stress and strain and other office safety and injury risk. Nevertheless, ergonomic workstation corrections don't necessarily help improve shallow breathing habits, which correlate to poor circulation and lung function.

For those who have never heard of shallow breathing, it's easy to illustrate. Simply slump over and breathe normally. Now sit up straight and breath. You know instantly that you're taking in more air when you're not slumped over. Most of us learned to sit up straight in school when we were kids. During that time, teachers were mostly focused on healthy spine development and good air intake that kept our brain well oxygenated, focused, and alert.

During my professional career, like many of you, I've worked within office environments and know a thing or two about workspace ergonomics, air ventilation systems, and the MERT (Medical Emergency Response Team) response process to react to employee health emergencies. When working for a large corporation, you gain a lot of insight, experience, and perspective on workspace stress, injuries, and toxic air environments. And you come to see how these things may or may not be related and take a toll on health.

I recall as an MERT member responding when an employee complained of a heart or breathing problem. And I recall him or her leaving in an ambulance.

Some employees were even found dead in their office cubes. I understand that these things happen, but what was shocking was the age, frequency, and number of affected office employees. When forty- to fifty-year-olds leave in an ambulance or you see a few of them drop dead, you know this is not from the scourges of aging or living a hard lifestyle. It appeared these deaths were mostly caused by bad habits and overweight condition and likely related to a stressful work environment.

When you work for long periods of time at a desk each day, it is important to practice frequent stretch and walk breaks. Also consider when you're off work not taking those office habits home. "While doing a bit of extra work at home may seem like a good short-term fix, if it becomes a regular part of your evening routine then it can lead to problems such as back and neck problems, as well as stress-related illness. This is especially the case if you're using handheld devices and not thinking about your posture" (Maur 2012).

When unhealthy lifestyle habits and environment are not conducive to good health, illness and disease can become life-threatening.

Professor Beverly Hunt, medical director of Lifeblood, said, "Our research has uncovered a ticking time-bomb with some nine million office workers and countless young gamers putting themselves at risk of a potentially fatal blood clot." The article quoting Hunt went on to say, "The human body is designed for the 'caveman' lifestyle; active, agile and constantly mobile. Instead we have become increasingly sedentary, obstructing the body's ability to function as it should" (Smith 2012). As gamer and cell phone movie viewing and social media and telecommuter technologies advance, so do sedentary habits, and health risks increase.

Early signs of a sedentary person with unhealthy lung function can sometimes be obvious by simply being aware of shortness of breath during conversation.

However, a person with poor lung function who appears fit may not be obvious or easy to identify until vitals are taken by a medical doctor. If a person talks to you and can hardly finish a sentence before running short of breath, this is a good indicator of weakened lung function caused by any number of bad habit(s) or environmental or medical condition factor(s). Physical appearance and energy levels are often good indicators of how healthy a person is in general.

Because a sedentary lifestyle, poor posture, and unhealthy work or home air environment can condition lungs for poor breathing function, one may experience shortness of breath, lack energy, or feel tired all the time and not look or feel well. And these unhealthy attributes will not motivate someone to exercise or move more, unless poor breathing function, health condition, or environmental air quality is addressed.

Shallow breathing can be caused by anxiety, stress, lifestyle, and environment, including a medical condition that causes hyperventilation and rapid breathing. "The average person takes between eight and sixteen breaths per minute. Rapid shallow breathing, also called tachypnea, occurs when you take more breaths than normal in a given minute. When a person breathes rapidly, it's sometimes known as hyperventilation … Rapid shallow breathing can be caused by infections, choking, blood clots, diabetic ketoacidosis, heart failure, or asthma" (Kahn 2016).

Shallow, irregular, and rapid breathing patterns can occur in people who appear healthy and may or may not be considered sedentary people. And a polluted living and work environment may be the cause of such symptoms. According to researcher Diane Gold of the Harvard School of Public Health, air pollution can cause a clinically significant increase in symptoms such as shallow breathing, cardiac issues, and sleep apnea risk. "You are at a 13% higher risk of having shallow breathing or stopping breathing for at least 10 seconds if pollution goes from the lower range to the higher range of pollution for that city" (Doheny 2010).

So at what air pollutant level is shallow breathing and sleep apnea most likely to occur for those sensitive to unhealthy air conditions?

If days are hot with little air movement, air pollutants are more likely to cause respiratory problems the closer you are to sea level. On these types of days, it is prudent to monitor news and radio stations for air quality indicators. EPA air quality standards and warnings for major cities within the United States can also easily be found at airnow.gov. If carbon monoxide levels exceed 9 ppm in eight hours or 35 ppm for one hour, for example, these levels are considered harmful to health and environment (EPA 2016). Consider limiting your exposure outdoors when air quality hits these marks.

How Does Shallow Breathing Impact Lung Function and Overall Health?

Recall that the average person takes between eight and sixteen breaths per minute. Shallow breathing is when our exchange of oxygen and carbon dioxide in the lungs lacks full inspiration and expiration, causing rapid breathing. This also means our *lung reserve (residual airspace)* is mostly void of oxygen. That airspace is the unused reserve or residual lung volume and capacity not exercised at rest and partially or fully used during exercise activity or during physical work.

In order to relate to unused lung capacity, I'd like to have you perform a simple breathing exercise. It will help you understand the difference between reserve lung space and vital lung capacity.

Vital lung capacity is the maximum amount of air a person can expel after full inspiration. That's pretty easy to relate to. But how about residual space?

Take in a deep breath, then forcefully exhale as much air from your lungs as possible and continue to push air. Don't stop pushing air even though you feel no more air can come out.

More continues to come out.

Keep pushing; you can push more.

You can actually continue to push and squeeze more air out of your lungs than you thought possible through forceful and concentrated effort. After ten seconds of continued lung exhalation at a consistent purge, you now know you have a fairly large lung reserve space that's not used during rest.

Lung capacity is the total air volume you're able to inspire and expire, which includes lung reserve, also referred to as residual lung space or capacity.

Increased Lung Capacity Improves Physical Performance and Health

Science shows us "some of the conditions that benefit the most from deep breathing exercises include, insomnia, headaches, migraines, heart disease, back pain, balancing pH, high blood pressure, emphysema, improving sports performance, unspecified chronic pain, adrenal fatigue, depression, anxiety disorders, panic attacks, PTSD, MS, food sensitivities, chemical sensitivities, fibromyalgia and arthritis. However, there probably isn't any condition that wouldn't benefit in some way, particularly if it is accompanied by pain and stress. I personally find deep breathing to be the most effective form of stress relief, next to exercising" (Perkins 2015).

Also, "oxygen is a natural, powerful cleanser, oxygen therapy is used to cleanse the body of bacteria, viruses, and toxins. Just by learning and practicing deep breathing techniques it is possible to vastly increase the available oxygen in the body to cleanse it. Mostly we shallow breathe. The trick is to remember to do it frequently, at any time" (Norma 2010).

How does shallow breathing specifically influence blood pressure? Since the heart's action is involuntary, it can only respond to demand on the heart. If the heart senses a drop in oxygen in the body, then the heart will work harder and pump more blood. This is one way in which blood pressure increases. We know high blood pressure that is continuous during rest is not healthy for us.

The involuntary blood pressure and heart rate response *does not* require the lungs take in more air while sedentary, or at rest. The heart and blood pressure will increase without exercise to meet our metabolic, cellular, and biological systems' functional needs. However, when blood pressure and heart rate remain elevated for too long, health risk increases.

I have a blood pressure cuff and take my pulse frequently to ensure my cardiopulmonary and circulatory systems are functioning well (chapter 9, "Health Risk Prediction and Prevention"). As a matter of fact, I considered vitals important enough that I took them and covered the results during every client consultation. Blood pressure, heart rate, and body weight baselines can be plotted and compared to future results and, if applicable, prompted me to refer a client to seek the opinion of a medical doctor—especially when vitals indicated a high health risk could accompany a significant lifestyle change.

How Do Healthy Lungs and Activity Support a Good Immune System?

Although our direct focus here is not on our lymphatic (immune) system, it plays a supporting role to the circulatory system in removing harmful foreign particles, bacteria, and dead or dying cells. This system reacts to the oxidative cellular response, pathogens and parasites, and any number of toxin possibilities that would attempt to attack the body.

And keeping the body healthy requires the action of phagocyte cells, whose role it is to protect the body by consuming and removing waste, thereby filtering the blood via the lymphatic system's cleansing function. Whenever you move or perform breathing exercises, you also increase the action of waste removal through the body's lymphoid tissue or lymph system.

The lymph circulation system is separate from our arterial and venial blood circulation systems, with a specific filtering function and purpose. It actively removes toxins and waste products from blood circulation through the liver and kidneys. I must say, if you are unable to exercise daily or on the mend, it will be advantageous for you to apply deep-breathing exercises. A lymph system whose circulation is slowed down due to immobility retains toxins that must be filtered out of the body. And this can only be done through movement and activity or deep breathing exercise (Pick 2016).

Our circulatory systems and lung function are dependent on one another to cleanse the body, heal, get fit, and sustain good health. When one circulatory system underperforms, there is a stress relationship impact on another bodily function.

The environmental garbage we take in daily needs to be processed out of the body. It is healthy lung, cardio circulatory, and immune system functions that sustain a fit, healthy lifestyle and well-being.

Personal Fitness Challenge: "Breathe Deeply and Get Invigorated"

Spending a lot of time lying around after my surgeries was not only sapping my muscular strength and endurance; it was also sucking the life out of my lung capacity and body. At some point, I recalled an exercise physiology course long ago that analyzed lung, heart, and circulatory capacity function during rest and exercise. I recalled that performing physical tasks at varying efforts, intensities, and durations had a direct relationship to lung function, vitals, and oxygenated blood, along with working muscle performance, fat burning, and ill-health relationships.

The professor made it easy to see and relate to how immobility and bad habits would reduce lung function and increase health risk. And when performing physical work, the unconditioned person experienced elevated heart rate and blood pressure, along with rapid breathing, and required more frequent rest breaks.

When living a sedentary lifestyle, poor postural habits and shallow breathing are often the cause of unhealthy lung and circulatory function. When unhealthy habits continue, the risk of circulatory disease, stroke, and heart attack increase.

During 2004, after my first hip surgery, I focused on conditioning my lungs to improve their capacity and circulatory efficiencies. I began a regiment of deep-breathing exercises while bedridden to keep my lungs, heart, and circulatory and immune systems exercised and oxygenated. To this day, I continue deep-breathing exercises while walking, weight lifting, and at rest and prior to sleep.

I know that some wonder why I'd practice deep-breathing exercises during my daily walks. After all, walking is aerobic, and you're already taking in more air than a body at rest. Although this is true, I know I can always take in more, as demonstrated during the forceful lung exhalation of residual airspace.

For example, I often walk at 50 to 70 percent of *aerobic intensity of effort* (see chapters 3 and 18). I'm cognizant that, during low-intensity walks, I'm not expanding my lungs as much as I do when walking at 70 percent intensity up hills. In order to exercise more of my vital lung capacity, I willfully force the useless air out of the residual lung space by consciously making an effort to take in more air while walking. Taking in more air hastens repair of cellular damage and toxin removal and assists in burning more body fat weight.

The functioning lung-gas exchange becomes optimized when full (vital) lung capacity is flush with fresh oxygenated air. "During exercise, your body consumes large amounts of oxygen. In fact, this is part of what helps you to lose weight. The more oxygen your body consumes, the harder that you're working out. It's one reason that you typically lose a lot of weight when you first start working out" (FitDay 2016).

It is known that deep-breathing exercise, when done correctly, ensures the residual lung volume is exercised. However, "to make sure adequate air gets into the lungs, we need to breathe slow and deeply. Even when we exhale deeply some air is still in the lungs (about 1,000 ml) and is called residual volume. This air isn't useful for gas exchange. There are certain types of diseases of the lung where residual volume builds up because the person cannot fully empty the lungs. This means that the vital capacity is also reduced because their lungs are filled with useless air" (Boundless 2016).

Through my years of participating in sport and individual activities such as football, baseball, weight training, track-and-field events, karate, jujitsu, and yoga, deep-breathing exercises was a standard practice during warm-up and cool down.

Grand master martial artists, yogis, and meditative specialists around the world understand the benefits of deep breathing for health; healing; and focused energy of the mind, body, and spirit. Deep-breathing exercises is practiced religiously for all types of self-healing, focus, and spiritual benefits.

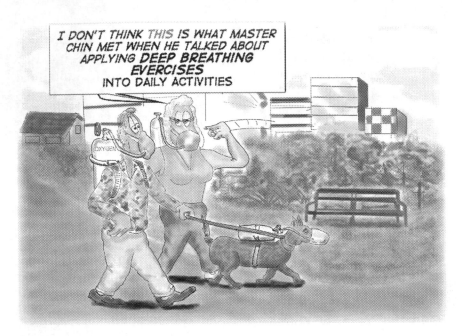

To find breathing exercise instruction and techniques, look for yoga, tai chi, or martial artist practitioners or other meditation and relaxation experts online, at libraries, within educational institutions, and among local businesses.

At a minimum, if you're unable to exercise for a long period of time, I highly recommend you apply deep-breathing exercise to keep lung capacity, cardiopulmonary, and immune system functions and metabolism well maintained. Applying deep-breathing exercise during a recovery period will support toxin removal and tissue repair, minimize weight gain, and expedite a speedy recovery.

Apply Deep-Breathing Exercise When Seated, When at Rest, While Walking, and Prior to Sleep

Learn how to apply the same deep-breathing exercise I used during recovery and put this exercise to practice right now.

While sitting up straight or standing, inhale deeply. Imagine filling your lungs from the bottom up. Inhale slowly through your nose for a count of six to eight seconds, hold the inflated lungs for a few seconds, and then spend a longer period of time expelling the air through your mouth.

During full vital capacity inhalation and exhalation, don't rush it. Otherwise, you'll feel like you're hyperventilating.

Work toward repeating this breathing technique four to six times. It may take up to three to five minutes to complete the exercise. I often incorporate deep-breathing exercise during my five-minute stretch warm-up and cooldown before and after exercising in a gym and then additionally while watching television or discretely at a business meeting or while attending church.

Use correct posture during breathing exercises. Ensure that you don't lean forward and reduce the chest cavity area and that your head remains slightly tilted upward during the exercise. This will ensure you are sitting or standing straight. Focus on a tight abdominal cavity during exhalation (also great as an ab and core toning exercise).

Repeat deep-breathing exercise as many times throughout the day as possible. Eventually, your involuntary vitals systems will improve. Your body will then become conditioned to take in more oxygen. You'll sleep better at night and look more rested and feel energized throughout the day.

Breathing technique while walking – Apply the same breathing technique as you would while sitting, standing, or lying down. Then work to increase or decrease breathing patterns based on walking intensity and duration. If you are conditioned to walk frequently, your lung capacity is most likely well conditioned. However, you can take in more air when you're mindful and want to do it. But if at any time deep-breathing exercise causes a feeling of hyperventilation, you are overbreathing. If you feel light-headed or dizzy, breathe normal and slow down to a snail's crawl until the light-headed feeling goes away.

Your goal is not to hyperventilate and pass out. When the time is right, focus again on deep-breathing exercise. Because walking requires greater oxygen uptake than being at rest, deep breathing during walks takes more focus. With focus, you'll learn to pace your breathing rhythm and develop a level of comfort with it. The point is, you can find a walk cadence and breathing rhythm with greater oxygen intake that works well for you. It's simply a matter of practice. But it is wise to first practice breathing technique seated or just before bedtime prior to taking it on the road.

If applying breathing exercise prior to sleep, lie flat without a pillow and go through the breathing technique as if sitting in a chair or standing. This is very relaxing and will aid in your ability to fall asleep while conditioning the lungs.

Deep breathing is also good to practice before a big interview or a public speaking engagement. It energizes the mind and body, reduces postural stress, and relaxes the whole body and brain for better delivery of message while calming the nerves.

Remember, it's easy to get lazy at breathing.

Keep in mind that, regardless of physical or health adversity and mobility challenge, anyone can benefit from deep-breathing exercise.

Chapter 17

Longevity Secrets Divulged

Nature provides what we need to live happy, healthy, and productive long lives.

—MirrorAthlete Principled Fitness and
Healthy Lifestyle Philosophy

It's no secret Westerners pay billions of dollars a year for products and services that unnaturally stimulate weight loss, enhance physical performance, and promise fountain-of-youth results. By now, you understand that any physical progress gained from man-made products and services that offer quick results is often short-lived and increases health risk because these products are not true to nature and don't change bad habits into better ones.

As you've learned, industrial segments within our marketplace are not interested in decreasing diet fads, products and services related to antiaging, and fitness- and performance-enhancement gimmicks. There's no money in it for them. Regardless, after reading previous chapters, you also understand there is no need to shell out your hard-earned cash for any man-made product in order to achieve a healthy lifestyle change goal.

Let's examine how living a life without man-made conveniences and antiaging, diet, and fitness gimmicks can keep us healthier and living longer. Simply by studying a culture absent of Western influence, it becomes clear how living a healthier lifestyle can heal us mentally, physically, and spiritually.

On the Greek island of Ikaria, data shows a population of around ten thousand. It also tells us these people are three times more likely to live past the age of ninety when compared to those of us in America. Along with measurably longer life spans, the islanders of Ikaria have little need of medical attention in comparison to other nearby islanders within the region of Sardinia's Nuoro province, where they live on a remote mountainous terrain island surrounded by the Aegean Sea. I wondered what longevity secrets they possessed and why a neighboring island didn't share the same benefits. As I compared the two island cultures, the questions I had were answered fairly quickly.

"*National Geographic* writer Dan Buettner, specializes in reporting on what he calls 'blue zones'—pockets where populations manage to avoid succumbing to debilitating modern health scourges like type 2 diabetes, heart disease, and cancer" (Philpott 2012).

Although some argue these longevity results are attributable to superior genetics, it appears the islanders' unique lifestyle and environment are more likely the cause.

For a decade Buettner's sponsored project was to study places "where people live the longest"; this grew out of studies with his partners, Dr. Gianni Pes of the University of Sassari in Italy and Dr. Michel Poulain, a Belgian demographer. "After gathering all the data, Poulain and his colleagues at the University of Athens concluded that people on Ikaria were, in fact, reaching the age of 90 at two and a half times the rate Americans ... We do know from reliable data that people on Ikaria are outliving those on surrounding islands (a control group, of sorts)" (Buettner 2012).

There is much healthy lifestyle and antiaging wisdom to be gained by studying remote cultures and then comparing the data attained from those studies to that of Western culture. In other words, if you want to increase healthy lifespan beyond ninety years, study cultures absent of Western influence.

How does the old adage go—when in Rome, do as the Romans do (or in this case, as the Ikarian people do). Data from the remote island reveals many distinct differences in the way the islanders live and the way most of the world lives. They have strong family bonds and morals and value family, friendships, and religious gatherings. They also walk daily to get work done, which includes harvesting and gathering a balanced, organic island diet. They also live in a relaxed environment free of many modern conveniences, toxins, and pollutants.

What can this culture teach us about disease prevention and antiaging? An amazing data point that is hard to ignore plagues our culture. "Among the islanders over 90 (~1/3rd of their population) there is virtually no Alzheimer's disease or other dementia. In the United States more than 40 percent of people over 90 suffer some form of this devastating ailment" (Garland 2010). The takeaway—this island population has not been exposed in a significant way to outside influences.

The questions I had after diving into this unique culture were many: How do the islanders live, work, and play or spend their leisurely time? How do their diet, exercise activity, and environment differ from ours? After all, our habits and behavior are greatly influenced by environment and culture.

Nearly all of the fruits and vegetables on Ikaria are personally grown and sold at the local marketplace and void of chemical herbicides, pesticides, and fertilizers. The islanders' Mediterranean diet is low in saturated fats mostly found in meats and dairy products. They eat meat on an average five times per month and consume significant amounts of potatoes because of the mountainous supporting terrain that yields them. They eat mostly whole foods—grain, fruit, fish, and vegetables. Approximately 150 of the greens grown on this island are said to have ten times the antioxidants of red wine. The main cooking oil is olive oil, which is used liberally *unheated* with many of their meals.

The island study shows unique food sources only found on this island and very beneficial to health. For example, Ikarian honey is an excellent antioxidant, as is all honey. But it is interesting to note that our honey does not appear to be as beneficial as the honey harvested on the island. Maybe it has to do with Ikaria's unique selection of herbs, pine trees, and other unique flora. Buettner's team of demographic and medical researchers, funded by AARP and *National Geographic*, state, "The local honey contains antibacterial, anticancer and anti-inflammatory properties. (Unfortunately, the health benefits of Ikarian honey do not extend to American honey, as far as we know)" (Buettner 2009).

Also the islander's sourdough bread has high counts of complex carbohydrates. When these complex carbohydrates are included in diets, it seems to be beneficial for those with diabetes. This benefit occurs because the sourdough carbohydrates improve the glucose metabolism, which helps to sustain lean body mass and aids in prevention of type 2 diabetes.

General research on sourdough health benefits confirms the fact. "'With the sourdough, the subjects' blood sugar levels were lower for a similar rise in blood insulin,' said [Professor Terry] Graham ... 'What was even more interesting was that this positive effect remained during their second meal and lasted even hours after. This shows that what you have for breakfast influences how your body will respond to lunch'" (University of Guelph 2008).

Most of Ikaria's elderly over ninety state they drank goat milk all of their lives. This milk, in comparison to other milk, is easier on the digestive system. Goat's milk is rich in tryptophan, which lowers blood pressure, includes antibacterial compounds, and thwarts depression. L-tryptophan can be found within many supplements, protein mixes, and animal products.

The people of Ikaria drink plenty of chamomile and seasonal herb mixes, also known as mountain teas (marjoram, wild mint, sage, and dandelion leaves) with mild diuretic properties. These teas and herbs are also considered excellent antioxidants. It has long been established that teas support lowering blood pressure and also reduce the risk of heart disease. Ikarians also drink on average two to three cups of coffee a day. "Researchers hypothesize that Greek coffee may be more beneficial than other coffee drinks because it has a moderate amount of caffeine and is rich in antioxidants and polyphenols. They also suggest that when coffee is boiled it retains more of the healthful chemical compounds than when it is filtered or prepared by other methods" (Sesana 2013).

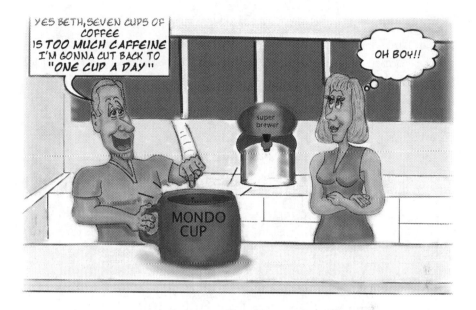

In the past, coffee has gotten a bad rap. But now science is showing us that three to five or more cups of coffee per day can provide us with many health benefits—reduced chance of stroke, heart attack, diabetes, cancer, and Parkinson's and Alzheimer's disease (Pace 2013).

"Of course, it may not be only what they're eating, it may also be what they're not eating. Are they doing something positive, or is it the absence of something negative?" (Buettner 2012). In developed countries there is access to all types of convenience and processed foods. On this remote island, that has not been the case. However, imported snack products are beginning to find their way into the local villages. Some children have a preference for Western snacks over some of the traditional foods. It is not known how this will impact these people over the long term.

Does the health and longevity prevalent on Ikaria have anything to do with walking activity and social gatherings?

There is a big difference in the way cultures view and value walking activity. Whereas the islanders walk to gather food and interact with others out of necessity, we *mostly* do not. And this is what makes their daily activities and lifestyle uniquely different than ours.

They have very few personal luxuries, such as cars, public transportation, and technological advancements. And every purposeful trip on foot sustains their way of life, allowing them to socially interact with family members and neighbors in distant villages. They are rarely left alone, especially when they take that day's walk to catch fish and bring it back to the village.

Although I'm an advocate of daily walking exercise, I'm not suggesting you walk to a local fishing spot to get your exercise. But I have a similar take on a *like* activity that provides similar aerobic benefits within any environmental setting. Since most don't live on a remote island, it's hard to replicate the way the islanders live. However with a few lifestyle modifications and habit changes you can leverage a similar lifestyle to receive similar benefits.

In today's world of technological advancement, the internet's social chat rooms, movies, and game time plug-ins have reprioritized our youth's time, moving them away from healthy habits (including daily exercise activity). By ungodly design, Western technology, convenience foods, and sedentary habits have caused more people to become overweight and obese—causing epidemic-like illnesses and disease conditions like no other time in modern history. That's why comparing cultural lifestyles and disease and mortality rate data is so valuable. We can learn how to reverse engineer the obesity and related disease problems by studying people who have little-to-no disease and are active beyond the age of ninety.

The island people also show how important it is to participate in religious and community events within peaceful and joyful surroundings. For example, when people attend community gatherings they appear healthier and happier and seem to live longer. There are pockets of places within the United States outside the island study that appear to confirm this claim.

It is observed that, within Ikaria's Greek Orthodox culture, the islanders gather for regular social and spiritual activities. And in comparison to a place within the United States, another religious culture shows us a connection to healthy longevity. For instance in Loma Linda, California, there is a "population of Seventh-day Adventists in which most of the adherents' life expectancy exceeded the American average by about a decade" (Buettner 2012).

We know through social and demographic studies that time spent in family-friendly settings and at such events—including spiritual reflection—can help us unwind and destress and have a positive influence on behavior. Unfortunately, within many westernized places, the marketplace technologies distract us—especially our youth.

When healthy habit change plays second fiddle to the likes of Pokémon Go (a recent game innovation phenomenon and obsession played on cell phones) or a plethora of hours spent instant messaging and texting and in social chat rooms or on any number of online applications and movie viewing, what is the likely result? You got it—unhealthy, sedentary habits. And if these habits become obsessions, increased physical and mental health risks become the new norm. Thereafter, a behavioral therapist, psychologist, medical doctor, and other specialists may be of service to help reverse the course.

To further relate to the Ikaria lifestyle, another data point shows the islanders live with less employer stress compared to us. Their philosophy is that work will eventually get done, so why worry about it? Unlike us, these people don't spend countless hours worrying about their employers' timelines. This philosophical difference is said to reduce anxiety and stress, improve worker attitude, and increase production. Like Latino siestas, Ikarians relax the mind and body during midday naps.

Midday naps have been valued by Eastern cultures for thousands of years. The practice is also valued by many Western corporate wellness groups for good reason. It is a relaxing de-stressor that appears to improve production goals, health, and well-being. Business organizations that offer these midday relaxation programs often refer to them as "power naps." It is said that power naps can minimize risk of heart attack, decrease blood pressure, and even reduce arthritis, wrinkly skin, and other such ailments.

But the islanders' expectations and that of Western employers differ in that we must meet and often exceed employers' expectations. In many cases, Western employees take work home with them, which is very different than the Ikaria work philosophy.

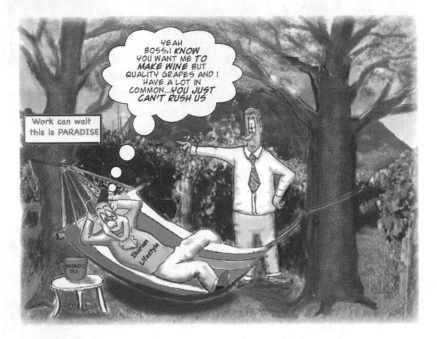

It's no secret our culture makes living an islander lifestyle challenging because of our "I want it now" expectation. Regardless, if you're ready to make a healthy lifestyle change, my advice is to leverage a little time toward an Ikarian habit to achieve similar wellness and longevity benefits.

No matter who you are, where you live, or what physical challenges you may face, you now know the Western culture's quick-results secrets are no secret at all. And sustaining good health and fitness levels for life requires mindful effort and applying a *principled fitness and healthy lifestyle plan* that works for you.

Personal Fitness Challenge: "Mobilize the Body and Heal Naturally"

I used a cane, crutches, and a wheelchair during long periods of time before and after THR (total hip replacement) and after bone graft surgery to save the other hip. Throughout these surgeries and recovery periods, I stayed motivated to participate in low-intensity exercise the best way I knew how.

The long recovery periods between surgeries were anything but easy. It proved to be very challenging physically and mentally because of a prior back injuries and degenerative vertebrae disease.

While waiting on surgeries, I also began to rely too much on pharmaceuticals to control pain, which often trumped the natural release of brain-body feel-good chemicals. I needed to find a way during recovery to become more mobile, while decreasing pain naturally, in order to lose weight. I understood that increasing low-intensity aerobic exercise would eventually reduce my body pain and need for pain medication. *But getting to this point was anything but easy.*

I know you're wondering how one can get more mobile while struggling through a challenging healing process. From introspection, I can say that regardless of pain and mobility challenge, the motivation to heal sooner rather than later is going to be different for someone else.

One major overriding factor *I believe* keeps many people from healing sooner rather than later is when the doctor's exercise and mobility plan is completely ignored. This is not so hard to understand. The temporary or permanent loss of mobility, increased pain, and feeling out of sorts creates varying levels of pain, anxiety, and depression. And with too much time on your hands, internalizing the meaning of disabling circumstances has a way of discouraging even the best recovery plan. Expeditious recoveries after injury are dependent on following the doctor's orders and internal drivers that keep you motivated to work on the healing process.

Like many who've experienced long-term limited mobility after injury, I fell into a life-changing situation. Until my hip injury and disease diagnosis, I was considered by most an elite athlete, bodybuilder, soldier, jack of all trades, community leader, technician, business entrepreneur, and fitness consultant for many years. Little did I know how much the ordeal would change my life.

Like I had with the decades-old back injuries that still plague me today, I eventually learned how to work around two bad hips and back issues by accepting a tolerable amount of total body pain. For example, from 2003 to 2008, I experienced daily chronic muscle spasm and pain in both my upper body and lower body at a pain level of six to seven on a scale of ten, with ten being the worst pain possible. Today is much different. I'm able to manage an acceptable level of pain with intermittent pain spikes and muscle spasms during and after exercise activity.

I continue to lift weights and walk long distances. How do I do this? I adjust my walking pace and rest (daily siestas), which I refer to as "decompression" when needed. And on days when I'm doing strength training, I lift safe weight ranges that require limited range of motion on select pieces of equipment. In addition, I perform stretching exercises before, during, and after workouts, which helps to improve range of motion, blood circulation, and pain alleviation. One thing about chronic pain, like tinnitus (continuous ringing of the ear), once you have it, it's not likely to go away but can be managed effectively, for life without medication in some cases.

Through customized exercise programming, I'm able to lessen the resistive forces on my neck, back, hips, and knees while sustaining an efficient metabolism, healthy body weight, and muscle mass retention. However, if I wasn't mindful of pain centers throughout my body, I'd likely aggravate my injuries, reinjure myself, or cause unacceptable weight-bearing joint pain.

Leveraging a modified strength-training routine to maintain muscle mass and avoid causing further injury is a very important concept to get right. That is, during strength training, if it hurts, modify the exercise in a way that it doesn't cause unacceptable pain. Challenge yourself to exercise differently.

Although my exercise and pain management program works for me, as mentioned previously, that does not mean it is right for you. As you'll truly understand after reading the next chapter, customized or relevant fitness programming is a unique prescription relative to the individual. No two fitness or healthy lifestyle change prescriptions, plans, or programs should be exactly alike if they are to be sustained long-term.

I've always followed the doctor's advice and recommendations for diet and exercise modifications. The difference in what I did versus what many patients won't do is that most don't attempt to go to a gym or move about on a city sidewalk and trail system using crutches, a walker, or a wheelchair to exercise postop.

With that being said, I didn't push pain to a point where I aggravated the healing process. To be honest, my efforts were not without pain. However, I understood my diagnosis and how increased mobility efforts *would heal me sooner rather than later* and *keep me healthy thereafter.* A properly managed pain and mobility plan relative to individual need—when applied correctly—*will* provide the motivation and willpower necessary to heal sooner rather than later and sustain increased mobility activity, *for life.*

Staying at home during physical recovery, in my opinion, is dreary, lonely, and a depressing ordeal. And if mobility exercise and/or just stepping outdoors is not a daily habit, the depression nemesis can bite hard.

Like many of you, I'm one of those people who have to constantly mobilize the body outdoors to feel well.

In another time, I was likely a nomadic wanderer or a MirrorAthlete warrior. Like those remote island people, I have a need to travel long distances to set camp, hunt, socialize, and gather things while connecting with God's green earth. I'm very aware of how important mobility is to the overall well-being of an encompassing being.

Going to the gym and walking outside using mobility aids was important to my recovery and my future outlook on life. I was motivated to move more and not concerned about hiding my physical weaknesses and handicap from others. Sure, this part of my life was somewhat embarrassing, especially when others witnessed my clumsy workouts and movements. But that was far better than the alternative—gaining more weight, losing strength and mobility, intolerable pain, increased depression, and more mind-numbing pills. That wasn't for me.

Some saw me as crazy to negotiate walking a busy suburban Californian sidewalk and trail system with walking aids—especially considering my slow response were I to need to move out of harm's way. After all, many cities throughout the nation don't prioritize resources for public sidewalks, trails, and pathway connections. And they certainly aren't up to ADA standards for wheelchair use. This is where a little preplanning to find the safest route in your hood is important, especially if you can't move quickly and have need to exercise outdoors.

Fortunately, the depression was short-lived because I chose to challenge myself physically on a daily basis. Does this mean I took unnecessary risks to expedite recovery? Yes I did. But my daily exercise was well planned, and it paid off in the long run. I thought, nothing ventured, nothing gained. For me, the benefits of getting outdoor mobility exercise far outweighed any risk of reinjury or accident.

During the time of my recovery, I reflected heavily on distant cultures and people who were essentially void of Western influences—places where people were happy, lived longer, and lived without disease. This led me later to discover those remote village people who lived well over ninety years of age. It became apparent that remote cultures could teach anyone a thing or two about abating or delaying the scourges of aging and healing naturally, while retaining mobility capability.

You'd think with our "$70 billion diet and $20 billion health-club industries in their efforts to persuade us that if we eat the right food or do the right workout, we'll be healthier, lose weight and live longer. But these strategies rarely work. Not because they're wrong-minded: it's a good idea for people to do any of these healthful activities. The problem is, it's difficult to change individual behaviors when community behaviors stay the same" (Philpott 2012).

During this time of reflection, I also began programming dual-purpose, or as I've often described it, *nomadic walking activity*. I needed to change my exercise habits and strength-training techniques. Exercising daily in a gym was not in my best fitness and health interest. I definitely didn't feel like I belonged there during postsurgery recovery. And I didn't feel my past exercise routine was compatible with my new lifestyle changes.

Through application of MirrorAthlete science principles, my daily habits and activities have changed dramatically over the last decade. For instance, I don't obsess about working out in a gym for hours to sustain desired fitness levels and results. And I no longer believe daily strength training, high-intensity interval training (HIIT), and high intensity aerobics is the gold standard to stay fit and feel and look well regardless of age—especially if you're not a competitive athlete.

I now walk seven days a week and hit an outdoor or indoor gym two to three times a week for strength training and to tone the body. Prior to the 2003 hip collapse and AVN disease diagnosis of both hips, I did a lot of heavy strength training with free weights in a gym and at home six days a week and ran and biked intensely three to four days a week. I rarely walked or warmed up prior to exercise. Nor did I often cool down with range-of-motion stretch exercises. I did often preach the importance of these things, however—my bad.

At that time, I found very little value in walking, hiking, or biking long distances. If you asked anyone who knew me prior to 2003, they'd likely say I didn't personally apply or prioritize low-intensity aerobic exercise. They'd be correct. I rarely walked anywhere over one to three miles and once in a while exercised on a treadmill, stair master, stationary bike, or rowing or cyclical machine, without consistency.

Today, I value walking so much it is a daily priority, and everything else is scheduled around it.

To this day, I continue a daily walking habit and have recruited good partners who've also experienced the benefits. By studying isolated people and contrasting lifestyles, I found that a greater appreciation for those cultural habits arose. These healthy places were mostly free of Western culture. It proved to me at some point that, if *healthy lifestyle literacy education* was taught in K–12 schools, a cultural shift to value those things would positively change behavior for the next generation. This is the reverse engineering needed to begin healing our nation's childhood obesity and related disease problems through adulthood.

I digress. So how do I motivate myself daily to continue a nomadic walking habit within a suburban environment that lacks sufficient public use trail systems and recreation facilities? I walk (hunt) and gather needed products and call it "dual-purpose walking activity," which simply requires a small backpack, one to three liters of water in it, and well-supported insole shoes and seasonal weather attire during inclement weather. Rain and snow do not stop me from walking daily. It's nothing but a thing—especially when you're prepared for it.

Once you're conditioned, dual-purpose walking is easy and fun. I hunt down a needed whole foods product found at a distant location, put it in my backpack, and bring it home. Dual-purpose walking activities may include walking to a destination like the local gym or a store or accessing a neighborhood trail or sidewalk system to catch a public transportation ride to a distant recreation location or city event or shopping center. The list goes on and on. This is my daily aerobic, fat-burning exercise of choice. And it gives me time to relax, get in touch with nature, pick up some healthy store-bought goods, or stop and do some strength training at an indoor or outdoor fitness facility. Then I plan for tomorrow as I walk home.

Believe me, I didn't start out walking eight to ten miles per day. And no, I'm not suggesting this become your starting point as a new activity goal. You first must condition yourself to walk longer distances each day if this becomes your low-impact aerobic exercise of choice. And before carrying any significant weight on your back, you start with no load and only a bottle of water in hand.

Most people who start a walking program are motivated to do so in a different way than what motivated me. I started low-impact aerobics in a wheelchair and then graduated to crutches and a cane and only traveled a few blocks from my front door to an empty church parking lot. After a period of time, I was able to travel up to a mile using those walking aids.

Inherently, people understand that walking, jogging, and biking have health and fitness benefits. When a spouse, family member, or friend sees the weight loss and increased fitness levels and fit appearance changes, they begin to believe they're capable of walking a mile or two to receive similar benefits. Often others will consider changing sedentary habits to participate in what they viewed previously as pointless. Often that old adage "to see is to believe" is absolutely true and necessary for some to change an unhealthy habit.

Walking can be a great social bonding opportunity if you have a dedicated partner or friend who commits to joining you once in a while. Conversations during walks also build better relationships among spouses and friends and this, in itself, is habit forming enough that you want to do it over again the next day.

However, remain mindful and don't expect anyone else to join you if he or she is not motivated or conditioned or mentally ready for it. I've had others look at me as if to say, "That's too far. Are you crazy? Use a car or call a cab." That's especially the case when they find out I went on an eighteen-miler that took five hours to complete. Instead of trying to convince others of the great health and fitness benefits, I choose to go it alone most the time because I've become addicted to the brain-body chemical release and meditative brain games I enjoy that keep me addicted to the habit. Until others experience those feel-good attributes, they have a hard time relating to it.

When someone does join you on a walk, it is important to walk within his or her physical ability. Believe me, the person will feel the habit-forming, natural chemical boost once he or she gets started. Let new walkers experience the walk in their own way and don't push them to cover long distances at a fast pace. I let them lead. I follow.

Just because a person looks fit does not mean he or she has the aerobic and muscular endurance capacity to walk the distances you're now capable of covering. Just because a person can walk a treadmill for forty-five minutes does not condition him or her in the same way you're able to walk long hours on the road, sidewalks, or trail systems. Likewise, you may find walking a treadmill or mountain hiking physically and mentally grueling because you've not conditioned targeted brain-muscle memory to perform that specific task or exercise. Think of the road as a piece of fitness equipment with different environmental and gravitational resistive settings with opposing and varying forces. For example, you have surface texture, elevation changes, weather, wind, air quality, traffic, and so on. For a good analogy, consider how hard it is to walk on beach sand as opposed to a flat, paved road.

Be sure to walk at a pace and distance your walking partner is comfortable with—especially if you enjoy the company. I know this will be tough for those conditioned to walk at a quick pace for long distances. The patience it takes to develop good walking partnerships will pay off in ways you have yet to experience. It's definitely worth the effort to bring good conversation on walks. Likewise, it's a bad idea to bring negative energy and bad attitudes.

When new partners participate in walking, select shorter distances and lower intensity of pace so they experience the physical and calming benefits. I often walk with those now conditioned to hoof it five to eight miles and stop midway for a cup of coffee and to enjoy a good conversation on my "fishing expeditions." I have multiple walking loops or walkabouts that circle back to the start point. After those walks, I often continue on and complete another four to six miles alone.

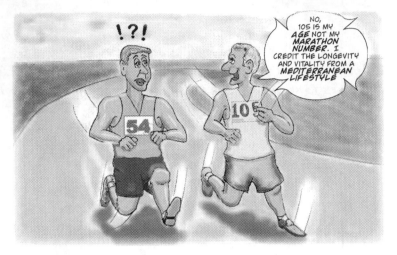

If you're serious about changing your lifestyle and tired of feeling broken, overweight, and unfit, MirrorAthlete's Principled Fit Healthy Lifestyle Philosophy can show anyone how to leverage healthy habits one step at a time. How does the old saying go? How do you eat an elephant? One bite at a time. Putting things into perspective, as applied in my case, it took years to achieve my mobility goal. But in most cases, people who want to focus on mobility improvements and increase fitness levels won't have to wait as long to see those changes—especially if they're not going through a physical recovery period.

Persistence in mobilizing the body sooner rather than later can put anyone into a well-being winners' circle and within a reasonable amount of time. You simply must believe you can improve upon any lifestyle change goal *you* set. And you know it is possible because the fit, healthy healing and lifestyle change truths are right in front of you.

For those of you who think you're too old to endure long walks and increase fitness levels, keep this motivating factor in mind. If an eighty- to ninety-year-old person can walk miles in a day on a remote island to fish, work all day in community gardens, and socialize at multiple events, you're capable of similar activities once you believe you're capable of doing the same things. You now know it is possible to live long, productive, fit, and healthy lifestyles because other cultures remind us how to do it—absent of Western influence.

The decision you need to make *now* is this: Are you ready to begin leveraging a healthier balance of good habits and behavior? Or will you continue the same course, at the expense of your health and well-being?

Chapter 18

Customized Fitness Programming

> Relevant exercise programming optimizes fitness and healthy lifestyle goals.
>
> —MirrorAthlete Principled Fitness and
> Healthy Lifestyle Philosophy

I've known many who've applied the same exercise programs for years and are happy to continue that course indefinitely. Others, like myself, use specialized exercise routines to prepare for seasonal recreation and sports activities and to set personal fitness goals.

Many exercise activities I participate in today are also the ones I enjoyed during childhood, which includes daily walks. As seasons come and go, I modify my personal fitness programs in advance, knowing which favored childhood activities I'll likely participate in.

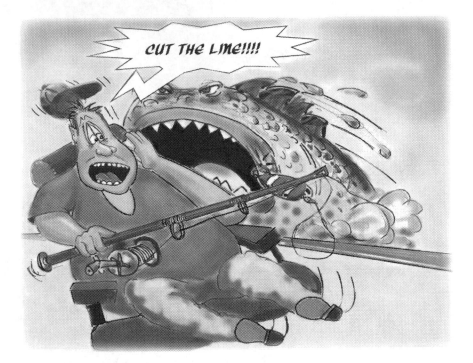

For example, a seasonal recreational activity may require the muscular endurance to land a large fish, or have enough upper body strength and flexibility to pull oneself out of the water onto a large tube towed by a boat, for those who enjoy that kind of thing. I know many of you think, *No problem*. But this muscular endurance task and others like it can be challenging when strength training has not been part of the fitness equation.

Last season, my wife and I were out boating with family and friends. We had a tube with a towrope attached to our boat. I was able to pull myself out of the water repeatedly to get on top of the tube prior to each ride without fail, whereas others my age and even thirty years younger struggled to achieve the task or could not do it at all.

For me, this is a fun watersport activity I enjoyed as a kid. I want to be able to physically do this as long as possible when the opportunity strikes. So just prior to boating season, I switch up my fitness program to focus more on upper body strength, muscular endurance, and midbody toning and flexibility exercises. My walking activities also increase to 70 to 80 percent aerobic intensity of effort as I negotiate more hills to lose the excess body fat gained after the first of the year.

To assist in customizing a daily fitness or seasonal recreational program, I've provided completed client form 13.1 "Tina's Healthy Habits Commitment Plan." And completed form 18.1 "Hank's Fitness Program & Tracking Record." Use these examples if needed to develop a personalized healthy habits and fitness plan (see appendix). However, recall that these client program examples are personalized. They're based on someone else's current medical history, fitness assessment, health condition, motivations, lifestyle preferences, environment, fitness levels, and activity aspirations. Instead of copying them, use them as a guideline to customize a relevant program that's right for you.

Like snowflakes, no two individuals are the same. Therefore, to achieve optimum fitness and performance results, personalized programming strategies must be relatable and applicable to each individual.

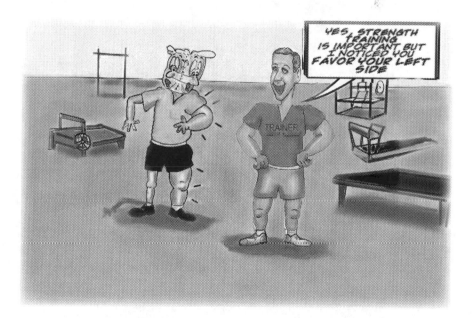

To plan, record, and track fitness results, feel free to magnify and copy blank forms 13.0 "Healthy Habits Commitment Plan" and 18.0 "Fitness Program & Tracking Record" (see appendix) and use them as a template to help develop your plan. Then apply the program. Also, refer back to the four previous client examples below to recall additional insight:

1. Marvin's primary fitness goal was cardio and muscular endurance (chapter 5, "Caloric Exchange: A Balancing Act").
2. Kate's primary fitness goal was weight loss (chapter 8, "All Fats Are Not Equal").
3. Tom's primarily fitness goal was strength gain (chapter 9, "Health Risk Prediction and Prevention").
4. Tina's healthy habit goal was weight loss (chapter 13, "Leveraging Healthy Habit Change").

Before getting into the various programming details and examples that follow, I've defined seventeen specific fitness terms to broaden your fitness knowledge base. These definitions are followed by a few thoughts on public use recreational resources found within many communities that can be used for little to no cost to increase fitness levels and achieve set results.

Fitness Programming Terminology

1 rep max (1RM). Lifting as heavy of a resistive weight or weight setting as possible one time at any exercise station.

aerobic exercise. Low- to medium-intensity exercise of long duration at a low rate of speed. During aerobic exercise, muscles prefer glucose and stored body fat fuel to continue exercise within an oxygenated cellular environment.

anaerobic exercise. High-intensity exercise of short duration and at a high rate of speed. During anaerobic exercise, muscles prefer glucose and stored muscle glycogen as a fuel source within a nonoxygenated cellular environment.

cross-training. An exercise or physical activity that conditions other muscle memory and coordination skill sets and may not be related to a primary fitness goal or competitive sport skill set.

effort. The strength, muscular, and cardio endurance and mental effort needed to complete work, perform a physical task, or achieve a fitness objective or goal.

force. Power necessary to move or counter an opposing resistance.

free weight lifting. Weighted plates on bars or dumbbells used at a free weight exercise station. Weight is typically added to a bar and secured by locking collars, and lifts are often assisted by a spotter.

intensity. A measurable amount of physical endurance, strength, force, or power.

intensity of effort. A performance measurement of effort applied to complete a physical task or activity, to get work done, or to achieve a fitness objective or goal—often measured as percentage of effort.

muscular endurance. The capacity of muscle to endure contractions repeatedly to stay in motion over a long period of time.

muscle memory. Activities that, when repeated frequently increase neuromuscular effort, whereas physical performance has a high level of coordinated efficiency and precision functionality. Once these connections are made by the brain and body, they last a lifetime but decrease in efficiency and precision without practice. The old adage, "practice makes perfect," is true.

power. The physical endurance and strength needed to equivocally counter or overcome an opposing force.

reps or repetitions. When a weight is repeatedly lifted more than once; completion of those repetitions is considered a set.

set. A programmed number of working muscle repetitions performed at an exercise station before rest equals one set.

strength. Capacity to overcome an opposing force with greater than equal force or power. Strength is often measured as lifting the heaviest weight one time and calculated using 1 rep max (1RM) formulae.

stationary or circuit weight-training equipment. Stationary exercise equipment targets specific muscle groups. The equipment is mechanically designed with cable-pulley or pivotal-hinge leverage systems with quick weight setting selections.

task-specific exercise. Conditioning the brain and body (*muscle memory*) specifically to achieve a fitness, physical performance, or activity goal or result.

Understanding the terminology above is an important component of developing a relevant fitness program and applying it successfully.

And just as important is having access to the resources necessary within a community to execute the fitness plan successfully. Without a plan and resources to apply it daily, increasing fitness levels and achieving set goals is going to be more challenging.

The other point I want to make clear is this: *It is not necessary to have financial means to achieve a fitness goal or live a healthier lifestyle.* This is especially true if it's understood that much can be accomplished outside of a gym using public use resources. These are resources that are not dependent on you paying someone hundreds of dollars for specialized services and products that don't work. Greater access to public transportation will help (though public transportation may no longer be of concern for many, with the inception of Uber and Lyft rides, for example). In either case, people can travel affordably to places that offer a healthier environment where they can perform exercise activity.

I highly recommend, if your city does not have a recreation center, adequate outdoor exercise gym, walking and biking trails, or public parks nearby that inspire exercise activity, lobby your city recreation and parks board and council. Tell them how important it is to prioritize, plan, budget, and develop these resources. It is true that a city's recreational amenities level out the health and financial disparity and other inequities that exist in all communities. These public use resources can be used at little to no cost and allow you to perform daily exercise activity on a tight household budget.

Just remember when you take your message to the city, make the case. *City recreation saves lives just like policing services do, but in different ways.* It is well established that public recreation programs that admit financially disparaged children for free help decrease juvenile mischief, drug use and the childhood obesity and related diseases now plaguing this nation. It is also acknowledged by experts that public recreation programs that support financially disparaged populations would decrease childhood and adult obesity and related diseases now plaguing this nation.

Regardless, if the place you call home makes you feel unsafe, anxious, depressed, sick, or isolated for lack of affordable or accessible recreational resources, or if it's just an unhealthy environment, it may be time to make a major lifestyle change. It's noteworthy to point out that those who have the means typically do just that. They leave and move to healthier city environments that offer multiple public use recreational amenities.

When cities provide recreation activities for the community, financial barriers are removed, behaviors change, and people are more motivated to value and live healthier lifestyles. As an economic benefit to communities, leisurely and discretionary income is repatriated back into the local economy. Healthy community development must prioritize city recreation resources for public use if cities hope to retain their tax base and sustain affordable city services for the long haul. The need for fit, healthy community environments is not a fad. It's what residents need and expect, and they will move to those places to age in place (National Recreation and Parks Conference 2015–2017). Such places make people feel safe and comfortable and offer activities in abundance for those of any age. Housing development, pedestrian pathways, and recreational activities have the ADA (American Disability Act) in mind. And in these places, anyone can expect to live independently and affordably in his or her home and community for as long as possible, hence *age in place.*

Rest assured—if your goal is to lose weight naturally and get more fit, you don't need to leave your community, have a gym membership, or beat yourself up performing high-intensity aerobic or anaerobic exercise. And you don't have to starve yourself or take unhealthy dietary products or purchase useless gimmicks.

I don't know any doctor who'd argue that beginning a daily walk habit or low-intensity recreational exercise is bad for anyone who wants to get fitter (unless a medical condition means such activity will increase health risk).

Even if you have partial use of your legs or are unable to use them at all, aerobic and anaerobic exercise benefits can be achieved through seated, upper-body stationary equipment. For example, seated endurance rope climber, arm pedal and stationary resistive strength-training equipment, and outdoor gyms are now very popular with stationary wheelchair fitness equipment and ADA access in mind (NRPA 2016, 2017).

Of course, if you have the means, fitness equipment can also be purchased in a home-use version. In addition, wheelchair or specialized bikes that are pedaled by hand are very popular and are used on roads, school tracks, city sidewalks, park pathways, and trail systems and in public plazas space.

As a fit healthy lifestyle consultant and through city council service, I know that unhealthy city development and environment is a detractor for those looking for places to age in place. Communities that don't invest in making neighborhoods safer—by providing adequate public transportation facilities; accessible, well-lit pedestrian walkways and parks; and indoor community recreation programming for active adults and working families—lose out. Failing to take these measures may mean cities losing a percentage of their housing tax base, as well as economic loss to small business. And individuals who don't have the means or the ability to choose to move will lose out too. Lack of access to affordable public use recreational facilities and transportation may likely mean the difference between success and failure when it comes to achieving a fitness goal and staying healthy.

As I learned while attending the OPRA (Oregon Parks and Recreation Association) November 2016 conference in Eugene, Oregon, the top three reasons boomers and retirees move away from a previous location are that they have a desire to live in a safe area with more recreational opportunities and away from cold extremes. They also spend on average $40,000 per year on leisurely recreational activities. As you can see, boomers, unlike those without financial means, have a choice of where they spend their money. But it is these resources from the largest and wealthiest group of people that provide public use recreational amenities for the less affluent.

Think about it. When a hundred boomers and retirees spend on average $4 million annually for leisurely activities, that should be an eye-opener for community leaders, economic developers, and recreation planners. I don't know too many cities that wouldn't want to repatriate those dollars back into the local economy. Unfortunately, too many politicians, city staff, and city boards and committees don't connect or relate to how public use recreational facilities and amenities sustain affordable city services and bring community together in a way that makes families want to age in place.

A word of advice to each community resident: Now you're aware, fitness programming success is greatly dependent on healthy city planning and development and public use recreation facilities, programs, and services. If community development doesn't put its residents' health, safety, and recreational needs first as a core city service, consider what a neighboring city has to offer and find a way to access those services or move to them.

I digress. Now what you've been waiting for.

To begin absorbing the customized fitness programming knowledge, it is necessary to relate to how muscle fiber types and fuel preference must be complementary to the exercise activity and fitness goal to achieve the desired result.

Muscle Fiber Types Have Food Fuel Preferences

A customized fitness program would not be complete without knowing how muscle fiber types function and what food fuels they prefer. The basics of this information were covered in chapter 3, "Muscles' Fuel Preference during Exercise." The following focus is to further illustrate how muscle fiber types prefer certain food and body storage fuels based on various intensities and types of exercise effort.

Here's a quick recap from chapter 3. Recall that our muscles are mostly comprised of slow- and fast-twitch fibers and a third type known as intermittent, consisting of a mix of those two muscle fiber types. Each fiber type has a specific food fuel need dependent on the intensity of physical effort.

For example, during high-intensity anaerobic exercise, fast-twitch muscles prefer blood glucose and stored glycogen, easily accessible within the liver and muscle tissue as an expedient energy source. Slow- to moderate-intensity aerobic exercise (slow-twitch fiber) prefers blood glucose and fuel from body fat reserves. Dietary proteins are mostly used to repair body tissues and not preferred fuels by muscle fiber during exercise.

It is also important to understand there are genetically gifted endurance and strength athletes with varying percentages of slow-twitch, intermittent, and fast-twitch muscle fiber composition.

Science shows us "human muscles contain a genetically determined mixture of both slow and fast fiber types. On average, we have about 50 percent slow twitch and 50 percent fast twitch fibers in most of the muscles used for movement ... Olympic sprinters have been shown to possess about 80 percent fast twitch fibers, while those who excel in marathons tend to have 80 percent slow twitch fibers" (Quinn and Fogoros 2018b).

Does this mean if you have an average fifty-fifty fiber type composition you can't be competitive as a world-class marathon runner or sprinter? No, it does not. Cross-training exercise techniques, sport-specific conditioning, and individual drive often and surprisingly trump the genetic advantage. I believe the athlete with heart and unyielding desire to win is the one to watch out for.

Simply reflect on Anthony Jerome "Spud" Webb, now a retired American NBA point guard. His basketball career lasted from 1985 to 1998. He was first drafted by the Detroit Pistons and stood only five foot seven. In 1986, Spud won the first NBA Slam Dunk Contest. He was only one of two athletes under six feet tall to win the competition. Webb trained Nate Robinson, five foot nine, of the New York Knicks twenty years later to perform the same feat. Robinson then proceeded to win the 2010 dunk contest held in Dallas, Texas.

The point is, never accept someone telling you you're too small or not fast or strong enough to achieve a competitive goal or dream. Believing with conviction and passion provides the willpower and heart necessary for some to succeed where others see impossible. Spud simply never saw himself as too short or not capable of competing with the height advantaged. The word *can't* was not in this former NBA star's vocabulary.

An Olympic bodybuilder, Olympic sprinter, and slam dunk competitor may certainly have genetically higher concentrations of fast-twitch muscle fiber compared to you and me. And that advantage may have helped those "like Spud" achieve winning feats regardless of physical size. However, I believe that, when you factor in a nondefeatist drive, it's those with the heart of a lion who are capable of beating the genetically gifted athlete.

Next, we'll define and analyze muscle fiber characteristics and energy exchange during exercise activity. Then we'll look at how a fuel source is preferred by the muscles when varying intensity of exercise effort is applied. We'll look at how to monitor and adjust intensity of effort to achieve the desired fitness and performance goal. And finally, we'll seek to understand how anyone can naturally gain an edge over a genetically gifted competitor.

Examining Muscle Fibers' Unique Energy Exchange Characteristics

When looking at fast-twitch muscle fiber under a microscope, the first thing you note is they're *white* in cellular appearance for lack of oxygenated myoglobin. The muscles myoglobin is similar to our blood's *red* pigmented hemoglobin, which carries iron and oxygen-binding proteins to nourish and energize cellular tissue.

"Because fast twitch fibers use anaerobic metabolism to create fuel, they are better at generating short bursts of strength or speed than slow muscles. However they fatigue more quickly" (Quinn and Fogoros 2018b), than do the other two types of muscle fiber, intermediate and slow-twitch fibers. Thinking about fast-twitch muscle fibers another way, during anaerobic activity, they can be conditioned to hold their breath longer under water (or without oxygen) but only for a very short period of time.

In all muscle fiber types, there is energy exchange that causes our muscles to contract and expand. And this synthesis occurs through ATP (adenosine triphosphate) energy production within the fibers' mitochondrial structure and often referred to as the muscle's powerhouse producer. This energy exchange causes muscle to contract and move us to get work done. ATP synthesis and muscular contractions occur at varying rates of speed, dependent on when the oxidative (aerobic) or glycolytic (anaerobic) energy conversion takes place and how much muscle fiber type neural innervation or muscular stimulation occurs (University of Washington 2011).

"In these [mitochondrial] structures, the potential energy in food is extracted and harvested within the energy-rich bonds of ATP (adenosine triphosphate), the unique energy currency of each cell." As intensity of physical effort increases, slow-twitch muscle fibers sequentially yield to intermittent and then fast-twitch muscle fibers, whose preferred anaerobic fuel during forceful activity is glucose and then glycogen. As fast-twitch muscle fibers fatigue through lactic acid buildup, they sequentially yield to intermittent and then slow-twitch muscle fibers as quick fuel sources are depleted. The slower rate of muscular intensity is fueled by fat reserve conversion to blood glucose (Katch and McArdle 1993).

Here's another way to look at muscle fatigue: When enough ATP by-product (lactic acid) is produced through forceful and fast exercise, fast-twitch muscle fibers' rate of contractions decreases. Then to continue activity at a slower pace, the intermittent and slow-twitch muscle fibers allow you to continue movement through walking, jogging, or a slower-paced run, fueled by the ATP energy exchange process.

Fat fuel can be thought of as a plentiful energy source compared to stored liver and muscle glycogen. For example, we know the body can survive without food for around thirty days or more because of fat fuel reserves. For most of us, we could go weeks without food. However, the survival reality is limited to two to four days when extreme environmental conditions present physiological and metabolic energy exchange challenges due to lack of hydration.

There have been many cases where people became lost or found in unfortunate circumstances and walked miles and survived to tell the tale—and lost a lot of body weight in the process. I attribute their survival to willpower, adequate hydration, and body fat reserves that provided the energy to walk the distance to civilization.

If one expected to set a fast pace under a similar survival scenario, a blood sugar fuel boost would be required. This is why we often see hikers and bikers eating trail mix or granola bars or consuming energy drinks on the go. These foods can be quickly absorbed and broken down into blood glucose to replenish blood sugar levels and muscle glycogen stores after a period of rest, enabling one to continue the faster-paced activity.

When the body works at high intensities to complete a physical task, it only has enough readily available blood glucose to fuel high-intensity muscular contractions for up to a maximum period of ten seconds. After this time and up to a period of three minutes, the fuel source switches to stored muscle glycogen. "In contrast, slow twitch fibers use a combination of glucose and fats for their energy supply. This is a much slower process and can be maintained with constant intensity for a continued time period" (Fitnessbeans 2014). And how well the cellular ATP and mitochondria function offsets or delays lactic acid buildup is predicated on physical condition, quick fuel storage capacity, intensity of aerobic effort, and energy exchange efficiency.

Building a Competitive Fitness Program to Beat a Competitor

Aside from fueling and conditioning muscle fiber to perform a task-specific exercise, clients also want to know how to gain a competitive advantage. This goal is important for some and not so much for others. Nevertheless, here's my take. To build a competitive advantage in your training program, I recommend researching your competitor's performance results. Also, consider similar training strategies and tactics. Note I said *similar*. Why do I point this out? Recall, no one person is wired the same genetically, physically, spiritually, or mentally. This uniqueness includes muscle fiber type percentages; energy exchange (along with muscle memory function coordinated with physical skill set efficiencies); and, don't forget, *heart*.

However, there are two consistent training principles that must not be overlooked if you're a serious competitor. That's training in a *similar* environment and using *similar* equipment and exercise technique. Train in a way that mirrors the training of a competing champion if you want to improve energy exchange and coordinated muscle memory efficiencies.

Once trained to efficiency, the muscle memory afterburners can be turned on and off as needed. For instance, your muscle memory doesn't forget how to ride a bike or throw a ball or sprint once it's developed. However ability to compete at a high level of play decreases without practice.

A good analogy of a winning competitor's success and failure rate is more relatable when the losing competitor understands how environment and relevant training practices result in a loss or win. For example, through examination of a winning race horse and jockey or a runner at a marathon event, we can better understand what contributed to the winning and losing result.

For instance, a replacement jockey may repeatedly lose races after a retired jockey placed first consistently on the same horse. What has caused this genetically gifted animal to lose repeatedly with a new jockey? After this analysis, we'll make a similar analytical comparison relative to a marathon runner. Then we'll use these examples in analogy and to explore how to be competitive in any sport.

At the horse races, bets are placed after bettors review horse profiles and performance histories. Those who bet on horse races, sports teams, and athletes know past and present performance stats of beast and human increase the odds of picking a winner. Horse race performance stats can be found in race programs, equestrian sport publications, and other associated trade articles with data on both rider and horse. Those stats are weighed and assessed by speculative gamblers, owners, and trainers well in advance of any race. Sports teams use player stats and data and study videos of competitors to adjust training tactics and to place bets just like those placed at the horse races. All trainers and professional athletes size up their competition in similar ways in order to train, achieve a competitive advantage, and win.

The rider and horse, like professional runners, must be in top mental and physical condition if they hope to win or place. Understand that the relationship between physical and mental coordination and muscle memory precision and performance efficiency is measured in hundredths of a second. This is why it's so important to understand past winning performance times and study a competitor's profile, stats, training environment, and actual training tactics to achieve a winning strategy.

Knowing this information prior to a sporting event can mean the difference between a win and a loss—a difference measured in less than a second. For instance, at the start of a horse race, the jockey initiates the signal for an explosive stride out of the gate. Then the horse is queued to canter to a gallop quickly. Then at some point, rider and horse accelerate and hold a set or variable race speed and stride to the finish line.

Likewise, a marathon runner must train the mind and body to coordinate and control conditioned muscle memory in a precise effort to run and sprint at the right times. He or she must be sure to avoid fatigue prior to the acceleration needed just before reaching the winning stretch and finish line. In both race scenarios (horse and runner), prior to the event, competitors must train in ways that are similar to the training of the "one to beat," within a winning timeline and in an environment that replicates the actual event.

If muscle memory is not conditioned or synchronized with physical body and mental effort, a genetic advantage may be of no advantage in any case. A last-minute jockey changeup before the race may cause a winning and genetically gifted horse to lose because of unsynchronized muscle memory coordination and/or speed changes signaled or communicated by the jockey. Under this scenario, the very signals the new jockey is employing in the hopes of winning may be what throws the horse off due to lack of synchronization.

Muscle movement coordination to accelerate and decelerate is not exact and, therefore, less efficient with a new jockey at the helm. It's not so much about physical conditioning in this case. The communicative precision via coordinated signaling cues has changed.

In the world of race cars, professional drivers experience the same time-sync inefficiencies in coordination of muscle memory—also known as motor skill. For instance, shifting gears to slow down or speed up indecisively and without precision can mean the difference between blowing an engine, crashing, or crossing the finish line within inches for the win.

For a runner, a negative performance may occur if environmental conditions are not part of the training program prior to the event. For example, when altitude, weather, and ground conditions of an event differ from the training environment, these differences have an effect on mental concentration. They can also affect muscle memory coordination when it comes to decisively choosing whether a moment calls to preserve energy, decelerate, or accelerate for the pass and win.

There are many teaching points any athlete in any profession could learn from these analogies and talking points. The key takeaway is that to gain a competitive advantage, study the competitor to beat. Then implement task-specific training with similar exercise in a like environment if you hope to be competitive and ultimately stand in the winner's circle.

Intensity of Effort Necessary to Achieve Personal Fitness Goals

If your fitness goal is simply to maintain a well-conditioned body, then apply daily aerobic and anaerobic exercise of low- to moderate-intensity. Through a balanced mix of exercise, you'll sustain an efficient metabolism, good range of motion, postural alignment, a healthy body weight, tone, and good strength and mobility relative to age throughout life.

However, outside of that norm, if your fitness goal is to become a competitive intramural racquetball player, for example, and you want to develop a muscular frame, program yourself to achieve both fitness goals. One way to do that is to train intensely with a racquetball partner no less than three days a week. On days you don't play racquetball, train anaerobically using heavy resistive weights and targeting muscle groups you want to develop. Then choose to take one to two days off a week from training. This allows for proper rest, repair, and restoration of muscles.

This type of exercise training is often referred to as cross-training—training that falls outside of a primary fitness or sports activity focus. Stimulating and conditioning motor skill coordination in various ways often helps a competitor achieve that extra winning edge. For instance, substitute a day of hard training to ride a bike, jog, kayak, or walk. This not only provides for muscle recovery time but may also provide an additional advantage by strengthening and balancing out other motor skill coordination not well conditioned.

Aside from restful exercise or leisurely activities, it's often the unique cross-training exercise seen in *American Ninja Warrior*, parkour, free running, and other similar high-intensity cross-training activities that can prepare you for and give you an advantage in the next competitive event. This is especially true if you're interested in competing in any number of competitive reality TV shows that require exceptional physical conditioning and gymnastic skillsets. Think *American Ninja Warrior*, *Steve Austin's Broken Skull Challenge*, *Survivor*, or any number of military-type boot camp competitions. Or if you're interested in a physically elite military career, obstacle course training will definitely provide the training necessary to become competitive in these specialized occupations.

Why Aerobics Enthusiasts Monitor Heart Rate to Burn More Fat

Fitness enthusiasts have used target heart rate (THR) to monitor intensity of aerobic exercise effort to stay within the fat-burning zone for decades.

Understanding how heart rate relates to the fat-burning zone is essential for those whose fitness goal is to lose body fat naturally. "Although it's technically true that exercising in the so-called 'fat burning zone' (at a lower intensity level of about 60% to 70% of maximum heart rate) does use a higher *percentage* of fat calories for fuel, the overall total calories burned is still fairly low. The reason is simple. Fat is a slow-burning fuel that requires oxygen to convert it to a usable energy, so it's great for long, steady, slow exercise, like backpacking, or cycling a long distance" (Quinn 2017).

Target heart rate can be determined through a simple mathematical formula easy to use and applied while exercising or at rest. Although there are more complex and more precise THR formulas, the *simple formula* will do. By applying THR formula and monitoring your heart rate, you can burn more fat calories during long endurance exercise activity. Why is this knowledge important? Exercise science shows a correlation between heart rate, intensity of aerobic effort, and muscle metabolism fuel preference.

If you don't want to calculate the simple formula or take a pulse count, you can purchase a pulse monitor. Or practice my nonscientific self-monitoring breathing technique soon to be shared. The self-monitored breathing technique is not scientific, but perceived breathing awareness and pace exertion will surely keep you within a fat-burning zone.

How to Calculate the Simple THR Formula Used to Monitor Heart Rate and Burn More Body Fat Weight

If you want to burn more body fat weight during exercise, you can use the simple THR (target heart rate) formula to keep exercise intensity within an efficient or optimum fat-burning zone through heart beat monitoring. All you need to do is plug an intensity of aerobic effort percentage into the simple THR formula. Then calculate your ten-second heart rate count baseline. This count will then be used to monitor actual HR (heart rate) during exercise to sustain a set intensity range of effort needed to burn more body fat.

To calculate heartbeat rate, first select the degree of intensity or exercise effort desired to achieve the fitness or training goal.

First choose and then insert an intensity of exercise effort percentage into the simple THR formula below:

- *50 to 60 percent* – Efficient intensity of exercise effort to burn body fat and experience weight loss
- *61 to 70 percent* – Optimum intensity of exercise effort to burn more body fat and experience increased weight loss
- *71 to 100 percent* – Increasing physical effort beyond 70 percent becomes more dependent on muscle glycogen and glucose fuel as exercise intensity increases past this point, whereas working metabolism becomes less dependent on fat to fuel the effort.

The simple THR formula calculates heartbeats per ten-second count. Now calculate your ten-second count: (220 [men] or 226 [women] – age) × intensity of aerobic effort %/6) = heartbeats per ten-second count.

Once you've made your calculation based on sex, age, and intensity of aerobic effort, you now have a ten-second heart rate count to monitor during exercise in order to burn more fat fuel and lose weight. You'll soon learn how to apply the ten-second count through a working example.

If your goal is to get in shape and lose body fat and you've been sedentary for a period of time and are overweight, select 35 through 50 percent intensity of aerobic exercise effort when beginning a daily exercise program. If you're conditioned to exercise and want to lose more body fat weight, chose 50 through 70 percent. If you're an elite or competitive individual who participates in intramural and professional sports, or simply wants to stay in the best shape possible and are not concerned about body fat weight, train at intensities of effort between 71 and 100 percent.

As promised, I'll show you a working example of how to calculate THR using the intensity of effort chosen and how to monitor the calculated ten-second HR during exercise to achieve your fitness goal.

1. Determine your maximum heart rate by taking 220 (men) or 226 (women) – your age. So, if you're a forty-year-old man, the calculation is: *220 – 40 = 180.*

2. Multiply the result (180 in our example) by 50 to 70 percent (the aerobic intensity of effort needed to burn fat at the minimum and optimum ranges): *180 × .50 or .70 = 90 or 126 beats per minute (BPM).*
3. Divide the beats per minute by six: 90 or 126/6 = 15 or 21 beats per ten-second pulse count.
4. If you know your fat-burning range is between 90 and 126 BPM, then a ten-second pulse rate can be monitored during exercise. For example, increase or decrease intensity of exercise effort as needed to stay within the set fat-burning THR range of 15–21 beats/ten seconds.

"These calculations provide only estimates of your heart rate maximum and cardiovascular work zone. To precisely determine your individual heart rate maximum, you would need to undergo physical testing, like in an exercise science lab" (Richey 2013).

Monitor pulse at the side of the neck or wrist during activity every fifteen minutes until the intensity of walk pace or activity effort is set within the THR range. Thereafter a set pace is established, and monitoring of heart rate becomes less frequent. Then perceived pace and breathing exertion may become a more intuitive practice, whereas monitoring or pulse check is no longer required to stay within the THR zone.

I recommend that when beginning a walk or aerobic exercise routine, you calculate a lower intensity of aerobic effort into the simple formula. This will provide a safe range to begin burning fat and further condition and coordinate muscle groups and circulatory function to achieve an advanced aerobic physical condition. As you become better conditioned, recalculate your THR. If your goal is to burn more total calories or condition the body for high-intensity muscular endurance activities and improve cardiovascular capacity, then recalculate the THR at higher percentages.

If you're walking, jogging, or participating in high-impact aerobic dance and having problems catching your breath or if you can't speak well, you're likely exercising at an unconditioned physical capacity and may be well over 70 to 80 percent THR. Listen to your body. If it hurts or it becomes too difficult to breathe or talk, slow down or stop the activity!

Keep in mind that any physical activity that gets you up and moving causes more oxygen to be taken in, improves blood circulation, and is of health benefit (recall chapter 16, "Don't Take Breathing for Granted"). When you begin aerobic exercise after living a sedentary lifestyle, you may not be able to perform at a 35–50 percent intensity of effort for long durations. Don't let this discourage short walks or other low-impact exercise activities. I've talked to clients who believed that, if exercise couldn't be performed at 50 percent intensity of THR, there was little benefit. Therefore, they'd quit before even getting started.

This is misguided thinking and a mistake if the fitness goal is to burn body fat, reduce body weight, alleviate joint pain, and get fitter. Any form of low-impact daily aerobics improves energy exchange, which directly correlates with improved body tone, oxygen exchange, lung capacity, cardiovascular circulation, and immune system function and increased mobility, flexibility, and muscular endurance. All of this leads to body fat weight loss.

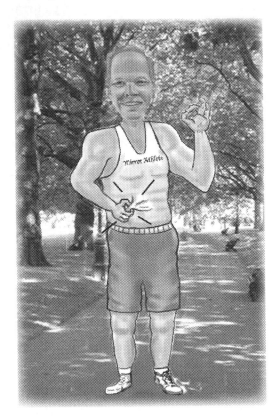

If in doubt, remember that *low-impact aerobics offer significant fitness benefits*. Simply recall the mitochondria energy exchange truths. As the body gets in increasingly better condition through aerobic exercise, so too will the ATP mitochondrial fat-burning energy conversion and exchange improve. "The good news is that they [mitochondria] increase in number and activity, by as much as 50%, in just a matter of days to weeks in response to regular aerobic exercise in adults of all ages" (Weil 2014). Once your body becomes conditioned to endure low-impact aerobic exercise, the mitochondria powerhouse energy exchange becomes more efficient at using glucose, glycogen, and body fat fuel.

Now let's use walking exercise to illustrate my nonscientific breathing and pace method to stay within the fat-burning zone. This allows you to check in without using a heart rate monitor or calculating the simple formula or taking a pulse count.

Simply put, if you can't carry on a conversation without struggling to take in air, you're walk pace is too intense. Slow down! If you're walking alone, try reciting anything verbally to get an idea of whether you're out of breath and pushing yourself too hard. (Yeah, I know I'm asking you to talk to yourself. You can be discrete about it if you're worried what others might think as you cross paths.) Regardless, if breathing is too easy, pick up the pace and walk with purpose.

Another measure is, if you have to open your mouth to breath, you may be working too hard. If you're not close to opening your mouth, pick up the pace a little. If you must keep your mouth open because of habit, you'll have to use the speaking or monitored heart rate count to adjust your walk pace. Again, if you feel like you're going to pass out, slow down, rest, and then readjust the intensity of effort and walk pace.

I easily achieve greater than 80 percent intensity of effort when I am negotiating six- to eight-degree sloped hills at a set pace of 3.8 to 4 miles per hour. I prefer ramping up or down intensities of physical effort in changing elevations (hills), as opposed to flat land walking on a daily basis to stay in excellent cardio and muscular endurance shape. Rolling terrain seems to challenge my brain and body to exert more physical effort and burn more total calories. Also when exercising at a high-endurance rate, I focus on breathing through my nose. Once my mouth opens, I slow down. My breathing technique and the lactic acid buildup in my thighs tell me when my heart rate is likely above the optimum fat-burning range (greater than 70 percent THR). I often confirm this by taking a pulse count at the side of my neck and then adjust pace accordingly. This ramping up and down of aerobic pace sustains a well-conditioned circulatory system while burning more body fat.

I rarely push beyond an 80 percent to 85 percent effort of exercise intensity, or THR. I know that, at 70 percent intensity, I'm optimizing my fat-burning furnace. And at greater than this, I begin to burn more carbohydrates than fat and increase total calorie burn from a mix of available fuel sources.

You now know with certainty that there is a direct correlation between type of exercise activity, intensity of effort, and muscle fuel preference within a set THR range.

How to Program and Benefit from Anaerobic Exercise

Anaerobic exercise is characteristic of high-intensity activities of short duration, where maximum speed, force, and power are required to prepare for a specific task. Examples include power lifting, sprinting, long jumping, javelin throwing, shot put, bodybuilding, and boxing, to name a few.

Anaerobic activities are fairly easy to spot because the effort necessary to perform them occurs within a very short period of time and does not use or optimize the fat-burning furnace. When intensity of exercise effort reaches 80 to 100 percent THR or intensity of physical effort, the caloric fuel preference by working muscle, as we previously learned, shifts toward approximately 80 percent carbohydrates and 10 to 20 percent fat fuel requirement (chapter 3, "Muscles' Fuel Preference during Exercise").

Many weight lifters believe if they pump iron at high levels of intensities, they'll build muscle and lose body fat equally. We know exercise science shows us this is partially correct. However, if your goal is to burn more body fat weight and your THR is greater than 80 percent throughout a strength-training program, you'll burn more glucose and muscle glycogen until lactic acid forces you to slow down. Once again, muscle is ready to contract at a low or high rate of speed and dependent on fuel store availability.

I've personally programmed myself and clients for *circuit weight training* (soon to be covered), where THR never falls below 90 percent intensity of effort. Circuit weight training can be an extremely fast-paced workout when competitive conditioning is the objective. I've often built programs like this for athletes who were interested in cross-training exercise in which high-intensity effort is needed to optimize explosive and forceful speed and strength for competitive sport play.

Train to Optimize Speed, Strength, and Muscle Bulk Development

If you want to develop more strength and bulk for the chest, arms, buttocks, and upper legs, the first step in muscle building is to determine each muscle group's 1 rep max (1RM), which will allow you to assess progress. By calculating your 1RM, you establish a repetition baseline at each exercise station.

The 1RM has been used by trainers and other medical and fitness professionals to assess and prescribe strength-training and physical therapy programs post injury or surgery. "However, most prediction equations have been established from one or two exercises, usually the bench press and the squat, and may not be suitable to other exercises" (Kravitz, Nowicki, and Kinzey 2014).

I personally believe it's important to establish a 1RM baseline for each muscle group (chest, back, shoulders, abs, legs, calves, biceps, and triceps). Doing so is especially important if you're interested in recording strength and muscle bulk development and performance gains and then developing a plan to advance to the next level.

The 1RM represents the most you can lift one time per exercise station. For example, if you want to maximize strength and development of muscular bulk, then calculate intensity of strength effort at equal or greater to 80 percent of 1RM—or work toward that goal. Evidence suggests this is optimal for maximizing strength and muscular endurance gains, whilst helping to improve bone mineral density (Fisher et al. 2011, 147).

To make the 1RM math simple, let's apply it to the bench press with a resistive weight setting of 100 pounds. In this example, 100 pounds is the most weight one can lift one time at the bench press station. Now, calculate 100 pounds at 80 percent intensity of 1RM effort. To do so you'll multiple one hundred pounds by 80 percent ($100 \times .80 = 80$). You should be using an 80-pound setting during the bench press activity. So plan to achieve lifting that amount of weight repeatedly four to six times at the station to complete one set. This may require reducing the eighty pounds to sixty or seventy pounds if you're having a hard time squeezing out the fourth repetition. This training technique allows you to maximize strength gains.

In the previous example, six repetitions at seventy pounds to complete one set on the bench press is the goal. I've programmed clients to begin training at less than 80 percent 1RM until repetitive muscle endurance and strength improves—especially when a client is barely able to squeeze off three reps at 80 percent 1RM. In other words, the client could squeeze out three reps at 80 percent of 1RM but not four.

A 1RM must be set to achieve four to six repetitions wherein the fifth or sixth repetition is challenging but not impossible to achieve. Once you've achieved or exceeded the sixth rep, increase the weight by five pounds and rep out no less than four to six repetitions per set. Then once able to rep off the 100 pounds x four repetitions – set a new 1RM and repeat the process. This sequence of muscle conditioning is used to further increase strength and muscle bulk development.

If you're looking to improve muscular endurance and speed, once you're conditioned, take no more than a one-minute rest break between reps per set at each weight lifting station. Perform no less than eight to ten repetitions at equal to or greater than 80 percent 1RM and repeat the exercise for two to four sets at each weight station or exercise set.

Why do I choose eight to ten repetitions to failure? I've learned forceful reps up to eight to ten per set at equal to or greater than 80 percent 1RM generates the best neuromuscular stimulant response to improve both aerobic and anaerobic innervation of muscle for competitive sports at a high level of intramural play.

Recall that programming for any fitness goal must consider body type, current health condition, medical history, balance, postural alignment, flexibility, lifestyle, environment, and individual fitness goals.

For example, my 1RM for leg strength exercise is often set at 50 to 70 percent due to previous back and hip injuries. *Fitness programming logic under this scenario* holds that unnecessary aggravation that increases unwanted risk to preexisting injury serves no purpose if the goal is to sustain an active lifestyle, lose weight, and enjoy life to the fullest. I've also referred to this lifestyle principle as "aging gracefully."

On the opposite end of the fitness spectrum, if your goal is to train seasonally as a competitive sprinter, then you may want to consider increasing leg exercise repetitions indoors by performing circuit weight-training sessions at twelve to fifteen reps per set and lifting the heaviest amount possible to failure. This will condition the leg muscles for explosive starts/takeoffs and sprint force acceleration of short durations to the finish line.

For elite athletes, the 1RM setting at a resistive weight-training station may be 85 to 90 percent of repetitive lifts to failure per set. In other words, the competitive athlete often lifts at whatever 1RM setting allows him or her to barely squeeze off twelve to fifteen repetitions per set at each leg exercise station, where the last reps feel unbearable because of lactic acid buildup and muscle fatigue.

Programming intended to train an athlete for high-intensity sprints requires that the athlete endure a daily routine that conditions him or her to be competitive in the appropriate environment. For instance, sprinting programs should include indoor anaerobic exercise conditioning, as well as timed hundred-yard sprinting exercises on a track no fewer than four days a week. If a track event is to occur at high altitudes, high-altitude training is a must. Athletes now have access to specialized masks that simulate high altitudes at sea level. This equipment allows them to condition their lungs and circulatory systems in an environment similar to that of the event they're training for. If you're going to compete at high altitudes, seek professional sports trainers with expertise in this area.

Aside from increased muscular endurance, strength, and muscle bulk, another physiologic benefit occurs as a result of strength training's influence on the body's metabolic and hormonal systems.

How Anaerobic Exercise Influences the Body's Hormonal Systems

Strength training and lifting technique play a significant role in increasing natural GH production following exercise. "The magnitude of hormonal response is related to the amount of muscle tissue stimulated… Exercise variables contributing to GH release include intensity, load, rest interval, and the amount of muscle mass utilized" (Marks and Kravitz n.d.). Also see chapter 15, "Antiaging and Physical Performance-Enhancement Truths."

If you want to increase GH naturally to sustain bulk and strength and to enhance physical and sexual performance, your fitness program should work toward 80 percent or greater of a 1RM strength-training exercise.

A word of caution—be patient as you increase your 1RM per set. Listen to your body and back off or increase effort as needed. Recalculate 1RM weekly. If increased resistive loads make you feel bad or cause unbearable pain, stop the activity and reassess the training program and follow up with a personal trainer, coach, or sports medicine doctor or primary care physician as needed. Otherwise, you may experience a serious musculoskeletal injury.

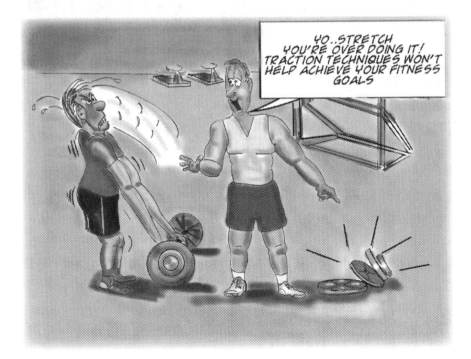

Stationary Circuit Weight Training May Be for You

Here's how to program a simple stationary circuit weight-training program that may or may not include free weights. Select six to ten different stationary pieces of equipment in a gym. Plan at minimum to exercise chest, back, arms, abs, and legs at separate stations to complete one circuit. For example, set your 1RM and perform eight to ten reps at each station. Once you're doing more than ten reps per station, increase your 1RM percent to get back within an eight to ten rep count per station. And rest no longer than two minutes between each set at each station. Work up to completing one to three full station circuits per session. Regardless of how many sets are complete, finish the circuit(s) within thirty minutes and call it good. You can only accomplish more sets and circuits from that point forward.

For those of you who currently live a sedentary lifestyle and want to improve health and get into better shape, a daily fitness program could be as simple as that outlined below.

The American College of Sports Medicine provides resistive exercise guidelines (which I've listed here). In no way do I consider these guidelines alone a customized fitness program. As you're now aware, there's much more involved when fitness trainers and consultants develop, design, and apply a customized fitness and healthy lifestyle change program for each client. Nevertheless, when resistive exercises per ACSM guidelines are combined with daily aerobic exercise activity (in other words, walking, dance, jogging, biking, and the like) these recommendations can provide anyone at any age health, fitness, and longevity benefits.

Recommendations for participating in resistance exercise (ACSM 2014):

- Adults should train each major muscle group two or three days each week using a variety of exercises and equipment.
- Very light or light intensity is best for older persons or previously sedentary adults starting exercise.
- Two to four sets of each exercise will help adults improve strength and power.

- For each exercise, eight to twelve repetitions improve strength and power, ten to fifteen repetitions improve strength in persons who are middle age and older and starting exercise, and fifteen to twenty repetitions improve muscular endurance.
- Adults should wait at least forty-eight hours between resistance-training sessions.

When Customizing a Fitness Program, Don't Forget Intensity of Effort

You've learned that use of glucose and fat-burning muscle fuel occurs optimally at 50 percent to 70 percent THR during aerobic exercise. You've also learned that, during exercise that leads to greater than 70 percent to 79 percent THR and when applying a variety of anaerobic and aerobic exercises at varying intensities of effort, a transitional or intermittent muscle fuel and mix of glucose, muscle glycogen, and fat fuel is preferred. And finally, you've learned that glucose and muscle glycogen fuel are mostly preferred by working muscle at greater than the 80 percent THR threshold (or on a scale of one to ten, the perceived intensity of effort is intuitively translated as 8, which can be mathematically calculated and measured as 80 percent intensity of effort or 80 percent of 1RM).

Working muscle at higher reps and lower weight-resistance settings increases muscular endurance, toning, and aerobic benefit, while burning more body fat and calories *if resistive settings are less than 80 percent 1RM.* This requires rest time to be less than one to two minutes between exercise sets.

Exercising muscles at lower reps and increased resistive weight settings stimulates GH production, explosive speed, power, muscular strength, and bulk development and enhances physical and sexual performance. This type of exercise simultaneously burns more total carbohydrates or muscle glucose fuel *when resistive settings are greater than 80 percent 1RM.* Here again rest time is less than one to two minutes between exercise sets.

Rest *only* long enough to maintain a 50 percent to 70 percent THR during any type of exercise if your goal is also to burn more body fat.

Recall, you can use completed client forms 13.1 "Tina's Healthy Habits Commitment Plan and 18.1 "Hank's Fitness Program & Tracking Record" as guideline examples. Then plot your daily programs on blank client forms 13.0 "Healthy Habits Commitment Plan" and 18.0 "Fitness Program & Tracking Record" (see appendix)

When beginning any exercise session, you'll experience lactic acid buildup and muscle soreness if you've not exercised for a while and if you skip warm-up and cooldown exercises. The good news is that, when you do the same activity again, your muscles will start to get used to it. Allan H. Goldfarb, PhD, FACSM, professor, and exercise physiologist at the University of North Carolina, Greensboro, says, "You will actually have no soreness or less soreness because now you've strengthened the muscle or connective tissue" (Watson 2014).

Personal Fitness Challenge: "Patient Advocacy: A Powerful Skill Set"

I do believe that if I'd not had the fitness programming and client experience background, I'm not so sure I could have elevated my fitness levels to where I'm at today—especially given the chain of events that disabled me mentally and physically for a period of time. The exercise science knowledge and treatment referral skill sets were invaluable when it came to planning and programming my way out of a long-term immobility situation.

For many, including myself, knowing how to advocate for specialized medical treatment referrals was something more or less learned on the fly. Nevertheless, it's a necessary skill set, which can be useful at any point in time. It can be particularly useful when you're mentally, physically, and spiritually broken.

Here's how I advocated and received related and timely referrals to needed medical resources. I was relentless at setting New Year's resolutions and personal commitments, which included resolving to follow through on appointments and to analyze and learn medical terminology and to understand my diagnosis. Then I researched various treatment options after each physician consultation. After comparing physician notes, I'd advocate for an insured or uninsured treatment option that I believed was best for me.

I can't overemphasize the importance of having a handle on medical terminology and advocating for the best referrals and treatment plans possible. If you're not representing your best health interests or don't have a family member advocating on your behalf, then a health maintenance organization's (HMO's) policy may put cost savings before your best interests—even if *unbeknownst to you*, the insured patient, there is a better option under the plan. I've found that, when I represent my medical and health interests, I've received the best health care and the best-covered treatment options available.

However, one word of advice—arrogance, ignorance, loudness, and pushiness get you nowhere. Learn to be humble, respectful, and attentive in two-way communication with your doctor. Do your due diligence by understanding what your health policy covers first. If you don't understand your coverage, simply call the underwriter of the policy (HMO patient services can help with this). If you have coverage for a preferred treatment option and it's related and applicable to healing what ails you, doctors will almost always buy off on a self-referral if it makes sense under policy guidelines. This has been my personal experience.

However, respecting the physician's medical skill sets and listening with a keen ear works best. Regardless, if you believe your primary care physician is not acting in your best interests or appears to have a chip on his or her shoulder, request through patient services to be reassigned a new one. Three strikes you're out is my model. If, by the third visit with a doctor, I feel uncomfortable or not valued as a patient and as if I'm not receiving the care I need and deserve, I request a new primary care physician. Keep in mind, going this route can take up to six months to have a new primary care physician assigned. This step should not be taken lightly. And I've only had to use this tactic once.

Due diligence and timely action with prepared material in hand, including questions ready for the doctor, almost always gets the attention, time, focus, and referred services you need and deserve. This is why the patient must fully understand his or her medical history and have a grasp on some of the medical terminology—not unlike understanding fitness and healthy habit programming terminology and the process of prescribing a fit, healthy lifestyle program. But if all of this does not work out to your advantage and you feel you're going backward, you have the "right to fire" your primary care provider, just like you would a personal trainer or lifestyle coach who didn't meet expectations.

In the event you fired your primary care provider and are awaiting reassignment, if you can't wait for referred treatment, go to emergency and request the referral there. Full disclosure, I've used this tactic more than once, and it cost me out of pocket. In my opinion, it was worth every penny.

Time is of the essence when it comes to serious injury and health issues. This is why you must be prepared to advocate for medical resources and to receive treatment in a timely manner. And if you're incapable of doing so, a loved one must be designated to do it for you through durable power of attorney (DPA). This is simply a legal document that authorizes someone to act on your behalf for all health and treatment decisions and to make payments.

Learn how to tell your story or write it down so a family member can advocate on your behalf. This story may include past treating physician history, diagnosis, therapies, prescriptions, allergies to foods, and medications, for example. Doing so helps ensure that precious time is not wasted in delayed treatment or receiving unnecessary services that may cause more harm than good.

Years ago, I resolved to frequent my primary care physician and self-refer to get the pain management resources I needed to heal sooner rather than later. My personal fitness goals at first were to lose body weight and increase my walking distances while applying better pain management practices. The next three years after the first surgery were extremely challenging because of previous back injury and pain complications. Regardless, I got through it with a supportive family and timely treatment referrals.

Over time, I continued to improve in aerobic duration, strength, and flexibility in preparation for a second hip surgery. Mobility and stretching exercises, although painful, helped to alleviate pain through improved oxygenated blood circulation and increased flexibility, which aided in repair of soft tissue damage and maintenance of musculoskeletal range of motion.

Because I allowed myself to fall into an obese state initially after the surgeries, my cardio and muscular endurance suffered. However, I vowed after the first surgery to program daily aerobic exercise as soon as possible. The exercise plan required a modified walking routine starting at 35 percent THR. My mobility equipment of choice was limited to a wheelchair and later to crutches and a cane. It took me six weeks once I set the aerobic pace to achieve a 50 percent THR using mobility aids up to and throughout a one-mile walk loop.

I also included strength-training exercises, which I performed on stationary equipment at 50 percent 1RM daily. Wednesdays and Sundays were set as days of rest. I worked up to eight to twelve reps for two sets at each stationary weight station, focusing on upper body strength and muscular endurance using low resistive weight settings.

Prior to and after working out, I included five to ten minutes of stretching exercise on a floor mat during warm-ups and cooldowns. These stretch exercises were prescribed during physical therapy sessions to increase my range of motion to help reduce radiating nerve pain.

Today, I walk daily between 70 to 85 percent THR (about nineteen to twenty-five beats per ten-second pulse count). By changing my walk pace and the terrain, I control the endurance effort and fat-burning and cardio benefits. With that said, I still continue to manage varying levels of acute and chronic body pain. The hip and back pain is manageable if I don't push myself beyond a certain point.

I visit a doctor frequently and lie down throughout the day to recharge and decompress my back. I'm definitely in touch with how my mind, body, and spirit respond to increased physical and mental stress and adjust daily work activity and exercise and rest accordingly— gauged by perceived pain level.

By requesting referrals through my primary care physician, I was able to expedite relevant treatment by medical specialists early on. Thereafter, I integrated and applied the doctor's prescription into my customized fitness program and further modified it. For example, my hip and back pain was a result of painful walking posture. Through self-referral, I saw a podiatrist and received custom insoles for my shoes, which corrected poor foot posture, reduced weight-bearing pain throughout my body, and removed a severe limp. Ownership in the referral process allowed me to advance to the next aerobic fitness level and live a more active lifestyle.

My recommendation to those of you with physical challenges or those who are recovering from injury or disease is this: Don't depend on others to tell your medical history or the story of your injury, disease, or pain if you're capable of doing so yourself. I understand that taking care of the self medically is not something we're educated on or trained to do. But I believe it's a necessary skill set if one expects to live life to the fullest and age gracefully with full mobility intact.

Today, I continue to walk six to seven days a week, averaging sixty miles per week. Which includes hiking to some of my favorite target shooting places in the great Northwest.

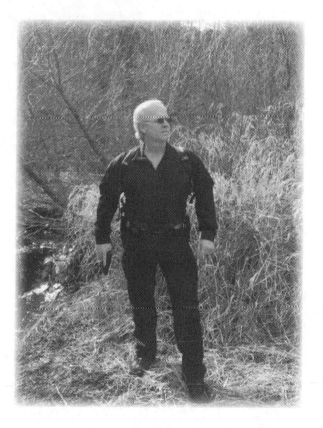

I also incorporate strength training between walking activity. I've walked freely without mobility aids since 2008. I've donated to those in need the walkers, wheelchairs, and crutches I once depended on for years.

I can tell you from personal experience that learning to advocate and self-refer for preferred and relevant medical treatment, as well exercising daily, become more important in the process of staying on the mend. And staying on the mend also requires applying predictive and preventative health maintenance practices, as discussed in chapter 9.

In doing these things, you'll become addicted to the healthy lifestyle habits you incorporate. And I guarantee you'll live life to *your* fullest potential.

Conclusion

Since we don't have a national fitness policy that mandates resources toward ill-health prevention and fit, healthy lifestyle education, this important education will continue to be left out of K–12 school curriculums, and future generations will suffer for lack of it in more than one way.

Today's reality is that more of us are living an unhealthy lifestyle. And it's taking a toll on families, the workforce, the health care system, and quality of life experiences.

"About half of all American adults—117 million individuals—have one or more preventable chronic diseases that relate to poor quality dietary patterns and physical inactivity, including cardiovascular diseases, hypertension, type 2 diabetes, and diet-related cancers. More than two-thirds of adults and nearly one-third of children and youth are overweight or obese. These devastating health problems have persisted for decades, strained U.S. health care costs, and focused the attention of our health care system on disease treatment rather than prevention" (DGAC 2015).

"These high rates of overweight and obesity and chronic disease … come not only with increased health risks, but also at high cost. In 2008, the medical costs associated with obesity were estimated to be $147 billion. In 2012, the total estimated cost of diagnosed diabetes was $245 billion, including $176 billion in direct medical costs and $69 billion in decreased Productivity" (US Department of Health and Human Services 2015).

"The 2015 DGAC (Dietary Guideline Advisory Committee) hopes that its report will aid in developing public policies that aim to establish a 'culture of health' at individual and population levels and, in so doing, make healthy lifestyle choices easy, accessible, affordable and normative-both at home and away from home" (DGAC 2015).

Regardless of the DGAC's good intentions to establish a "culture of health," if those good intentions don't begin within our K–12 schools, a significant reverse in childhood obesity and significant decrease in associated chronic disease will not likely be seen over the decades to come. Nor will the escalating health care costs and declining national productivity change much over the same time period in my opinion.

Although ill-health prevention and healthy lifestyle education for our K–12 students is the right thing to do, the reality of developing public policies that legislate those resources into our children's classrooms will not likely be a national priority anytime soon. Who knows? Maybe the US Department of Education, the US Department of Agriculture, the US Department of Health and Human Services, and the Centers for Disease Control and Prevention will surprise us all.

Until that perfect storm occurs—if it ever does—communities can rally together and prioritize and lobby for more neighborhood sidewalks, more paths and trail systems, and more safe walking connections to and from schools. They can encourage municipalities to provide more public use gathering places, parks, outdoor activity facilities such as outdoor fitness centers and BMX obstacle bike courses, etc., and recreational facilities with indoor activities that inspire community to come together and motivate individuals to become more physically active and fit. Kids who grow up in such communities will grow into adults and raise families that also value the same things. When communities educate children on healthy lifestyle and ill-health prevention, the health and productivity of the next generation and future communities benefit. In my opinion, this is the right way to establish a "culture of health."

I know many community residents don't have access to affordable fitness and recreation facilities and don't have the resources to travel or access such things. However, with a little ingenuity and innovation as described throughout the book, anyone—including your children, through you—can learn how to create a customized fit, healthy lifestyle program with the right knowledge in hand and at little cost. It's still working for me at age 59 and it will work for you. Believe!

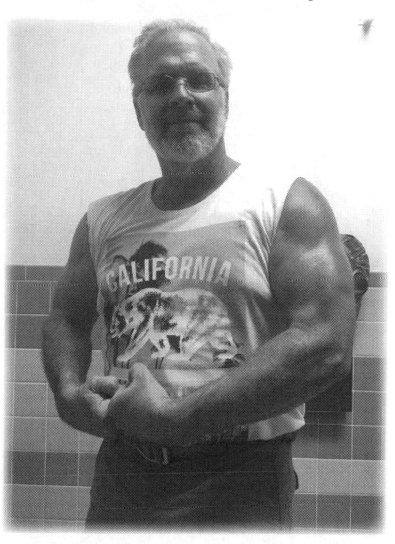

How you change your lifestyle and gather the resources you need to improve your *Ageless MirrorAthlete*™ image and share it with your family and friends is up to you. The difference now is you've heard from a consumer safety advocate and fit, healthy lifestyle coach sharing truthful information you can relate to and apply now—one step at a time!

Now get 'er done!

Appendix

Cooking Fats and Smoke Point (SP) Data

Oil/Fat 1 tbsp	Calorie per serving	Chol	SFA%	MUFA%	Omega-9 fatty acid%	PUFA%	Omega-3 fatty acid%	Omega-6 fatty acid%	Omega 6:3 Ratio	Smoke Point Temps
Avocado oil	124	0	11.6%	70.6%	67.9%	13.5%	1.0%	12.5%	13.1:1	400°F
Butter	102	31 mg	62%	29%	24.6%	4%	.4%	3.4%	8.6:1	250–300°F
Canola oil	124	0	7%	55%	61.7%	33%	9.1%	19%	2.1:1	400°F
Extra virgin coconut oil	120	0	86.5%	5.8%	5.8%	1.8%	0%	1.8%	No omega-3 present	350°F
Corn oil	122	0	13%	24%	27.3%	59%	1.16%	53%	46.1:1	450°F
Cottonseed oil	120	0	25.9%	17.8%	17%	51.9%	53.3%	12.7%	.2:1	420°F
Extra virgin olive Oil	119	0	13%	74%	71.3%	8%	.8%	9.8%	12.8:1	375°F
Lard	115	12.2 mg	40%	45%	41.2%	11%	1.0%	10.2%	10.2:1	370°F
Palm oil	120	0	49.3%	37%	36.6%	9.3%	.2%	36.6%	45.9:1	455°F

									No omega-3 present	450°F
Peanut oil	119	0	17%	46%	44.8%	32%	0%	3.2%	No omega-3 present	450°F
Safflower	120	0	7.5%	75.2%	74.8%	12.8%	.1%	12.7%	127:1	510°F
Soybean	120	0	15.3%	22.7%	22.6%	57.3%	7%	50.3%	7.1:1	460°F
Sunflower	120	0	13%	51.5%	46%	23%	.9%	35.3%	39.4:1	440°F
Major fatty acid identifier	PUFA omega-3 fatty acids: alpha-linolenic acid (ALA), also known as essential LNA; eicosapentaenoic acid (EPA); docosahexaenoic acid (DHA)				PUFA omega-6 fatty acids: essential linoleic acid (LA), also once known as vitamin F (for fat); gamma-linolenic acid (GLA); arachidonic Acid (AA)				MUFA omega-9: oleic, mead, and erucic acid	

Note: For each oil serving identified in the table, the total of unsaturated fatty acids plus that of saturated fatty acids will not add up to 100 percent. This is because each oil or animal fat has a miniscule amount of other nutrients within it. (The table data was adapted and consolidated from NutriStrategy 2015, The Conscious Life 2016, and Whitney et al. 1987, H2–H65).

Form 5.1. Daily Caloric Expenditure Worksheet: "Marvin's" Worksheet Example

Energy systems caloric needs	BMR men/ women caloric cost factor 1.0 and 0.9 kcal/ kg/hr.	Body weight (BW) in pounds	Convert body weight to kilograms BW/2.2kg	Hours of activity	BMR daily energy cost	+ RMR daily energy cost	+ EMR daily energy cost	Daily caloric cost
BMR (sleep)	See form 5.3 1.0	175 lb.	79.55 kg	8 hrs.	636 cal	0	0	SubT kcals 636 cal
Refer to the client example in chapter 5, "Caloric Exchange: A Balancing Act" – Calculating Marvin's 8-hour BMR caloric energy requirement during sleep; Table 5.1, Estimated Caloric Intake Requirement per Day, Age, and Activity; and Table 5.2 Caloric Energy Cost per Activity per Minute.								
RMR (daily activity)	See Activity Table 5.2, approximates 2.0 kcals/kg/hr. (light activity) 2.0 kcals × 79.55kg × 14 hrs. = 2227.4 kcals	79.55kg	14hrs	636	2227.4	0	SubT kcals 2863	
EMR (exercise activity)	See Activity Table 5.2, approximates 11.d kcals/kg/hr. (jog/run) @ 6 mph) 11.3 kcals × 79.55kg × 2hrs = 1356 kcals	79.55kg	2hrs	636	2227	1356	Total kcals 4220	

Form 5.2. Daily Caloric Expenditure Worksheet

Energy systems caloric needs	BMR men/ women caloric cost factor 1.0 and 0.9 kcal/ kg/hr.	Body weight (BW) in pounds	Convert body weight to kilograms BW/2.2kg	Hours of activity	BMR daily energy cost	+ RMR daily energy cost	+ EMR daily energy cost	Daily caloric cost
BMR (sleep)								SubT kcals
Refer to *Ageless MirrorAthlete: Overweight and Unfit No More*, chapter 5.								
RMR (daily activity)								SubT kcals
EMR (exercise activity)								Total kcals

Form 5.3. Simple Body Mass Index (BMI) Worksheet: "Marvin's" Worksheet Example

---

To calculate men or women's BMI, divide weight in pounds by height in inches squared (in this case, Marvin's) and multiply that by 703. The formula is:

body weight in pounds/height in inches squared × 703

For example (using Marvin's stats):

175lb./(5' 10" [70"]^2) × 703

175/(70 × 70 = 4,900) = .0357 × 703 = 25.10% body fat

Refer to Chapter 5, "Caloric Exchange: A Balancing Act"

Date	Body weight (pounds)	Height in (inches)	Height in inches squared (e.g. 70 × 70)	Body weight divided by inches squared (e.g. 175/ 4900)	Multiplied by 703	Equals Body Fat %	BMI Standard
1 Jan	175 lb.	70"	4,900	.0357	25.09	25.10%	~Normal

Table 5.3. BMI Standards

BMI below 18.5 is considered underweight.
BMI between 18.5 and 24.9 is normal weight.
BMI between 25.0 and 29.9 is overweight
BMI of 30.0 and above considered obese.
BMI of 40.0 + extremely high obesity.

Form 5.4. Simple Body Mass Index (BMI) Worksheet

<table>
<tr><td colspan="8">To calculate men or women's BMI,
(Refer to *Ageless MirrorAthlete: Overweight and Unfit No More*, chapter 5.)</td></tr>
<tr><td colspan="8">**Chapter 5, "Caloric Exchange: A Balancing Act"**</td></tr>
<tr><td>Date</td><td>Body wt. in pounds</td><td>Height in Inches</td><td>Height in Inches Squared (70 x 70)</td><td>Then body wt. divided by inches squared</td><td>Then Multiplied by 703</td><td>Equals Body Fat %</td><td>BMI Standard</td></tr>
<tr><td></td><td></td><td></td><td></td><td></td><td></td><td></td><td></td></tr>
<tr><td></td><td></td><td></td><td></td><td></td><td></td><td></td><td></td></tr>
<tr><td></td><td></td><td></td><td></td><td></td><td></td><td></td><td></td></tr>
<tr><td></td><td></td><td></td><td></td><td></td><td></td><td></td><td></td></tr>
<tr><td colspan="8">Table 5.3. BMI Standard

BMI below 18.5 considered underweight.
BMI between 18.5 and 24.9 is normal weight.
BMI between 25.0 and 29.9 is overweight
BMI of 30.0 and above considered obese.
BMI of 40.0 + extremely high obesity.</td></tr>
</table>

Form 10.0 MirrorAthlete Pick a Favorite Healthy Meal

Foods	Date	Fats	Carbs	Proteins	Calories
B = Breakfast, L= Lunch, D= Dinner					
Daily macronutrient "g" sub totals					
Daily calorie sub totals					
(Macronutrient "calorie" balance %s)					
Day's meals avg. macronutrient balance %					

Macronutrient grams to calorie conversion: 1g fat = 9 cal, 1g carbohydrate = 4 cal. 1g protein = 4 Cal
Macronutrient Calorie % calculation: (fat cal/tot cal = fat cal %) + (carb cal/tot cal = carb cal %) + (protein cal/tot cal = protein cal %) = 100% calorie intake
Macronutrient Balance: Adults (19 years and older)—fats 20–35%, carbohydrates 45–65%, proteins 10–35%
Other Terms: (g = grams; c or cal = calories; carbs = carbohydrates)

Nutritional Analysis:
Food caloric totals (add meal calorie subtotals) _____ day's total calories
Your allowed calories/day _____ calories/day (see note below)
Net calories under or over _____ calories
Day's meals average macronutrient balance by %: Fats intake: __% (daily fats 20–35% nutritional guidelines), carbohydrate intake: __% (daily carbs 45–65% nutritional guidelines), protein intake: __% (daily protein 10–35% nutritional guidelines). Did you meet the nutritional macronutrient balance guidelines?
Instructions: Plan to write to fourteen of your favorite daily meal plans on pieces of paper and then fold them in half. Put them in a box, mix it up, and pick one for the next day's random meal plan. Then put it back in box for the next day's drawing. This practice takes the decision making out of what your next day's favorite meals will look like and allows you to prep meals in advance.
Note: (Refer to tables and forms found in *Ageless Mirror Athlete: Overweight and Unfit No More*, chapters 5 and 10.)

Form 10.1. MirrorAthlete Pick a Favorite Healthy Meal: Marc's Worksheet for One Day

Foods	Date	Fats	Carbs	Proteins	Calories
B = Breakfast					
2 cups of raisin bran	1 Jan	3.12g	85.48g	9.74g	409 cal
2 cups of 1% milk	1 Jan	4.7g	24.36g	16.44g	205 cal
Snacks					
Snacks					
Daily macronutrient "g" sub totals		7.82g	109.84g	26.18g	143.84 g
Daily calorie sub totals		70.38c	439.36c	104.72c	614 c
(Macronutrient "calorie" balance %s)		11.5%	71.5%	17.0%	100%

Macronutrient grams to calorie conversion: 1g fat = 9 cal. 1g carbohydrate = 4 cal. 1g protein = 4 Cal
Macronutrient Calorie % calculation: (fat cal/tot cal= fat cal %) + (carb cal/tot cal = carb cal %) + (protein cal/tot cal = protein cal %) = 100% calorie intake
Macronutrient Balance: Adults (19 years and older)—fats 20–35%, carbohydrates 45–65%, proteins 10–35%
Other Terms: (g = grams; c or cal = calories; carbs = carbohydrates)

Foods	Date	Fats	Carbs	Proteins	Calories
L = Lunch					
¼ lb. hamburger patty	1 Jan	20.21g	0g	29.2g	299 cal
1 slice American Cheese	1 Jan	7.39g	1.97g	5.37g	96 cal
2 slices multigrain wheat bread	1 Jan	2g	24g	5.2g	135 cal
1 cup low-fat fruit yogurt	1 Jan	1.5g	29g	5g	145 cal
1 tbsp mayonnaise	1 Jan	10g	0.1g	0.1g	94 cal

Protein bar (1 serving) (You can find protein and meal replacement bars @ 150–300 cal/serving)	9g	23g	30g	290 cal
Daily Macro Nutrient "g" Sub Totals	50g	78.1g	74.9g	203 g
Daily Calorie Sub Totals	450c	312.3c	300c	1,062 c
(Macronutrient "Calorie" balance %'s)	42.4%	29.4%	28.25%	100%

***Macronutrient grams to calorie conversion:** 1g fat = 9 cal, 1g carbohydrate = 4 cal, 1g protein = 4 Cal*
***Macronutrient Calorie % calculation:** (fat cal/tot cal= fat cal %) + (carb cal/tot cal = carb cal %) + (protein cal/tot cal = protein cal %) = 100% calorie intake*
***Macronutrient Balance:** Adults (19 years and older)—fats 20–35%, carbohydrates 45–65%, proteins 10–35%*
***Other Terms:** (g = grams; c or cal = calories; carbs = carbohydrates)*

Foods	Date	Fats g	Carbs	Proteins	Calories
D= Dinner					
Large potato	Jan 1	.37g	57.97g	6.2g	260 cal
8-oz. 20% lean sirloin	Jan 1	14g	0g	66g	394 cal
2 tbsp sour cream	Jan 1	6.04g	1.22g	.92g	62 cal
2 cups broccoli	Jan 1	.68g	12.08g	3.14g	62 cal
Drink two 3.5-oz. glass red wine	Jan 1	0g	5.6g	0g	170 cal
1g of alcohol = 7 calories	See alcohol serving link and beverage books for calories/drink http://caloriecount.about.com/calories-wine-i14084 (citation)				
Total - 17g of alcohol in 7 oz.					
Daily macronutrient "g" sub totals	21.09g	76.87g	76.26g	174.22 g
Daily calorie sub totals	190c	307.48c	305.04c	802.52 c
(Macronutrient "calorie" balance %s)	23.7%	38.3%	38%	100%
Day's meals avg. macronutrient balance %	25.86%	46.4%	27.75	100%

Macronutrient grams to calorie conversion: 1g fat = 9 cal, 1g carbohydrate = 4 cal, 1g protein = 4 Cal

Macronutrient Calorie % calculation: (fat cal/tot cal= fat cal %) + (carb cal/tot cal = carb cal %) + (protein cal/tot cal = protein cal %) = 100% calorie intake

Macronutrient Balance: Adults (19 years and older)—fats 20–35%, carbohydrates 45–65%, proteins 10–35%

Other Terms: *(g = grams; c or cal = calories; carbs = carbohydrates)*

Calories Analysis:

Food caloric totals (add meal calorie subtotals): 2,479 day's total calories
Marc's "personal fitness challenge": Calories intake/day 3,000 calories/day (if I want to lose weight without increasing exercise activity).
Net Calories under or over: 521 calories. (I can eat more calories this day or accept additional weight loss).

Day's meals average macronutrient balance by %: Fats intake: 25.86% (daily fats 20–35% nutritional guideline), carbohydrate intake: 46.4% (daily carbs 45–65% nutritional guideline), protein intake: 27.75% (daily protein 10–35% nutritional guideline). Did you meet the nutritional macronutrient balance guidelines? Yes.
Net carbs: sugar alcohols, fiber, and glycerin are not included in food calculations.

Form 13.0. Healthy Habits Commitment Plan

Healthy Habits Commitment Plan *MirrorAthlete.com* Client: _____ Age: __ Sex: __ Wt.: __ Ht.: __ Fitness Goal: Wt. Loss__ Muscle Bulk __ Muscle Endurance __ Tone __ Cross-train __						See healthy habits (HH) defined below
Choose healthy habit practices & frequency	**Daily**	**Weekly**	**Month**	**Quarterly**	**Weight & Date**	**"Leveraging healthy change" through healthy habit commitment**
Small meal & snacks					‾‾‾	CH13; HH 1, 8
Drink 12–16 oz. water with meal					‾‾‾	CH13; HH 1, 4
Food portion control					‾‾‾	CH10, 13; HH 6, 8
Grazing, or 6–8 meals a day					‾‾‾	CH13; HH 1, 8
Make meal last 20 minutes					‾‾‾	CH13; HH 4, 7
Leave meal table						CH13; HH 3, 5, 10
2–3 L of H2O/day						CH13; HH 4
Habitual vices						CH13; HH 3
3–4 fruits & vegs						CH13, HH 2, 8
V&M supplement						CH13; HH 2, 8
3 bal meals/day						CH10, 13; HH 3, 8
Food after 8 p.m.						CH13; HH 11
Eat fried foods						CH13; HH 8, 9
Eat baked goods						CH13; HH 8, 10
Restaurants						CH13; HH 8, 9, 10
Fast foods						CH13; HH 8, 9

No leftovers						CH13; HH 12
Exercise program						CH5, 13, 18; HH 13
Cert. fit trainer						CH13; HH 13, 14
Annual checkup						CH9; 13; HH 13, 14

Form 13.1. Tina's Healthy Habits Commitment Plan

Healthy Habits Commitment Plan *MirrorAthlete.com* Client: <u>Tina</u> Age: <u>44</u> Sex: <u>F</u> Wt.: <u>144</u> Ht.: <u>5' 3"</u> Fitness Goal: Wt. Loss <u>X</u> Muscle Bulk__ Muscle Endurance__ Tone <u>X</u> Cross-train ___						**See Healthy Habits (HH) Defined Below**
Choose healthy habit practices & frequency	**Daily**	**Weekly**	**Month**	**Quarterly**	**Weight & Date**	**"Leveraging healthy change" through healthy habit commitment**
Small meal & snacks					144 1 Jan	CH13; HH 1, 8 – Not interested in small meals and snacks between the main meals
Drink 12–16 oz. water with meal	X				140 30 Jan	CH13; HH 1, 4 – Drink 1–2 glasses of water at each meal
Food portion control	X				137 18 Feb	CH10, 13; HH 6, 8 – Form 10 Pick a Favorite Healthy Meal – Cut food portion's in half 5 days/week
Grazing, or 6–8 meals a day					133 1 Mar	CH13; HH 1, 8 – Not interested in grazing or multiple small meals daily
Make meal last 20 minutes	X				130 27 Mar	CH13; HH 4, 7 – Slow down food consumption rate
Leave meal table			*Fit*	*Goal*	*Complete*	CH13; HH 3, 5, 10 – Can resist eating more food
2–3 L of H2O/day	X					CH13; HH 4 – Commits to drinking 2 liters of water daily
Habitual vices				X		CH13; HH3 – Agrees to give up beer calories for 3 months
3–4 fruits & vegs						CH13; HH 2, 8 – Non commit: cost and inconvenience
V&M supplement	X					CH13; HH 2, 8 – Agrees to take a daily V&M

3 bal meals/day	X					CH10, 13; HH 8, 3
Food after 8 p.m.	X					CH13; HH 11 – Allowed limited fruits or vegetables
Eat fried foods		X				CH13; HH 8, 9 – No more than 1 serving every 2 weeks
Eat baked goods		X				CH13; HH 8, 10 – 1–2 servings every 2 weeks
Restaurants			X			CH13; HH 8, 9, 10 – Not more than 1–2/month patronage
Fast foods			X			CH13; HH 8, 9 – Eat at a fast food place once a month
No leftovers	X					CH13; HH 12 – Agree to freeze leftovers
Exercise program	X					CH5, 13, 18; HH 13 – Walk 5 days/week, 30–60 min
Cert. fit trainer		X				CH13; HH 13, 14 – I was consultant from Jan 1–Mar 18
Annual checkup				X		CH9, 13; HH 13, 14 – Checkup within 3 months

(Form 18) Client Name:'

Fitness Program and Tracking Record

MirrorAthlete.com

Age: ____ Sex: ___ Wt.: ____ Ht.: _____

Fitness Goal: Wt. Loss ____ Muscle Strength___ Muscle Endurance___ Tone ____ Cross-train ____ Other___

"Ch. 3, "Muscles' Fuel Preferences During Exercise"; Ch. 18, "Customized Fitness Programming"

MirrorAthlete Weekly Exercise Program/Tracker

Exercise Program	Programmed Sets	Programmed Reps	Intensity of Anaerobic Effort 1RM (10–100%)	Equip. Wt. (lb.)	Actual Performance Weekly Averages		Comments 1–5 reps = Strength 8–12 Reps = Cross-training 15–20 reps = Endurance
Aerobic Activity:			10–100% 1RM Intensity of Strength Effort		50–70% THR Intensity of Aerobic Effort		50–70%THR Fat-Burning Zone and 85–100%1RM Optimum Strength and Bulk Development
					Sets	Reps	

MirrorAthlete Customized Fitness Program

Daily Exercise Activity	Daily	Frequency/Week	Bi-Weekly	Sets	Reps	Weight (lb.)	Endurance Intensity%	Strength Intensity%	Strength-Aerobics: 1RM wt. lifted one time to determine strength intensity% desired Example: 1RM @ 250lbs × .8 = 200lb. repetitions/set

(Form 18.1) Client Name: Hank

Fitness Program & Tracking Record

MirrorAthlete.com

Age: _54__ Sex: _M_ Wt.: _200__ Ht.: _5' 11"

Fitness Goal: Wt. Loss ____ Muscle Strength _X_ Muscle Endurance
_X_ Tone ____ Cross-train _X_ Other____

"Ch. 3, "Muscles Fuel
Preferences During
Exercise"; Ch. 18,
"Customized Fitness
Programming"

MirrorAthlete Weekly Exercise Program/Tracker

Exercise Program	Programmed Sets	Programmed Reps	Intensity of Anaerobic Effort 1RM (10–100%)	Equip. Wt. (lb.)	Actual Performance Weekly Averages		Comments 1–5 reps = Strength 8–12 Reps = Cross-training 15–20 reps = Endurance
Aerobic activity: walking			60-80% 1RM Intensity of Strength Effort		50–70 % THR Intensity of Aerobic Effort		1.5 to 3 hours daily @ ~4.0 mph, or 8–12 miles daily. 50%THR = 14 HR/10 sec. 70% THR = 19 HR/10 sec
					Sets	Reps	
Bench press	3	4–6	80%	200	2	6	chest strength focus
Seated shoulder press	2	8–12	70%	105	2	15	Shoulder endurance focus
Pulley back rows	2	6–8	60%	105	3	8	Back cross-training focus
Seated bicep curl	3	4–6	80%	80	2	6	Bicep bulk & strength focus
Seated triceps press	3	8–12	60%	60	3	10	Triceps endurance focus
Seated leg extender	2-3	8–12	80%	160	2	10	Leg endurance focus

Another Way to Record Custom Fitness Programming as Follows

Daily Exercise Activity	Daily	Frequency/Week	Bi-Weekly	Sets	Reps	Weight (lb.)	Endurance Intensity%	Strength Intensity%	Strength-Aerobics: 1RM Wt. lifted one time to determine strength Intensity% desired Example: 1RM @ 250 lb. × .8 = 200 lb. repetitions/set
Walking	X						70%		Goal: Walk no less than 1 hour/day. Choose flat/hills to increase intensity.
Bench		2		3	6-8	200		80%	80% of 250lbs 1RM=200lbs
Shoulder		2		2	6-8	105		70%	70% of 150lbs 1RM=105lbs
Back		2		3	6-8	105		60%	60% of 180lbs 1RM=105lbs
Bicep		2		3	4-6	80		80%	80% of 100lbs 1RM=80lbs
Triceps		3		3	8-12	60		60%	60% of 100lbs 1RM=60lbs
Legs		3		4	8-12	160		80%	80% of 200lbs 1RM=160
Note:	Leg exercises: 2 set quads and 2 set hamstrings. Rest cycles between sets, 2 minutes.								

References

Abbamonte, Lee. 2013. "Why You Should Get Over Steroids in Professional Sports." Lee Abbamonte (website), January 16, 2013. Accessed November 26, 2013.

Admin. 2014. "Well Being for Women." Wellbeingforwomen (website). September 22, 2014, Accessed June 17, 2018.

American College of Sports Medicine (ACSM). n.d. "ACSM Issues New Recommendations on Quantity and Quality of Exercise." ACSM (website). Accessed August 10, 2014.

American Heart Association. 2013. "Good vs. Bad Cholesterol." American Heart Association, Inc., May 1, 2013. Accessed February 3, 2014.

American Obesity Treatment Association. n.d. "Treatment and Behavior." American Obesity Treatment Association (website). Accessed March 28, 2014.

Anderman, Robbie Hanna. 2011. "Obama's Deregulation of GMO Crops." *Tikkun*, May 27, 2011. Accessed May 3, 2014.

Alliance for Natural Health USA (ANH-USA). 2012. "You Think HFCS Drinks Are Dangerous, Mr. Mayor? Why Do You Think Diet Drinks Are Better?" ANH-USA (website), June 5, 2012. Accessed January 6, 2014.

American Psychological Association (APA). 2012. "What You Need to Know about Willpower: The Psychological Science of Self-Control." APA (website), February 2012. Accessed June 4, 2014.

Australian Olive Association. n.d. "Health Effects of Rancid Oils." Australian Olive Association (website).

Avena, Nicole M., Pedro Rada, and Bartley G. Hoebel. 2009. "Sugar and Fat Bingeing Have Notable Differences in Addictive-like

Behavior." *The Journal of Nutrition* 139, no. 3 (March): 623–28. The American Institute of Nutrition (website), January 21, 2014.

Baillie-Hamilton, Paula F. 2002. "Chemical Toxins: A Hypothesis to Explain the Global Obesity Epidemic." *The Journal of Alternative and Complementary Medicine* 8, no. 2: 185–92. Print.

Beelen, M., A. Zorenc, B. Pennings, J. M. Senden, H. Kuipers, and L. J. Van Loon. 2011. "Impact of Protein Coingestion on Muscle Protein Synthesis during Continuous Endurance Type Exercise." *NCBI* 300, no. 6: E945–54. Print.

Beil, Laura. 2011. "The Dangers of Supplements: Special Report." *Men's Health Magazine: Men's Guide to Fitness, Health, Weight Loss, Nutrition, Sex, Style and Guy Wisdom.* Men's Health Magazine (website), June 22, 2011. Accessed June 3, 2013.

Benbrook, Charles, PhD. 2009. *Critical Issue Report: The First Thirteen Years.* Rep. The Organic Center (website), November 2009. Accessed May 3, 2014.

Benson, Jonathan. 2013. "The Structural Rigidity of Trans Fats, and Why They Are so Dangerous for Your Health." *Natural News.* Natural News Network (website), May 4, 2013. Accessed January 21, 2014.

Bernard, John. 2012. *Business at the Speed of Now: Fire up Your People, Thrill Your Customers, and Crush Your Competitors.* Hoboken, NJ: Wiley. Print.

Bhasin, Shalender, Glenn R. Cunningham, Frances J. Hayes, Alvin M. Matsumoto, Peter J. Snyder, Ronald S. Swerdloff, and Victor M. Montori. 2010. "Testosterone Therapy in Men with Androgen Deficiency Syndromes: An Endocrine Society Clinical Practice Guideline." *The Journal of Clinical Endocrinology and Metabolism* 95, no. 6:2, 536–559.

Bihari, Michael, MD. 2013. "How Does the Affordable Care Act Address Prevention?" *Health Insurance.* About.com, 24 April 2013. Accessed November 26, 2013.

Blamire, John, Professor. 2005. "Components of Cells the Macromolecules and Triglycerides." Exploring Life @ BIOdotEDU (website). Accessed February 3, 2014.

Bosch, Laurentine Ten. n.d. "Top 10 Food Additives to Avoid." *Hungry for Change.* Food Matters (website). Accessed April 9, 2018.

Botanical-Online. 2014. "Mediterranean Diet Foods." *Botanical Online.* Accessed March 3, 2014.

Boundless. n.d. "Lung Capacity and Volume." Boundless (website). Accessed June 15, 2014.

Boundless. n.d. "Response to Stress by Adrenal Hormones." Boundless (website). Accessed June 4, 2014.

Bowen, R. 2006. "Growth Hormone (Somatotropin)." *Pathophysiology of the Endocrine System.* Colorado State University (website), December 24, 2006. Accessed June 4, 2014.

Buettner, Dan. 2009. "Live More Good Years." *AARP* (website), September/October 2009. Accessed July 3, 2014.

———. 2012. "The Island Where People Forget to Die." *The New York Times*, October 24, 2012. Accessed July 3, 2014.

Bustamante, Lisa, Debbie Howe-Tennant, and Christina Ramo. 1996. "The Behavioral Approach." Suny Corland (website). Accessed March 28, 2014. Suny Cortland.edu.

Calorie Lab. 2000–2014. "Butter & Margarine Calorie Counter." *CalorieLab.* Calorie Lab Inc., (website). Accessed January 22, 2014.

Cave, Simone. 2010 "Snack Attack: 'Grazing' Used to Be King, but Now Experts Say It Slows Metabolism, and Can Cause Tooth Decay and Diabetes." *MailOnline.* Associated Newspapers Ltd., June 29, 2010. Accessed 14 April 2014.CDC (Centers for Disease Control and Prevention). 2011a. "Adult BMI Calculator: English." CDC (website), May 4, 2011. Accessed May 20, 2013.

———. 2011b. "Vitamins and Minerals." CDC (website), February 23, 2011. Accessed April 14, 2014.

———. 2012. "Food Groups." CDC (website), September 27, 2012. Accessed May 20, 2013.

———. 2013. "Adult BMI Calculator: English." CDC (website), October 24, 2013. Accessed December 12, 2013.

———. 2016. "Well-being Concepts." CDC (website), May 31, 2016. Accessed March 21. 2018.

———. n.d. "Health-Related Quality of Life (HRQOL) –Well-being Concepts." CDC (website). Accessed October 19, 2015.

Cell Biolabs. 2014. "Lipid Peroxidation." Cell Biolabs, Inc. (website). Accessed March 2014.

Celli, Beth. 2014. "Importance of Cholesterol in the Body." LIVESTRONG.COM, January 15, 2014. Accessed February 3, 2014.

Center for Reintegration. n.d. "Healthy Lifestyle." The Center for Reintegration (website). Accessed April 27, 2013.

Cherny, Melody. 2012. "Don't Eat Like a Caveman." *Food Safety News*. Marler Clark, January 2 2012. Accessed November 26, 2013.

Christensen, Stephen Allen, Dr. 2010. "The Health Benefits of Evening Primrose Oil." *Suite,* January 18, 2010. Accessed March 5, 2014.

———. 2011. "What Percentage of Your Diet Should Be Complex Carbs?" LIVESTRONG.COM, July 29, 2011. Accessed November 26, 2013.

Chudler, Eric H., PhD. n.d. "Neurotransmitters and Neuroactive Peptides." *Neuroscience For Kids*. Accessed 4 June 2014.

Churchward-Venne, Tyler A., Nicholas A. Burd, and Stuart M. Phillips. 2012. "Nutritional Regulation of Muscle Protein Synthesis with Resistance Exercise: Strategies to Enhance Anabolism." *Nutritional Regulation of Muscle Protein Synthesis with Resistance Exercise: Strategies to Enhance Anabolism* 9, no. 40. *Nutrition and Metabolism*. BioMed Central Ltd, 17 May 2012. Accessed 26 September 2013.

Cloud, John. 2009. "Why Exercise Won't Make You Thin." Editorial. *Time*, August 9, 2009. Accessed May 3, 2013.Corbin, Lori. 2011. "Are Celebrity Weight Loss Products worth Buying?" ABC, May 25, 2011. Accessed November 26, 2013.

Corleone, Jill. 2014 "What Are the Health Benefits of Eating Pumpkin Puree?" *LIVESTRONG.COM*. Demand Media, Inc., January 11, 2014. Accessed May 3, 2014.

Cummins, Ronnie, and Katherine Paul. 2014. "Did Monsanto Win Prop 37? Round One in the Food Fight of Our Lives." AlterNet (website). Accessed May 3, 2014.

Curtis, C., R. Meer, and S. Misner. 2006. "Food Additives – Are They Safe?" *Food Safety, Preparation and Storage Tips*. The University of Arizona Cooperative Extension, Department of Nutritional Sciences. Accessed January 21, 2014.

Daussin, Frédéric N., Joffrey Zoll, Elodie Ponsot, Stéphane P. Dufour, Stéphane Doutreleau, Evelyne Lonsdorfer, Renée Ventura-Clapier, Bertrand Mettauer, François Piquard, Bernard Geny, and Ruddy Richard. 2008. "Training at High Exercise Intensity Promotes

Qualitative Adaptations of Mitochondrial Function in Human Skeletal Muscle." *American Physiology Society*, February 16, 2008. Accessed May 3, 2013.

Davis, Jeanie Lerche. 2006. "How Antioxidants Work: Preventing Free Radical Damage and Oxidation." *WebMD*, April 22, 2006. Accessed May 3, 2014.

De Vendômois, J. S., F. Roullier, D. Cellier, and G. E. Séralini. 2009. "A Comparison of the Effects of Three GM Corn Varieties on Mammalian Health." *International Journal of Bilogical Sciences* 5, no. 7 (December 10): 706–26. Accessed May 3, 2014.

Deccan Chronicle. 2017. "Overheating of Oil Can Cause Cancer: Study." Deccan Chronicle (website). February 15, 2017. Accessed April 7, 2018.

Deckelbaum, Richard J., Dr., and Dr. Christine L. Williams. 2001. "Childhood Obesity: The Health Issue." *Obesity a Research Journal* 9, S11: 239S–43S. Accessed June 3, 2013.

DeGrande, Barbara. 2009. "Supersize Me – How Fast Food Destroys Our Health." Suite101.com, October 14, 2009. Accessed May 20, 2013.

Deike, John. 2014. "Shopping Guide Helps Consumers Dodge Genetically-Engineered Foods." *EcoWatch*, February 19, 2014. Accessed April 27, 2018.

Del Monte, Vince. 2013. "Fitness Modeling." *Ask Men*. Accessed November 26, 2013.

DeNoon, Daniel J. 2002. "Growth Hormone Linked to Cancer." *WebMD*, July 25, 2002. Accessed April 30, 2018.

Depression Wiki. n.d. "Serotonin." In *Neurotransmitters*. Wikia. Accessed 4 June 2014.

Dietary Guidelines Advisory Committee (DGAC). 2015. "Scientific Report of the 2015 Dietary Guidelines Advisory Committee." Rep. no. First Print. USDA United States Department of Agriculture, Feb 2015. Accessed May 3, 2018.

Dickler, Jessica. 2012. "Family Health Care Costs to Exceed $20,000 This Year." CNN Money (website), March 29, 2012. Accessed October 29, 2015.

DOW AgroSciences LLC. n.d. "Monosaturated Fats in the North American Diet." Omega-9 Oils Heart Trustmark. Print.

Dryden-Edwards, Roxanne, MD. n.d. "Binge Eating Disorder." MedicineNet.com. Accessed 28 March 2014.

Dugdale, David C. and David Zieve, eds. 2011. "Electrolytes: MedlinePlus Medical Encyclopedia." U.S National Library of Medicine, September 20, 2011. Accessed May 3, 2013.

Dworkin-McDaniel, Norine. 2012. "7 Ways to Kick a Food Addiction." *For Women of Style and Substance MORE*. Accessed January 6, 2014.

Eat Right. 2014. "Do Carbohydrates Cause Weight Gain?" Eat Right: Academy of Nutrition and Dietetics. Accessed February 3, 2014.

Eberstein, Jacueline A., RN. n.d. "Controlled Carbohydrate Nutrition." Controlled Carbohydrate Nutrition (website). Accessed February 3, 2014.

Elements Database. 2015. "Complex Carbohydrates." Elements Database Periodic Table. Accessed November 14, 2015.

Emery, David. 1999. "Aspartame Warning." (Aspartame [NutraSweet] Warning.) About.com, February 20, 1999. Accessed January 6, 2014.

Envita Medical Center. n.d. "The Important Role Oxygen Plays in Cancer Treatment." Envita Medical Center (website). Accessed June 3, 2018.

EPA (Environmental Protection Agency). 2012. "National Ambient Air Quality Standards (NAAQS)." EPA (website), December 14, 2012. Accessed June 15, 2014.

Epstein, Samuel S. 1999. "Monsanto's Genetically Modified Milk Ruled Unsafe by the United Nations." *Cancer Prevention Coalition*. Preventcancer.com, August 18, 1999. Accessed May 3, 2014.

European Hydration Institute. n.d. "Hydration." European Hydration Institute (website), Accessed May 3, 2013.

Fairchild, Su, MD. 2012. "Dr. Fairchild's Guide to Healthy Cooking Oils. *Healthy Cooking Oils*. December 7, 2012. Accessed April 7, 2018.

FatSecret. 2014. "Food Database and Calorie Counter – Vegetable Oil." *Fatsecret*. FatSecret, Accessed 22 January 2014.Fisher, James, James Steele, Stewart Bruce-Low, and Dave Smith. 2011. "Evidence-Based Resistance Training Recommendations." *Medicina Sportiva* 15, no. 3: 147–62. Print.

FitAtMidlife. 2018. "Macronutrients and Calories." *Fit at Midlife*. February 4, 2018. Accessed April 6, 2018.

FitDay. 2011. "Nutrition Info For: Beef Stew with Potatoes and Vegetables (including Carrots, Broccoli, And/or Dark-green Leafy), Tomato-based Sauce." *FitDay*. Accessed February 24, 2014.

————. n.d. "The Difference between Polyunsaturated Fat and Trans Fat." *FitDay*. Accessed April 5, 2018.

————. n.d. "Understanding Oxygen Consumption Rate during Exercise." *FitDay*. Accessed June 15, 2014.

FitnessBeans. n.d. "Muscle Fibers: Fast Twitch Versus Slow Twitch." *FitnessBeans*. Accessed August 10, 2014.FTC (Federal Trade Commission). n.d. "Consumer Information, Dietary Supplements." FTC Consumer Protection Agency, Accessed June 3, 2013.

Garland, Wayne, Dr. 2010. "World's Healthiest Diet: In a Bottle." *Ask Dr. Garland*, May 18, 2010. Accessed July 3, 2014.

Geib, Aurora. 2012. "Aspartame Withdrawal and Side Effects Explained – Here's How to Protect Yourself." NaturalNews.com, March 2, 2012. Accessed April 4, 2018.Georgetown University. n.d. "Body / Mind / Spirit – Framing the Issue." *National Center for Cultural Competence*. Georgetown University. Accessed October 19, 2015.

Gerrig, Richard J., and Philip G. Zimbardo. 2002. "Glossary of Psychological Terms." From *Psychology and Life*. Boston, MA: Allyn and Bacon by Pearson Education. Reprinted by Permission of the Publisher. On American Psychological Association (website). Accessed March 28, 2014.

George Mateljan Foundation. 2014. "What Are Cold Pressed Oils?" *The World's Healthiest Foods*. Accessed March 3, 2014.

Ghigo, E., E. Arvat, J. Bellone, J. Ramunni, and F. Camanni. 1993. "Neurotransmitter Control of Growth Hormone Secretion in Humans." *The Journal of Pediatric Endocrinology* 6, no. 3–4: 263–66. National Center for Biotechnology Information. Accessed June 4, 2014.

Gordon, Anne, RN. 2013. "Lyme Disease, Morgellons Disease, and GMO Foods, All Connected?" GreenMedInfo.com, June 7, 2013. Accessed May 3, 2014.Griffin, Morgan R. n.d. "Obesity Epidemic 'Astronomical.'" *WebMD*. Accessed October 19, 2015.

Grogan, Martha, M.D. 2012. "Does Grass-fed Beef Have Any Heart-health Benefits That Other Types of Beef Don't?" Mayo Clinic

Mayo Foundation for Medical Education and Research, January 25, 2012. Accessed May 3, 2014.

Guppy, Paul. 2011. "Collective Bargaining and the Influence of Public-sector Unions in Washington State." Washington Policy Center (website), February. Accessed November 26, 2013.

Hajhashemi, V., G. Vaseghi, M. Pourfarzam, and A. Abdollahi. 2010. "Are Antioxidants Helpful for Disease Prevention?" *Research in Pharmaceutical Science* 5, no. 1: 1–8. Print.

Halper, Elizabeth, PhD. 2013. "What Is Behavior Modification?" LIVESTRONG.COM, August 16, 2013. Accessed March 28, 2014.

Han, Gunsoo, PhD, Wisung Ko, PhD, and Byungjun Cho, PhD. 2012. "Relationships Among Hydrostatic Weighing, BMI and Skin Fold Results of College Students." *Journal of Physical Therapy Science* 24, no. 9: 791. Print.

Harris, Bill, Dr. In Food Insight. 2011. "Food Insight Interviews Dr. Bill Harris on Omega-3 and Omega-6 Fatty Acids." International Food Information Council Foundation (website), December. Accessed July 21, 2013.

Harvard School of Public Health. 2014. "Shining the Spotlight on Trans Fats." Harvard School of Public Health. The President and Fellows of Harvard College. Accessed January 21, 2014.

Harvard University. 2011. "Benefits of Exercise – Reduces Stress, Anxiety and Helps Fight Depression, from Harvard Men's Health Watch." Harvard Health Publishing, Harvard Medical School (website), February. Accessed June 4, 2014.

HealthStatus. n.d. "Calories Burned Calculator." HealthStatus.com. Accessed May 20, 2013.

Henley, Sherry, and Scottie Misner. 1999. "Fats and Cholesterol in the Diet." The University of Arizona. Cooperative Extension, College of Agriculture and Life Sciences (website), August. Accessed February 3, 2014.

Hertz-Picciotto, Irva. 2012. "Study Finds High Exposure to Food-borne Toxins." UC Davis Health, November 13, 2012. Accessed January 6, 2014.

US Department of Health and Human Services (HHS) and USDA (US Department of Agriculture). 2010. "Dietary Guidelines for Americans, 2010." Health.gov (website). Accessed 31 March 2018.

Hill, James O., PhD, and Frederick L. Trowbridge, MD. 1998. "Childhood Obesity: Future Directions and Research Priorities." *Pediatrics 65* os 101, no. 3: 570–74. American Academy of Pediatrics. Accessed June 3, 2013.

Ho, Wee Peng. n.d. "Anti-Inflammatory Diet: How to Choose the Right Cooking Oil." *The Conscious Life*. Accessed March 3, 2014.

Hoffman, Matthew, MD. n.d. "Low Testosterone: How to Talk to Your Doctor." *WebMD*. Accessed June 4, 2014.

Health Resources and Services Administration (HRSA). n.d. "Health Literacy." HRSA (website). Accessed October 19, 2015.

Harvard School of Public Health (HSPS). 2014. "Antioxidants: Beyond the Hype." Harvard School of Public Health (website). Accessed May 3, 2014.

Hsu, Stacy. 2012. "Find Right Footwear for Best Posture, Health, Doctor Says." *Taipei Times*, August 15, 2012. Accessed May 3, 2013.

———. 2013. "Find Right Footwear for Best Posture, Health, Doctor Says." *Taipei Times*. Accessed November 26, 2013.

Hyman, Mark, MD. 2011. "Food Addiction: Could It Explain Why 70 Percent of Americans Are Fat?" *HuffPost. The Blog*, November 17, 2011. Accessed April 5, 2018.

Individuals with Disabilities Education Act (IDEA). 2013 "Burning Fat: Myths and Facts." IDEA Health and Fitness Association (website). Accessed May 3, 2013.

———. "Burning Fat: Myths and Facts." *IDEA Health and Fitness Association*. Accessed March 29, 2018.

Inness-Brown, Victoria, MA. 2008. "Aspartame Study: 67% of Female Rats Developed Visible Tumors." *InfoWars*, September 15, 2008. Accessed January 6, 2014.

Internicola, Doreen. 2013. "Fitness after 65 Is No One-size-fits-all Endeavor." *Chicago Tribune* and Reuters, April 8, 2013. Accessed April 27, 2013.

K, Norma. 2010. "Killing Bacteria, Pathogens, Viruses, and Toxins Naturally," *Green Planet*, August 21, 2010. Accessed September 25, 2013.

Kahn, April. 2012. "What Causes Rapid Shallow Breathing?" *Healthline*, July 17, 2012. Accessed June 15, 2014.

Katch, Frank I., and William D. McArdle. "Biology and Chemistry Basics." *In Introduction to Nutrition, Exercise, and Health.* Philadelphia: Lea & Febiger, 1993, 11. Print.

———. "Energy for Exercise." In *Introduction to Nutrition, Exercise, and Health.* Philadelphia: Lea & Febiger, 1993, 169+. Print.

———. "Evaluation of Body Composition." In *Introduction to Nutrition, Exercise, and Health.* Philadelphia: Lea & Febiger, 1993, 233–58. Print.

———. "Modification of Eating and Exercise Behaviors." In *Introduction to Nutrition, Exercise, and Health.* Philadelphia: Lea & Febiger, 1993, 301–14. Print.

Katie – Wellness Mama. 2014. "Why You Should Never Eat Vegetable Oil or Margarine" *Wellness Mama.* Accessed March 3, 2014.

Komisar, Harriet. 2013. *The Effects of Rising Health Care Costs on Middle-Class Economic Security.* Part of Middle Class Security Project: An Initiative of the AARP Public Policy Institute. Rep. no. 74. AARP. Print. AARP (American Association of Retired Persons) (website), January. Accessed April 29, 2013.

Kotz, Deborah. 2013. "Energy Drinks: FDA Issues Warning on DMAA." Boston.com, April 11, 2013. Accessed May 6, 2018.

Kralova Lesna, I., P. Suchanek, J. Kovar, P. Stavek, and R. Poledne. 2008. "Replacement of Dietary Saturated FAs by PUFAs in Diet and Reverse Cholesterol Transport." *Journal of Lipid Research* 49: 2,414–418. ASBMB (American Society for Biochemistry and Molecular Biology) (website). Accessed March 2014.

Kravitz, Len, PhD, Kenneth Nowicki, MS, and Stephen J. Kinzey, PhD. n.d. "1 RM Max Strength Testing." University of New Mexico (website). Accessed August 10, 2014.

LA Times. 1985. "Genex Filed Suit Against Searle Over Aspartame." *Los Angeles Times.* Accessed April 4, 2018.

LaRose, Jessica G., Tricia M. Leahey, James O. Hill, and Rena R. Wing. 2013. "Differences in Motivations and Weight Loss Behaviors in Young Adults and Older Adults in the National Weight Control Registry." *Obesity a Research Journal* 21, no. 3: 449–53. Wiley Online Library. The Obesity Society, April 16, 2013. Accessed March 30, 2018.

Latini, G., F. Gallo, and L. Iughetti. 2010. "Toxic Environment and Obesity Pandemia: Is There a Relationship?" Abstract. *National*

Center for Biotechnology Information 36, no. 8, January 22, 2010. U.S. National Library of Medicine (website). Accessed May 20, 2013. Doi: 10.1186/1824-7288-36-8.

Layton, Julia. n.d. "How Calories Work." HowStuffWorks.com. Accessed July 15, 2013.

Lee, Haven. 2014. "What is a Pro-Oxidant?" Edited by Rachel Catherine Allen. *WiseGEEK*, April 11, 2014. Accessed May 3, 2014.

Lee, I. M., L. Djousse, H. D. Sesso, L. Wang, and J. E. Buring. 2010. "Physical Activity and Weight Gain Prevention." *JAMA: The Journal of the American Medical Association* 303, no. 12:1, 173–179. Print.

Lenzer, Jeanne. "Robert Coleman Atkins." *PMC* 326.7398 (2003): 1090. *National Center for Biotechnology Information*. BMJ Group, 17 May 2003. Accessed 19 October 2015.

Linus Pauling Institute. 2014. "Micronutrient Information Center – Essential Fatty Acids." Linus Pauling Institute at Oregon State University (website). Accessed March 3, 2014.

Lipman, Frank, Dr. 2010. "Where Do the Chemicals in Our Foods Come From?" Web log post. *Be Well: Dr. Frank Lipman's Daily Dose Blog*, June 7, 2010. Accessed March 31, 2018.

Little, Elaine. 2007. "Drinking Water Week: May 6–12, 2007." USPS (US Public Health Service Commissioned Corps) (website), May 2007. Accessed May 3, 2017, and November 26, 2013.

Lloyd, Janice. 2012. "High-carb Diet Is Linked to Early Alzheimer's." *USA Today*, October 17, 2012. Accessed March 30, 2018.

Macine Del Trasimeno. 2017. "History, Culture and Uses of Olive Oil. *Organic Olive Oil Production Consortium Macine Del Trasimeno.* Progetto Stormblock – Consorzio Olivicolo Macine Del Trasimeno. Accessed April 7, 2018.

Magee, Elaine, MPH, RD. n.d. "How Food Affects Your Moods." *WebMD*. Accessed March 28, 2014.

Marian, Conny. 2011. "How to Lose Fat on the Middle and Lower Abdominals." LIVESTRONG.COM, August 24, 2011. Accessed November 26, 2013.

Marks, Derek, M.S., and Len Kravitz, PhD. n.d. "Hormones and Resistance Exercise." University of New Mexico. (website). Accessed May 2, 2018. Unm.edu.

Maur, PA. 2012. "Health Risks of Out-of-office Work." *Health Hub*, June 19, 2012. Accessed June 15, 2014.

Mayo Clinic. 2011. "Red Wine and Resveratrol: Good for Your Heart?" Mayo Clinic Mayo Foundation for Medical Education and Research (website), March 4, 2011. Accessed January 6, 2014.

———. 2012. "Avascular Necrosis." Mayo Clinic Mayo Foundation for Medical Education and Research (website), May 4, 2012. Accessed May 3, 2014.

———. 2014. "Triglycerides: Why Do They Matter?" Mayo Clinic Mayo Foundation for Medical Education and Research (website). Accessed February 3, 2014.

———. 2017. "Weight Loss: Feel Full on Fewer Calories." Mayo Clinic Mayo Foundation for Medical Education and Research (website), January 20, 2017. Accessed March 31, 2018.

McCarthy, Tina. 2009. "13 Secret Toxins Lurking in Your Food, and How to Avoid Them." Alternet.com, August 10, 2009. Accessed January 6, 2014.

McMillen, Matt. 2012. "Low Testosterone: How Do You Know When Levels Are Too Low?" *WebMD*. Accessed June 4, 2014.

MedWatch. 2018. "MedWatch: The FDA Safety Information and Adverse Event Reporting Program." *U.S. Food and Drug Administration Home Page*. U.S. Department of Health and Human Services, April 3, 2018. Accessed April 3, 2018.

Mendiratta, Vibhu, Anamita Khan, and R. S. Solanki. 2008. "Avascular Necrosis: A Rare Complication of Steroid Therapy for Pemphigus." *Indian Journal of Dermatology* 53, no. 1: 28–30. *National Center for Biotechnology Information*. U.S. National Library of Medicine, June 28, 2005. Accessed June 4, 2014. Doi:10.4103/0019-5154.39739

Mercola, Joseph, Dr. 2002. "Aspartame: History of Fraud and Deception." *Mercola.com: Take Care of Your Health*. Mercola (website). Accessed April 4, 2018.

———. 2010. "The Label All Milk Drinkers Should Look Out For (Unless You Like Cancer)." Mercola (website), November 25, 2010. Accessed May 3, 2014.

———. 2012. "Major Trouble Ahead—If You Don't Fix This Deadly Deficiency." Mercola (website), January 12, 2012. Accessed July 20, 2013.

———. 2013. "Study: Both Exercise and Whey Augment Human Growth Hormone Production, Which Can Keep Your Body

Young." *Peak Fitness.* Mercola (website), February 1, 2013. Accessed June 4, 2014.

MirrorAthlete. 2018. "Mirror Athlete's Fitness Secrets!" Weblog post. Mirror Athlete, Inc. (website). Accessed May 24, 2018.

Mustang CrossFit. 2018. "The Paleo Diet." Mustang CrossFit. (website). Accessed March 31, 2018.

MyHealthNewsDaily. 2012. "3 Things You Need to Know about Eating Protein." *Fox News Health.* FOX News Network, LLC, August 31, 2012. Accessed April 6, 2018.

National Cancer Institute. 2014. "Antioxidants and Cancer Prevention: Fact Sheet." National Cancer Institute (website). Accessed May 3, 2014.

Natural Center for Cultural Competence (NCCC). n.d. "Framing the Issue" and "Holistic Health" in "Body/Mind/Spirit" NCCC (website). Accessed April 27, 2013.

Nelson, Nathan C. n.d. *The Free Radical Theory of Aging.* Department of Physics, Ohio State University. Accessed April 27, 2018.

New York Times. 1987. "Genex Chief Steps Down." *The New York Times,* January 6, 1987. Accessed January 6, 2014.

National Resources Defense Council (NRDC). n.d. "Toxic Chemicals." NRDC (website). Accessed December 12, 2013.

NutriStrategy. 2015. "Fats, Cooking Oils, and Fatty Acids." NutriStrategy (website). Accessed May 3, 2018.Oliver, Budda. 2008. "Indoor Air Quality vs. Outdoor Air Quality." *EzineArticles.* SparkNET, April 9, 2008. Accessed May 1, 2018.

Organic Trade Association. n.d. "GMOs 101." *Organic It's Worth It.* Ornish, Dean, Dr. 2011. "Cholesterol: The Good, the Bad and the Truth." *HuffPost. Healthy Living,* June 3, 2011. Accessed February 3, 2014. TheHuffingtonPost.com.

Orthomolecular.org. n.d. "Glycogen." Orthomolecular.org. Accessed May 3, 2013.

Pace, Julia. 2013. "New Findings on Coffee's Cardiovascular Benefits." *LifeExtension,* August. Accessed October 5, 2013.

Patient.co.uk. n.d. "The Pituitary Gland." *Patient.co.uk.* Egton Medical Information Systems Limited. Accessed June 4, 2014.

Peeples, Lynne. 2012. "Pesticide Use Proliferating With GMO Crops, Study Warns." *HuffPost. Green,* October 4, 2012. Accessed May 3, 2014.

Percia, Matthew, Shala Davis, PhD, FACSM, and Gregory Dwyer, PhD, FACSM. 2012. "Getting a Professional Fitness Assessment." American College of Sports Medicine Articles (website), January 10, 2012. Accessed November 26, 2013.

Perkins, Cynthia, M.Ed. 2012. "Deep Breathing Exercises." *No-Hype Holistic Health Solutions*. Accessed June 15, 2014.

Perry, Brian, Dr. n.d. "Eating Protein, Weight Loss, and the PYY Hormone." Drbrianperry.com. Accessed February 3, 2014.

Philpott, Tom. 2013. "Longest-Running GMO Safety Study Finds Tumors in Rats." *Mother Earth News*, April–May. Accessed May 3, 2014.

———. 2014. "What We Can Learn from the Greek-Island Diet and What We Already Know." *Mother Jones*. Mother Jones and the Foundation for National Progress, October 26, 2012. Accessed July 3, 2014.

Pick, Marcelle, OB/GYN, NP. n.d. "Deep Breathing—The Truly Essential Exercise." Marcelle Pick (website). Accessed June 15, 2014.

Policy and Medicine. 2010. "Pharmaceutical Marketing Lawsuits Slowing Considerably." Policy and Medicine (website), July 28, 2010. Accessed March 31, 2018.

Pomeroy, Ross. 2017. "Why French Fries Are More of a 'Superfood' Than Kale." RealClearScience.com (website), April 5, 2017. Accessed April 27, 2018.

Poulter, Sean. 2014. "Can GM Food Cause Immunity to Antibiotics?" *Mail Online*. Accessed May 3, 2014. Price, Maria Z. 2013. "What Is a Superfood?" *LIVESTRONG.COM*, August 16, 2013. Accessed May 3, 2014.

Public Health Law Center. 2010. "Trans Fat." Public Health Law Center at William Mitchell College of Law. Accessed June 27, 2013.

Quinn, Elizabeth, MS, BS. 2017. "Do You Really Burn More Calories Working in the Fat Burning Zone?" *Verywell Fit.*, October 16, 2017. Accessed May 30, 2018.

Quinn, Elizabeth, MS, BS, and Richard N. Fogoros. 2018a. "Eating and the Energy Pathway for Exercise." *Verywell Fit*, April 29, 2018. Accessed May 26, 2018.

———. 2018b. "What Are Slow and Fast Twitch Muscle Fibers?" *Verywell Fit*, February 24, 2018. Accessed May 30, 2018.

Rader Programs. n.d. "What Is Compulsive Overeating?" Rader Programs (website). Accessed March 28, 2014.

Reason. "What Is Anti-Aging?" *Fight Aging!* Fightaging.org, November 1, 2002. Accessed June 4, 2014.

Review, Kathleen M. Zelman, MPH, RD, LD, WebMD Expert. n.d. "Diet Review: The Caveman (Paleo) Diet." *WebMD.* Accessed May 20, 2013.

Rhone, Nedra. 2012. "Anti-aging Medicine Earns Converts and Critics." *The Atlanta Journal-Constitution*, September 24, 2012. Accessed June 4, 2014.

Richardson, Alicia. 2013. "What Is Oleic Acid?" LIVESTRONG. COM, August 16, 2013. Accessed March 3, 2014.

Richey, Kate. "Cardio Heart Formula." LIVESTRONG.COM, October 21, 2013. Accessed August 10, 2014.

Riley, Naomi Schaefer. 2011. "Why Unions Hurt Higher Education." *USA Today*, March 3, 2011. Accessed November 26, 2013.

Robert Wood Johnson Foundation. 2018. "The Childhood Obesity Epidemic." *Healthy Eating Research.* Robert Wood Johnson Foundation (website). Accessed March 31, 2018.

Rodale, Maria. 2013. "Oxygen: The Forgotten Nutrient." *HuffPost*, September 9, 2013. Accessed June 15, 2014.

Rodowicz, Kevin. 2009. "Chemical Engineering Innovation In Food Production." *Chemical Engineers in Action–Innovation.* AIChE (American Institute of Chemical Engineers) and Chemical Heritage Foundation, 2009. Accessed May 24, 2018.

Rosick, Edward R., DO, MPH, MS. 2004. "Why Aging Women Need Testosterone." *Life Extension Magazine*, April. Accessed June 4, 2014.

Rotella, Pam. 2006. "Healthy Fats, Essential Fatty Acids." PamRotella. com, June 1, 2006. Accessed February 3. 2014.

Roula Crews. 2012. "Body Fat Percentages & Lean Body Mass." *Roula Crews Wellness Coach.* Accessed June 27, 2013.

Sahlin, K., M. Mogensen, M. Bagger, M. Fernström, and P. K. Pedersen. 2006. "The Potential for Mitochondrial Fat Oxidation in Human Skeletal Muscle Influences Whole Body Fat Oxidation during Low-intensity Exercise." *American Physiology Society*, August 11, 2006. Accessed May 3, 2013.

SALOV. 2014. "Health Benefits of Olive Oil." *Filippo Berio.* SALOV North America Corp. Accessed February 24, 2014.

School Nutrition Association. 2014. "Implementation of the Healthy, Hunger-Free Kids Act." School Nutrition Association (website). Accessed May 3, 2014.

Schuab, Kimberly. 2013. "Crisco & Cholesterol." LIVESTRONG. COM, August 16, 2013. Accessed January 21, 2014.

Science Daily. 2013a. "Aerobic Exercise." *Science Daily.* Accessed November 26, 2013.

———. 2013b. "Top Four Reasons Why Diets Fail." *Science Daily,* January 3, 2013. Accessed November 16, 2013.

Scott, Jennifer R. 2009. "Calculate and Understand Your BMI." *Weight Loss.* About.com, September 28, 2009. Accessed May 20, 2013.

Sesana, Laura. 2013. "Greek Coffee May Be the Key to a Long, Healthy Life." *Washington Times Communities,* March 19, 2013. Accessed July 3, 2014.

ShamseNajabadi, Parvaneh, Amir Sabeti Dehkordi, and Olia Ahdeno. 2013. "Somato Types of Young Male Athletes and Non-Athlete Students." *International Research Journal of Applied Basic Science* 4, no. 4: 792–98. Accessed February 3, 2014.

Shomon, Mary. 2005. "Medical Students at Risk for Influence from Pharmaceutical Companies." *Thyroid Disease.* About.com, September 7, 2005. Accessed June 3, 2013.

Siddiqui, Imran. 2005. "Dopamine and Addiction." Paper for a course at Bryn Mawr College, Spring. Accessed January 6, 2014.

Smith, Rebecca. 2012. "Office Workers 'Doubling Risk of Blood Clots'" *The Telegraph,* May 15, 2012. Accessed June 15, 2014.

Snijders, M.C., L.G.H. Koren, H.S.M Kort, and J.E.M.H. Bronswijk. 2001. "Clean Indoor Air Increases Physical Independence: A Pilot Study." *Gerontechnology* 1, no. 2: 124–27. Print.

SourceWatch. 2013. "Aspartame." *SourceWatch.* Accessed January 6, 2014.

Spectrum Organic Products, Inc. n.d. "Liquid Oxidation: Rancidity and Healing of Oils." *Spectrum Essential News* 3, no. 5. Accessed March 4, 2014.

Sports Doctor, Inc. n.d. "Exercise and Air Pollution." *SportsDoctor.* Accessed June 15, 2014.

Sports Illustrated. 1998. "McGwire Uses Nutritional Supplement Banned in NFL." CNN Sports Illustrated/Associated Press, August 22, 1998. Accessed June 4, 2014.

Stein, Natalie. 2011. "A Description of Non Essential Fatty Acids." LIVESTRONG.COM, May 19, 2011. Accessed July 8, 2013.

Sullivan, Thomas. 2010. "Pharmaceutical Marketing Lawsuits Slowing Considerably." *Policy and Medicine*, July 28, 2010. Accessed June 3, 2013.

Suzuki, David, PhD. 2000. "Experimenting with Life." *YES!* Positive Futures Network, June 30, 2000. Accessed April 27, 2018.

Ten Bosch, Laurentine, Producer. 2013. "Ten Top Food Additives to Avoid." *Food Matters*. Accessed March 28, 2014.

TheLabRat.com. 2005. "Definition of Trans Fat." TheLabRat.com. Accessed January 21, 2014.

Thrasybule, Linda. 2012. "3 Things You Need to Know about Eating Protein." *Fox News*, August 31, 2012. Accessed July 8, 2013.

Tucker, Ross, PhD. 2010. "Fueled by Fat: Fat Burning 101." *Sports Scientists*, January 20, 2010. Accessed May 24, 2018.

Tuormaa, Tuula E. 1994. "The Adverse Effects of Food Additives on Health: A Review of the Literature with Special Emphasis on Childhood Hyperactivity." *The Journal of Orthomolecular Medicine* 9, no. 4. Orthomolecular.org. Accessed May 20, 2013.

Turner, Natasha, ND. 2012. "Seven Tips to Get the Most Out of Your Vitamins." Weblog post. *HuffPost Living*, May 17, 2012. Accessed January 6, 2014.

University of Maryland Medical Center (UMMC). 2011. "Omega-3 Fatty Acids." UMCA (website), May 10, 2011. Accessed July 20, 2013.

————. 2014. "Green Tea." UMC (website). Accessed May 3, 2014.

United States Congressional Senate. 1985. Proceedings and Debates. *Congressional Record*. 99th Cong., 1st sess. S. Doc. 58. Vol. 131. N.p.: GPO. Print. S5503, S5509-10.

University of Guelph. 2008. "Sourdough Bread Has Most Health Benefits, Prof Finds." University of Guelph (website), July 7, 2008. Accessed July 3, 2014.

University of Houston. n.d. "The 3 Somatotypes." University of Houston (website). Accessed February 3, 2014.

University of Minnesota. 2006. "New Study Shows Teenage Girls' Use of Diet Pills Doubles Over Five-Year Span." *Science Daily*, November 1, 2006. Accessed June 3, 2013.

University of Washington. 2011. "Muscle Fiber Types." University of Washington (website), January 27, 2011. Accessed August 10, 2014.

US Department of Labor. n.d. "Summary of the Major Laws of the Department of Labor." US Department of Labor (website). Accessed April 27, 2013.

US Department of Education. 2012. "U.S. Education Secretary Warns That Automatic Budget Cuts Would Hurt Children and Families." US Department of Education (website), July 25, 2012. Accessed November 26, 2013.

US Department of Labor (US DOL). n.d. "Summary of the Major Laws of the Department of Labor." US DOL (website). Accessed March 27, 2018.

US Senate Committee on Agriculture, Nutrition and Forestry. 2014. "2014 Farm Bill." US Senate Committee on Agriculture, Nutrition and Forestry (website), February 7, 2014. Accessed May 3, 2014.

US Department of Agriculture (USDA). 2008. "Table 4. Calories/Hour Expended in Common Physical Activities." *Dietary Guidelines for Americans 2005*. USDA, July 9, 2008. Accessed May 20, 2013.

―――. 2010. "USDA Announces Organic Agriculture Research and Extension Projects." USDA *National Institute of Food and Agriculture*, October 27, 2010. Accessed May 3, 2014.

―――. 2011. "Organic Certification | USDA." USDA (website), November 15, 2011. Accessed August 19, 2013.

―――. 2014. "National Organic Program." USDA, April 30, 2014. Accessed May 3, 2014.

―――. n.d. "Weight Management and Calories." USDA *Choose My Plate*, Choosemyplate.gov, Accessed July 15, 2013.USDA (United States Department of Agriculture) and USDHHS (United States Department of Health and Human Service). 2005. *Dietary Guidelines for Americans 2005*. 6th edition. Washington, DC: US Government Printing Office. DietaryGuidelines.gov. Accessed December 12, 2013.

―――. 2010. *Dietary Guidelines for Americans 2010*. 7th edition. Washington, DC: US Government Printing Office, December. DietaryGuidelines.gov. Accessed December 12, 2013.

————. 2015. *Dietary Guidelines for Americans 2015-2020*. 8th edition. Washington DC: US Government Printing Office. DietaryGuideline.gov. Accessed May 3, 2018.

US Department of Agriculture, Agricultural Marketing Service (USDA-AMS). 2013. "National Organic Program." USDA AMS (website), September 16, 2013. Accessed May 3, 2014.

US Food and Drug Administration (USFDA). 2013. "Tainted Products Marketed as Dietary Supplements." USFDA (website), October 29, 2013. Accessed December 20, 2013.

Vegan Society. 2014. "Essential Fatty Acids." The Vegan Society. Accessed February 3, 2014.Vigil, George. 2007. "Saturated Fats versus Partially Hydrogenated Vegetable Oils and Trans Fats." Wewantorganicfood.com, September 2, 2007. Accessed January 21, 2014.

US Department of Agriculture and Health and Human Services (USDA and HHS). USDA and HSS. *Dietary Guidelines for Americans 2010*, 7th Edition. Washington, DC: U.S. Government Printing Office, December 2010, December 2010. Accessed February 3, 2014.

Watson, Stephanie. n.d. "Managing Soar Muscles and Joint Pain." *WebMD*. Accessed August 10, 2014.

WebMD. 2010. "Air Pollution Significantly Increases Sleep Disorders." *WebMD*. Accessed June 15, 2014.

————. 2012. "High Protein, Low Carb Diets." *WebMD*. Accessed November 26, 2013.

————. 2013. "Vitamins and Minerals: How Much Should you Take?" *WebMD*. Accessed January 6, 2014.

————. 2014. "Understanding Cholesterol Numbers." *WebMD. Cholesterol & Triglycerides Health Center*. Accessed February 3, 2014.

————. n.d.a. "Atkins Diet." *WebMD*. Accessed May 20, 2013.

————. n.d.b. "FAQs About Dietary Supplements." *WebMD*. Accessed April 4, 2018.

————. n.d.c. "The Paleo Diet Review (Caveman Diet)." *WebMD*. Accessed December 11, 2013.

WeightLossForAll. 2018. "Great Sources of Simple Carbohydrate Foods – Weight Loss For All." WeightLossForAll (website), 2018. Accessed March 31, 2018.

Weil, Andrew. 2017. *8 Weeks to Optimum Health: A Proven Program for Taking Full Advantage of Your Body's Natural Healing Power.* London: Warner. Print.

Weil, Richard, MEd, CDE. n.d. "Aerobic Exercise Health & Fitness Benefits, Types, Programs and Routines." *MedicineNet.* Accessed August 10, 2014.

Weir, Kirsten. 2011. "The Exercise Effect." *American Psychological Association* 42, no. 11: 48. Print.

Wellwise. n.d. "Foods with Omega 6." *Wellwise.* Wellwise.org. Accessed March 4, 2014.

West, Greg. 2013. "FDA Ignores Health Risks Associated With Artificial Sweeteners." *Neon Tommy,* May 5, 2013. Accessed April 4, 2018.

Wheeler, Madelyn L., MS, RD, CDE, FADA, CD. n.d. "What Are Net Carbs?" *Diabetes Forecast the Healthy Living Magazine.* Forecast. diabetes.org. Accessed July 8, 2013.

Whitney, Eleanor Noss, Eva May Nunnelley, Hamilton, and Marie A. Boyle. 1987. "Table of Food Composition." *Understanding Nutrition.* Fourth ed. St. Paul: West Pub., H2–H65. Print.

World Health Organization (WHO). 2018a. "Genes and Human Disease." WHO (website). Accessed June 6, 2018.

———. 2018b. (World Health Organization). "Obesity and Overweight." WHO (website). Accessed June 6, 2018.

Wikipedia. n.d. "Lipid Peroxidation." *Wikipedia.* Accessed May 24, 2018.

———. "Omega 3, 6 and 9." *Wikipedia.* Accessed July 20, 2013.

Williams, Melvin H. 1988. "Chapter 2, Human Energy." In *Nutrition for Fitness and Sport.* Dubuque, IA: W.C. Brown, 30–44. Print.

Wilson, Lawrence, MD. 2009a. "Aspartame And Deadly Diet Foods." *Nutritional Balancing Science.* The Center for Development, November. Accessed January 6, 2014.

———. 2009b. "Food Habits and Addiction." *Nutritional Balancing Science.* The Center for Development, December. Accessed January 6, 2014.

Wilson, Reid. 2014. "Maine Becomes Second State to Require GMO Labels." *The Washington Post.* Accessed March 31, 2018.

Index

free radical damage, 196
free radical generators/activators, 211, 212, 213, 214, 219
free radical theory of aging, 196
free radicals, 196, 214, 215, 216–217
free running, 290
free weight lifting, 227, 270, 279, 301
Friedewald, William, 125

G

gamma-linolenic acid (GLA), 161
gardening, 189
G.D. Searle & Company, 103
GE seeds, 203, 204
genetic code, influence of on food choice, 77–78
genetically engineered (GE) foods, 86, 87, 163, 195, 197–198, 199, 201, 202, 203, 204, 205, 208, 211
genetically modified (GM or GMO) foods, 83, 85, 86, 118, 119, 194, 199–205, 207
Genex Corp., 103
GH (growth hormone), 232, 234–235, 240, 299–300, 302
ghee, 162
gimmicks, xxii, 3, 33, 41, 47, 49, 51, 54, 259, 281
glucagon, 28, 29–30
glucose, 27, 29, 30, 262, 278, 292, 295, 296, 302. *See also* blood glucose
glycerol, 123
glycogen, 27–28, 29, 30, 34, 278, 283, 285, 286, 292, 295, 296, 302

glycolysis, 29
goat milk, 262
Goldfarb, Allan H., 303
good health, defined, 7
gout, 45, 130
Greek Orthodox culture, longevity within, 264
green tea, as high antioxidant food, 219
GreenMedInfo.com, 110
growth hormone (GH), 232, 234–235, 240, 299–300, 302

H

habits. *See also* healthy habits; sedentary habits
    addictive cravings/habits, 91, 95–107, 108, 164–165, 167
    forming of, 164–176
    immobility habits, 248, 249
    leveraging healthy habit change, 177–193
    substitute addictive habits, 95–107
Hall, Janet, 105
Haney, Lee, 224
Harvard School of Public Health, 212
HDL cholesterol, 125, 126, 127, 128, 129, 151, 155
healing, xxiii, xxiv, 12, 23, 39, 54, 56, 94, 107, 108, 130, 174, 175, 191, 193, 212, 255, 267, 268, 270, 271, 274, 304
health care costs, 19–20, 88, 309, 310

high fructose corn syrup (HFCS), 120, 167, 205

high-carbohydrate diets, 42, 73, 124

high-glycemic-index foods, 45

high-intensity anaerobic exercise, 33, 36, 283

high-intensity interval training (HIIT) programs, 225, 270

high-protein diets/foods, 35, 40, 42, 43–44, 45, 72, 73, 97, 107, 130, 139, 150

hiking, 189, 244, 270, 273, 307

Hill, James, 86

"hitting the wall," 29, 33–34

Hoffman, Matthew, 239

holistic health, 2, 7

hormone chemicals, 231–233

hormone replacement therapy (HRT), 239–241

hormone therapy/treatment, 15, 234, 237, 238, 239–241

HR (heart rate), 47, 189, 232, 252, 254, 290–293, 295

human growth hormone (HGH), 234, 239

Hunt, Beverly, 249

hydration, 30, 31, 32, 190, 191, 192, 286

hydrocarbons, 245

hydrogenated fats, 110, 112

Hyman, Mark, 90, 112

hyperthyroidism, 233

hypothyroidism, 233

I

IGF-1 (Insulin-like-Growth Factor One), 208

Ikaria, 260–265

ill-health prevention, 11, 13, 15, 22, 23, 309, 310

immobility habits, 248, 249

immune system, 40, 77, 110, 215, 217, 218, 253, 254, 256, 294

the impossible, importance in believing impossible is possible, xxv

inflammatory bowel disease, 219

Inness-Brown, Victoria, 103–104

Institute of Medicine, 60

insulin management program, 101

intensity, defined, 279

intensity of effort, 35, 36, 42, 255, 279, 284, 289–290, 292, 293, 294, 295, 296, 297, 302–303

J

Jacobson, Michael F., 103

jogging, 9, 29, 62, 64, 65, 272, 286, 293, 301

Journal of Alzheimer's Disease, 45

jujitsu, 255

junk food, 6, 72, 164, 165

K

K-12 education, 14, 17, 59, 88, 209, 271, 309, 310

karate, 255

Kardashians, 47

Karp, Jason R., 36

Kessler, David, 111

Ketogenic "KETO" diet, 45

ketosis, 45, 76

kidney failure/damage/problems/disease, 45, 72, 76, 130–131, 203

Printed in the United States
By Bookmasters